Learning Imaging

Series Editors:

R. Ribes · A. Luna · P. Ros

José J. Muñoz · Ramón Ribes (Eds.)

Learning Vascular and Interventional Radiology

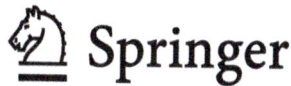 Springer

José J. Muñoz
Hospital Regional Carlos Haya
Avda. de Carlos Haya
29106 Málaga
Spain
jjmrc@telefonica.net

Ramón Ribes
Platero Martinez 19
14012 Córdoba
Spain
ribesb@gmail.com

ISBN 978-3-540-87996-1   ISBN 978-3-540-87997-8 (eBook)
DOI 10.1007/978-3-540-87997-8

Springer Heidelberg Dordrecht London New York

Library of Congress Control Number: 2010933079

Cover design: eStudio Calamar, Figueres/Berlin

Printed on acid-free paper

9 8 7 6 5 4 3 2 1

Springer is part of Springer Science+Business Media (www.springer.com)

"To Frutos Alvarez Gonzalez for his friendship and constant support in the Interventional Radiology Laboratory"

RAMÓN RIBES

"To Encarni, my wife, and to Álvaro, my son"

JOSÉ J. MUÑOZ

We thank John Giba for his contribution to the English edition of this manual

Preface

Interventional radiology is an exciting field, and interventional radiologists perform a huge variety of diagnostic and therapeutic procedures. Most interventional diagnostic procedures have been superseded by noninvasive methods, and the role of interventional radiologists has changed accordingly. Whereas traditionally interventional radiology involved diagnosis and a few therapeutic measures, nowadays it involves mostly interventional procedures planned using noninvasive diagnostic methods.

Interventional radiologists have to keep up with advances in noninvasive imaging techniques like conventional sonography, Doppler sonography, magnetic resonance imaging, MR angiography, cardiac MRI, multidetector CT, and CT angiography for treatment planning.

On the other hand, the number and variety of treatments that interventional radiologists perform continues to grow, supplanting or complementing other techniques traditionally performed by surgeons.

This teaching file aims to review our exciting field. We emphasize the two fundamental aspects that enable us to provide creative, agile solutions to our patients' problems: diagnosis and treatment.

Córdoba, March 2010   Ramón Ribes
Málaga, March 2010   José J. Muñoz

Contents

9   Biliary Interventions and Treatment of Focal Hepatic Lesions

CARLOS LANCIEGO and LORENZO GARCÍA

10   Percutaneous Genitourinary Interventions

ERNESTO SANTOS and JAVIER BLÁZQUEZ

Contributing Authors

José M. Abadal
Interventional Radiology Unit
Hospital Universitario Severo Ochoa
Avd. de Orellana s/n.
28911 Madrid
Spain

Lydia Alcalá
Clínica Las Nieves,
C/Carmelo Torres 2
23007 Jaén
Spain

Carlos Alonso
Clínica Quirón Málaga
C/José María Amado 23
29016 Málaga
Spain

Pedro J. Aranda
Cardiovascular Surgery Department
Complejo Hospitalario Carlos Haya
Avda. Carlos Haya s/n.
29010 Málaga
Spain

Iván Artero
Interventional Radiology Unit
Complejo Hospitalario Carlos Haya
Avda. Carlos Haya s/n.
29010 Málaga
Spain

Javier Blázquez
Interventional Radiology Unit
MD Anderson Oncological Center
Calle de Arturo Soria 270
28033 Madrid
Spain

Esther Boullosa
Interventional Radiology Unit
Complejo Hospitalario Universitario de Vigo
c/Pizarro 22
36204 Vigo
Spain

Marta Burrel
Interventional Radiology Unit
Hospital Clinic
C/Villarroel 170
08036 Barcelona
Spain

Joan Falcó
Corporació Sanitària Parc Taulí
Parc Taulí nº 1
08208 Sabadell
Spain

José R. Fortuño
Corporació Sanitària Parc Taulí
Parc Taulí nº 1
08208 Sabadell
Spain

Lorenzo García
Interventional Radiology Unit
Hospital Virgen de la Salud
Complejo Hospitalario Universitario de Toledo
Avda. Barber, 30
45004 Toledo
Spain

Álvaro Iglesias
Hospital Virgen del Rocío
Avda. Manuel Siurot s/n.
41013 Sevilla
Spain

Carlos Lanciego
Interventional Radiology Unit
Hospital Virgen de la Salud
Complejo Hospitalario Universitario de Toledo
Avda. Barber, 30
45004 Toledo
Spain

Antonio Luna
Clínica Las Nieves
C/Carmelo Torres 2
23007 Jaén
Spain

José J. Muñoz
Hospital Regional Carlos Haya
Avda. de Carlos Haya
29106 Málaga
Spain

Javier Peiró
Hospital Universitario Virgen Macarena
Avda. Dr. Fedriani 3
41071 Sevilla
Spain

Maribel Real
Interventional Radiology Unit
Hospital Clinic, C/Villarroel 170
08036 Barcelona
Spain

Ramón Ribes
Platero Martinez 19
14012 Córdoba
Spain

José Rodríguez
Interventional Radiology Unit
Complejo Hospitalario Carlos Haya
Avda. Carlos Haya s/n.
29010 Málaga
Spain

Ernesto Santos
Interventional Radiology Department
UPMC Presbyterian
200 Lothrop Street
Pittsburgh, PA 1521
USA

José Urbano
Interventional Radiology Unit
Fundación Jiménez Díaz (Clínica de la Concepción)
Avda. Reyes Católicos, 2
28040 Madrid
Spain

Fundamentals of Diagnostic Angiography

Iván Artero, José Rodríguez, and José J. Muñoz

J.J. Muñoz and R. Ribes, *Learning Vascular and Interventional Radiology*, Learning Imaging,
DOI: 10.1007/978-3-540-87997-8_1, © Springer-Verlag Berlin Heidelberg 2010

Case 1.1
■ Catheters, Guides, and Introducer Sheaths

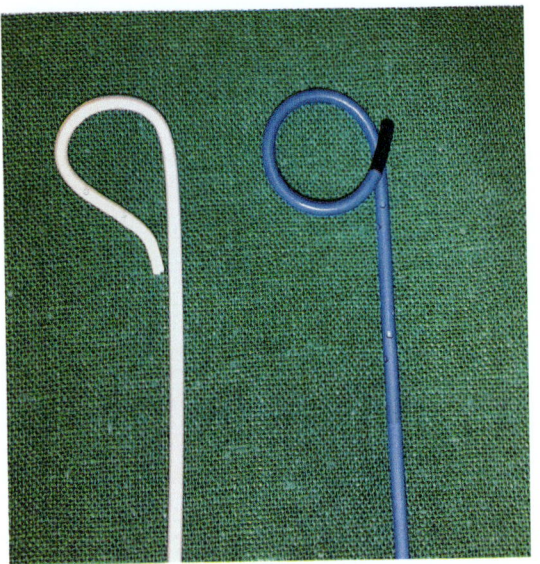

Fig. 1.1.1

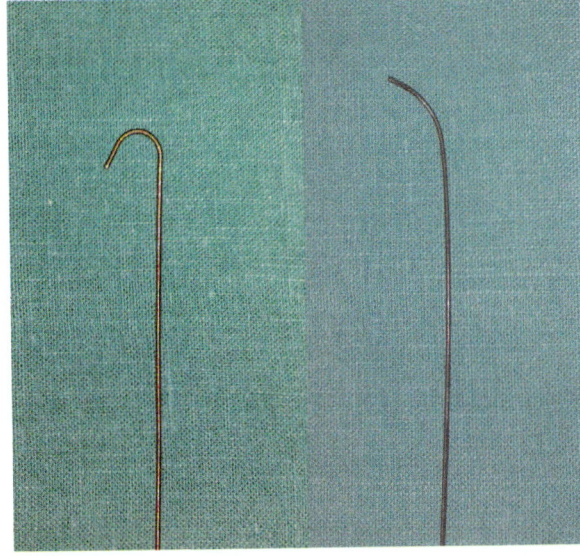

Fig. 1.1.2

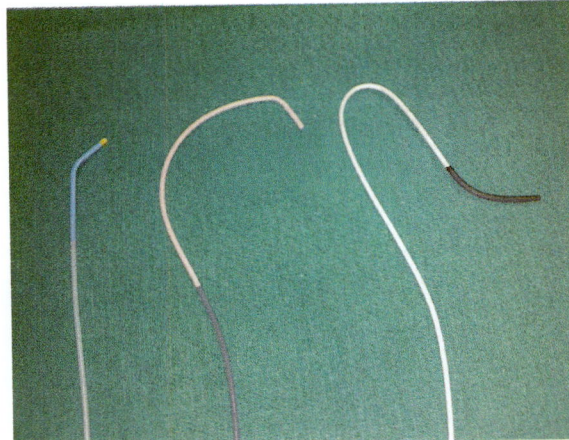

Fig. 1.1.3

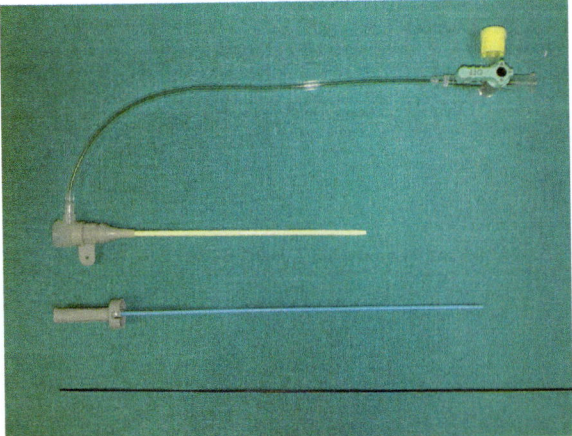

Fig. 1.1.4

Figure 1.1.1 From *left* to *right*, Neff catheter and pigtail catheter. Both are used for invasive diagnosis with injection of contrast agents through large arteries, so they have a multiperforated distal tip to enable high-flow injection

Figure 1.1.2 From *left* to *right*, distal tips of a conventional J-tipped guidewire and a curved-tip hydrophilic guidewire

Figure 1.1.3 From *left* to *right*, vertebral catheter, cobra catheter, and type I Simmons catheter. These catheters all have a preformed distal tip for selective catheterization; the choice of which one to use depends on the procedure

Figure 1.1.4 From *top* to *bottom*, introducer sheath, dilator, and guidewire

Comments

Guidewires and catheters are fundamental for any interventional procedure in vascular radiology. A wide range of catheters and guidewires are available; interventional radiologists should choose those that are best suited to the procedure and to their experience and training.

Each guidewire has a specific length, thickness, flexibility, composition, and maneuverability for the different purposes for which it was designed. In general, guidewires are devices that enable us to progress through a blood vessel, ureter, bile duct, or other organ; after they are introduced, they provide support for insertion of the catheter, stent, balloon, or other materials required for a specific diagnostic or therapeutic procedure. They normally have two tips: the anterior, which is flexible and has a shape preformed for its specific use, and the posterior, which is stiff and straight. Standard guidewires consist of an internal filament wrapped in very fine stainless steel thread. Hydrophilic guidewires are wrapped in certain polymers, which makes them easier to maneuver when wet; these are very useful for insertion through damaged or tortuous vessels, stenoses, etc. Guidewires are usually 0.035 or 0.038 in. in diameter and range from 125 to 150 cm in length. Micro-guidewires (0.014 or 0.018 in.) that enable navigation through very small vessels and microcatheter insertion are becoming increasingly more common. Exchange guidewires measuring up to three meters in length are necessary for changing catheters or other devices without the need to withdraw the guidewire from a determinate position.

Catheters are made of polyethylene, polyurethane, Teflon, or nylon. Like guidewires, catheters are shaped to facilitate the procedure for which they are designed. Catheters are normally described by their length, external diameter (measured in French (F) 3F = 1 mm), number and location of holes (multiperforated, with lateral holes …), and tip design (pigtail, cobra, Simmons…). The tip design is the most important characteristic because it enables us to enter into and maneuver through different ostia and vascular bifurcations, occlusions, stenoses, etc.

Introducer sheaths are catheters with a valve in one tip. They are shorter and thicker than the catheters that will be used during the procedure. Their main function is to maintain and protect the vascular access to enable material to be exchanged during the intervention. Introducer sheaths are color coded for size; like catheters, their diameter is measured in French, although in introducer sheaths, size refers to the internal diameter. Introducer sheaths consist of the sheath itself and a dilator, which as its name suggests, enables a progressive enlargement of the diameter between the guidewire and the introducer sheath.

Case 1.2

■

Seldinger Technique. Retrograde and Antegrade Approach Through the Femoral Artery

Comments

Figure 1.2.1 Cannulated needle and one-step needle

Figure 1.2.2 Diagram showing the Seldinger technique

Figure 1.2.3 US-guided vascular access. Color-Doppler shows the common femoral artery and the femoral vein in the upper half of the image. The lower half of the image shows the tip of the needle (*arrow*) as it enters the femoral artery

Figure 1.2.4 Atheromatous plaques in the common femoral artery help guide puncture under fluoroscopy

Retrograde access to the femoral artery is the vascular radiologist's basic approach to the arterial system for nearly any procedure, whether diagnostic or therapeutic.

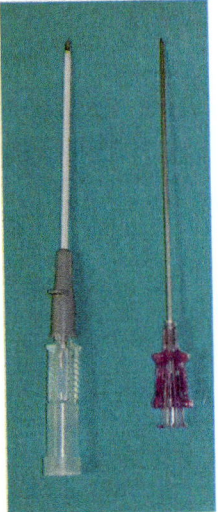

Fig. 1.2.1

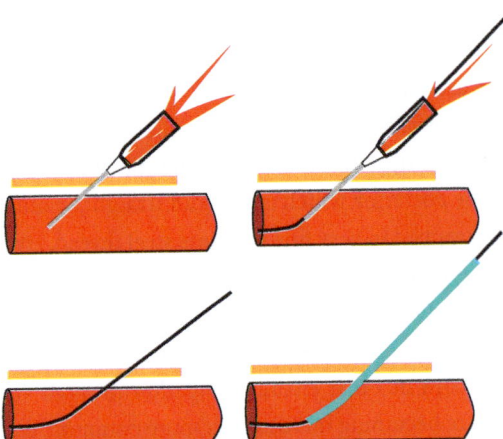

Fig. 1.2.2

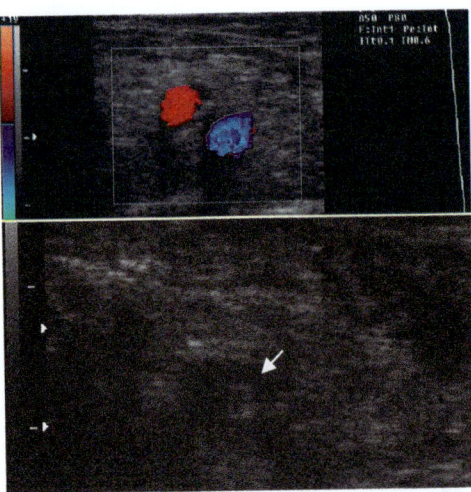

Fig. 1.2.3

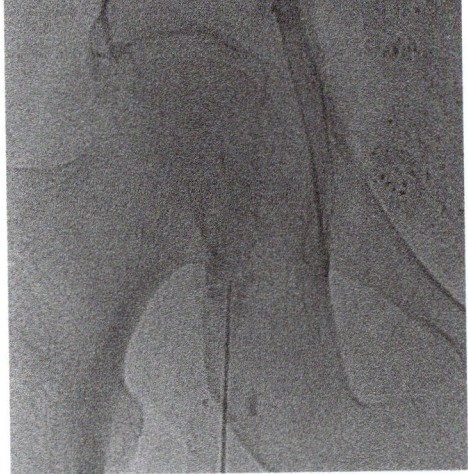

Fig. 1.2.4

In 1953, Sven-Ivar Seldinger first described percutaneous arterial catheterization using a needle, guidewire, and catheter. This technique consists of puncturing an artery, introducing the guidewire through it, and then using the guidewire to advance a catheter or introducer sheath through the artery.

The common femoral artery is usually the safest and simplest site to access the arterial system because it is wide, superficial artery that is normally disease-free and can be compressed against the femoral head to close the puncture site.

Classically, the inguinal fold is used as a reference for the puncture: the pulse is palpated cephalad to the fold and the skin is punctured caudal to it using a 45° angle toward the site where the pulse was palpated. These indications are imprecise in that the exact location of the artery varies with age, tissue laxity, and obesity; thus, it helps to locate the femoral head by fluoroscopy. Low puncture increases the risk of thrombosis, pseudoaneurysms, or arteriovenous fistulas; the risk of intra- or retro-peritoneal bleeding increases if the external iliac artery is punctured.

Local anesthesia at the puncture site is accomplished with local anesthetic such as 1 or 2% lidocaine; mixing this solution with injectable sodium bicarbonate eliminates the discomfort associated with the injection. We use 21–25G needles and aspirate intermittently to prevent intramuscular injection.

Certain procedures in vascular radiology (e.g., treatment of infrapopliteal vascular lesions) may require the antegrade approach to the common femoral artery. The principles underlying this approach are identical to those underlying the retrograde approach; however, the antegrade approach has a greater risk of complications, especially of arterial dissection. In these cases, arterial dissection favors arterial flow; thus, the risk of progression is greater and lower limb ischemia can develop.

Procedure Steps

1. Locate the femoral head fluoroscopically.
2. Palpate the femoral arterial pulse and choose the puncture site in function of whether a retrograde or antegrade approach is used.
3. Infiltrate local anesthetic.
4. Make a small incision in the skin.
5. Puncture the artery with a 16G Abbocath.
6. Withdraw the metallic guidewire from the Abbocath, check for adequate blood reflow and introduce the 0.035 guidewire.
7. Advance the guidewire and use fluoroscopy to check for correct placement.
8. Withdraw the Abbocath and introduce the introducer sheath.
9. Withdraw the dilator from the introducer sheath and check for adequate blood reflow.
10. Wash the introducer sheath with heparinized saline solution.

Equipment List

1. 10 and 20 mL syringes.
2. 21½G intramuscular needle.
3. Injectable 2% lidocaine solution.
4. Injectable 8.4% sodium bicarbonate solution.
5. 16G Abbocath.
6. 0.035 in. conventional curved-tip guidewire.
7. Valved introducer sheath.
8. Heparinized saline solution.
9. Scalpel blade.

Case 1.3
■
Brachial Arterial Access
with a Micropuncture System

Figure 1.3.1 Micropuncture kit, consisting of a 21G-needle, four French dilator/transitional introducer sheath, and 0.018 in. micro-guidewire

Figure 1.3.2 Palpation of the left brachial pulse and the moment of left brachial artery puncture with a 21G-needle from the micropuncture kit

Figure 1.3.3 Introduction of the dilator/exchange introducer sheath from the micropuncture kit over the 0.018 in. micro-guidewire

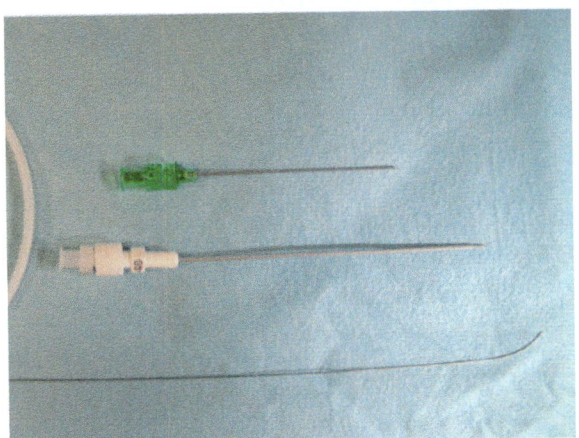

Fig. 1.3.1

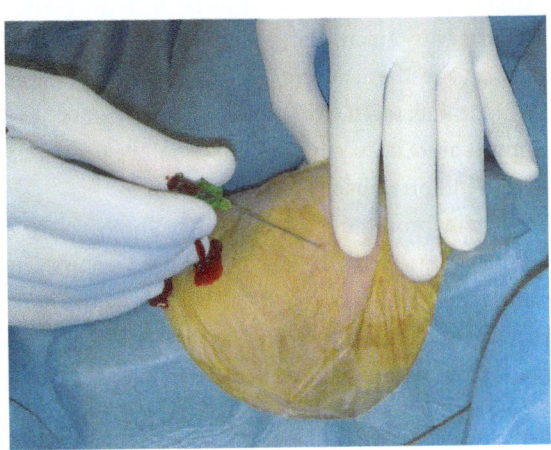

Fig. 1.3.2

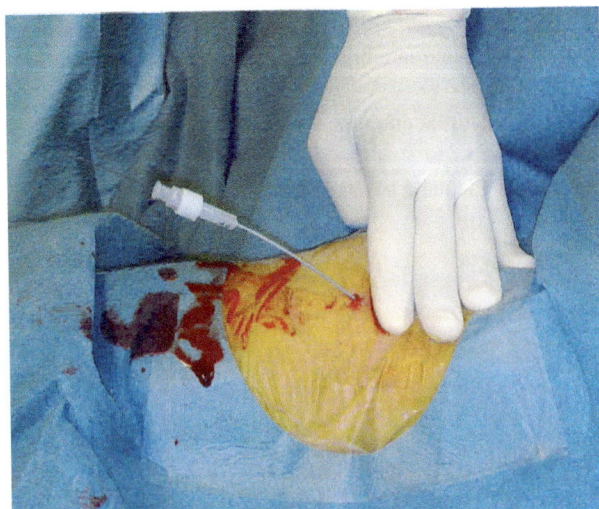

Fig. 1.3.3

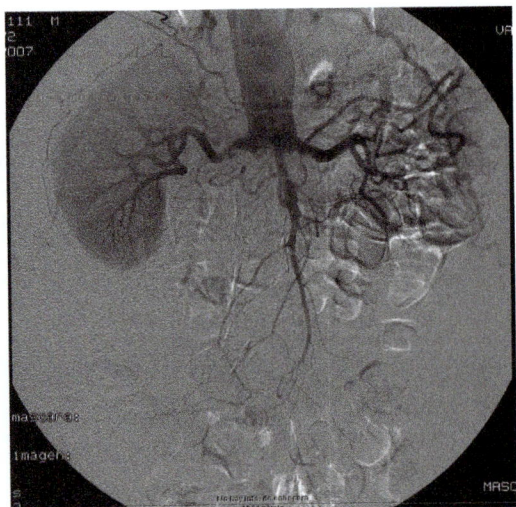

Fig. 1.3.4

Figure 1.3.4 Arteriogram with left brachial access in a 59-year-old male patient with Leriche syndrome showing complete occlusion of the infrarenal aorta

The brachial artery is accessed in the same w Wash the introducer sheath with heparinized saline sol ay as other arteries, i.e., using a needle, guidewire, and catheter, although its size and location entail certain particularities. The most distal portion of the artery, before its bifurcation into the cubital and radial arteries, is punctured cephalad through the antecubital fossa. The artery runs superficially at this point, so it can be loosely compressed against the deeper tendinous planes for palpation and puncture; moreover, after the procedure, hemostasis is easily achieved by compressing this point. The patient is placed in the supine position with the arm abducted. We always choose the left arm whenever possible to avoid crossing guidewires and catheters in the ostium where the other supraaortic trunks exit, which can lead to embolism.

We use micropuncture systems consisting of 21G needles, 0.018 in. guidewires, and a 4F transitional dilator, through which we introduce the conventional guidewire and introducer sheath. The diverse indications for brachial access include, in order of frequency, the absence of femoral pulses, the impossibility of femoral puncture due to prior surgery (femorofemoral by-pass), aortic occlusion (Leriche syndrome), a need to approach visceral stenoses or occlusions with a better angle (celiac trunk, superior mesenteric, occasionally renal arteries …), or the need to use two approaches to introduce aortic prostheses or to carry out complex revascularization techniques. Like femoral access, brachial access can be antegrade.

1. Palpate the humeral arterial pulse and choose the puncture site.
2. Infiltrate local anesthetic.
3. Make a small incision in the skin.
4. Puncture the artery with the micropuncture needle and introduce the micro-guidewire.
5. Withdraw the needle and replace it with a 4F introducer sheath.
6. Withdraw the micro-guidewire and transitional dilator and introduce the conventional guidewire.
7. Advance the guidewire and check for correct placement.
8. Withdraw the exchange sheath and introduce the 4F introducer sheath.
9. Withdraw the dilator from the introducer sheath and check for adequate blood reflow.
10. Wash the introducer sheath with heparinized saline solution.
11. Withdraw the metallic guidewire from the Abbocath, check for adequate blood reflow, and introduce the 0.035 guidewire.
12. Withdraw the Abbocath and introduce the introducer sheath.

1. 5 and 10 mL syringes; 25G hypodermic needle.
2. Injectable 2% lidocaine solution and 8.4% sodium bicarbonate solution.
3. Scalpel blade.
4. Micropuncture system.
5. 0.035 in. conventional curved-tip guidewire.
6. 4F valved introducer sheath.
7. Heparinized saline solution.

Case 1.4

■ Hemostasis Systems. Femoral Artery Closure with Angio-Seal Vascular Closure Device

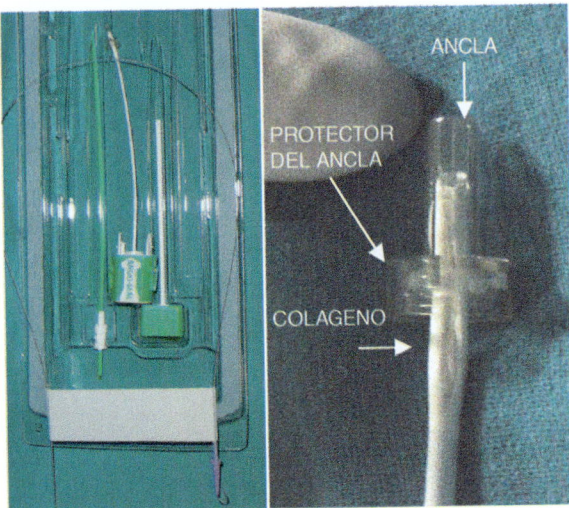

Fig. 1.4.1

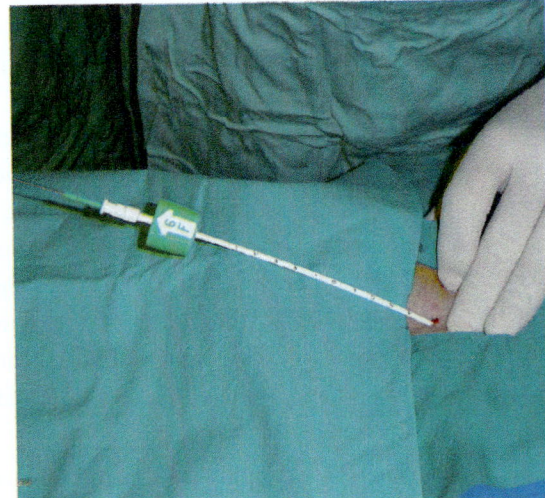

Fig. 1.4.2

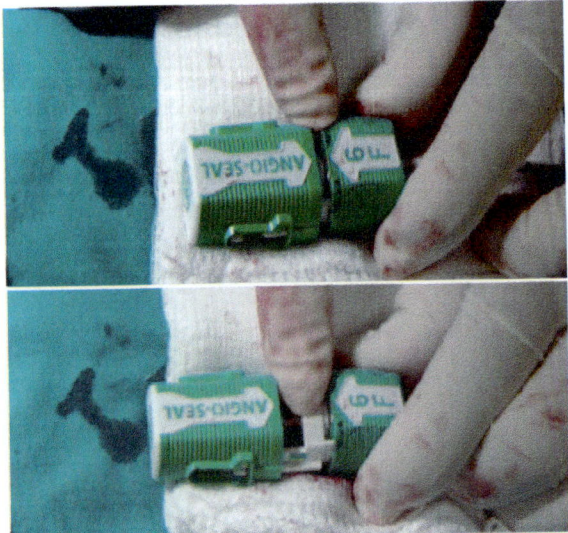

Fig. 1.4.3

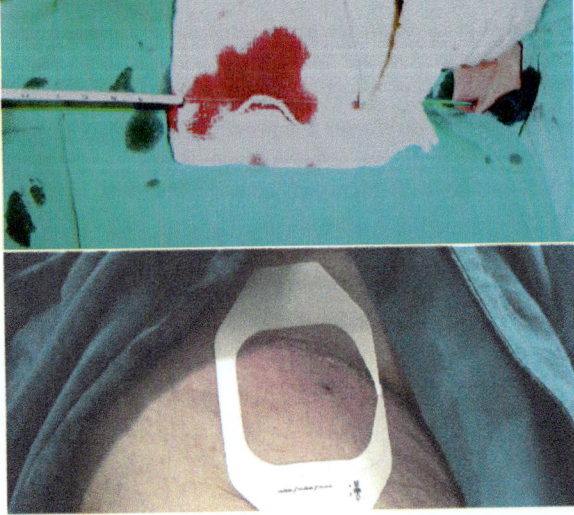

Fig. 1.4.4

Figure 1.4.1 The image on the *left* shows an arterial closure kit with Angio-Seal (St. Jude), consisting of a guidewire, dilator/introducer sheath, and collagen-introducing device. The image on the right shows the tip of the anchoring and collagen delivery device

Figure 1.4.2 Insertion of the specific Angio-Seal introducer sheath

Figure 1.4.3 Insertion (*upper image*) and separation (*lower image*) of the delivery device and the introducer sheath

Figure 1.4.4 Compaction of the collagen with the compaction tube (*upper image*). The *lower image* shows the immediate hemostasis at the puncture site

Manual compression after catheterization was the only available method of achieving hemostasis for over 50 years. This method was slow and required the physician's or nurse's time. Patients needed to be immobilized in a hospital environment for at least 24 h. Arterial hemostasis systems have been developed as an alternative to compression. These systems have the potential advantage of reducing the time to hemostasis and facilitating early patient mobilization. They are especially useful in patients in whom compression is very difficult (e.g., obese patients) as well as in those with altered hemostasis.

Arterial hemostasis systems can be divided into three categories:

- Those that place a collagen patch at the puncture site (Angio-Seal, Vaso-Seal…).
- Systems of percutaneous suturing of the artery (Perclose, Prostar…).
- External patches that accelerate hemostasis (Syvek patch, Closur…).

Each arterial closure system involves its own particular techniques, contraindications, complications, etc. The most common exclusion criteria for arterial closure systems are severe peripheral vascular disease, uncontrolled hypertension, puncture in sites other than the common femoral artery, arterial caliber less than 5 mm, hematoma, multiple punctures, or puncture of both arterial walls.

1. Introduce the guidewire and replace the valved introducer sheath with the specific Angio-Seal sheath.
2. Check that the sheath is correctly inserted in the artery with blood flow from one orifice of the dilator.
3. Withdraw the dilator and the guidewire.
4. Insert the collagen delivery device into the Angio-Seal introducer sheath until the two fit together.
5. Separate the collagen delivery device from the dilator to release the anchor inside the artery.
6. Tighten the suture that is attached to the anchor and to the collagen.
7. Compact the collagen in the external wall of the artery using the compaction tube.
8. Check for adequate hemostasis and cut the suture.

Angio-Seal arterial closure kit, consisting of:

1. 0.035 in. guidewire.
2. Specific introducer sheath and dilators for the Angio-Seal.
3. Delivery system for the anchor and collagen.
4. Scalpel blade.

Comments

Procedure Steps

Equipment List

Case 1.5
■
Complications of Vascular Access. Pseudoaneurysm of the Femoral Artery

Figure 1.5.1 Doppler color duplex US of the puncture area shows an image compatible with a pseudoaneurysm adjacent to the right common femoral artery. Note the characteristic helical flow inside the pseudoaneurysm

Figure 1.5.2 Pulsed Doppler US of the neck of the pseudoaneurysm shows high systolic velocities and turbulent flow

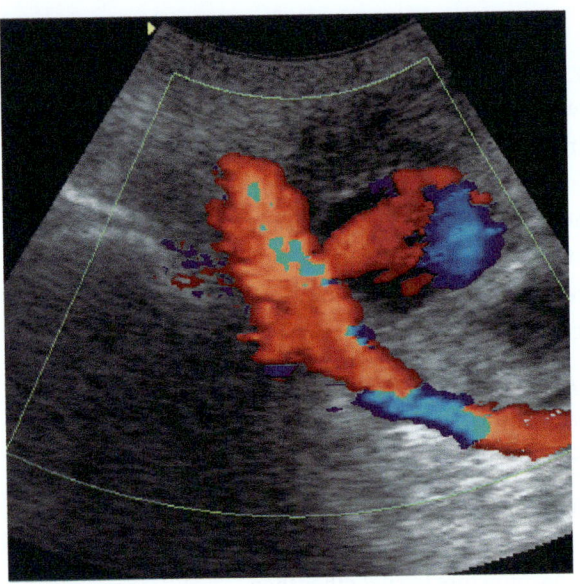

Fig. 1.5.1

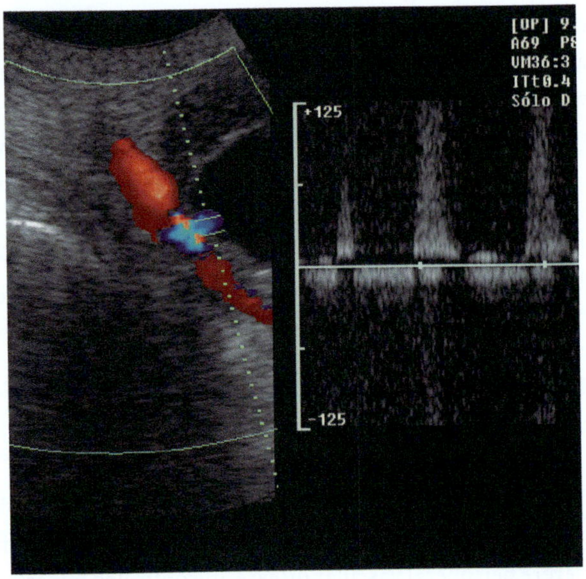

Fig. 1.5.2

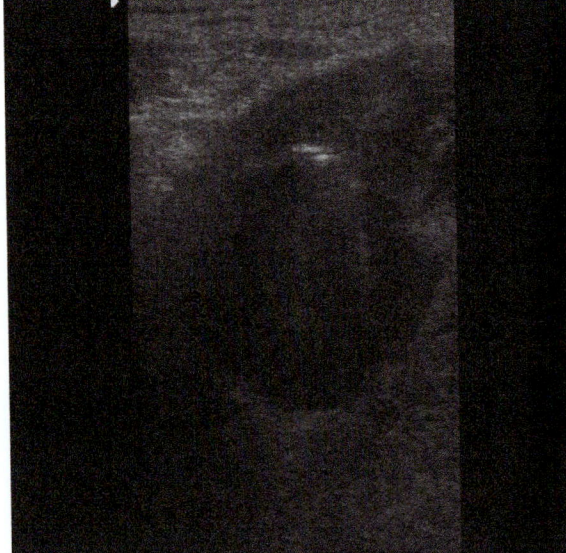

Fig. 1.5.3

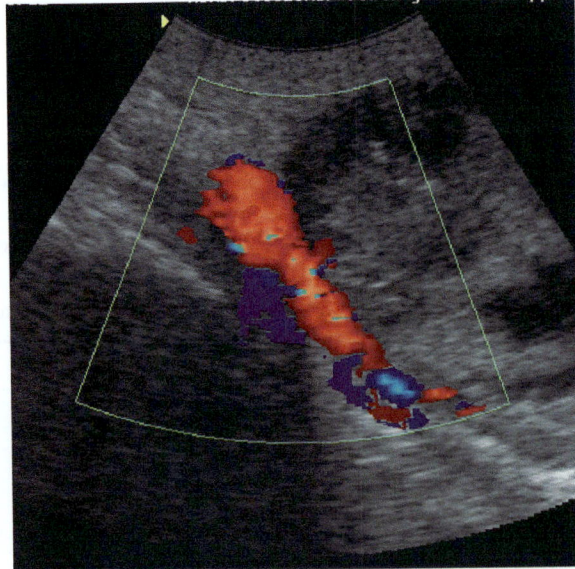

Fig. 1.5.4

Figure 1.5.3 US-guided puncture of the pseudoaneurysm: the needle tip is placed as far as possible from the neck prior to injecting thrombin

Figure 1.5.4 After thrombin injection, there is no flow inside the pseudoaneurysm

A 67-year-old man with a history of hypertension, hypercholesterolemia, and cardiac ischemia underwent heart catheterization and stenting of the anterior descending artery through the right femoral artery. Approximately, 24 h after the procedure, he experienced pain and extensive tumefaction around the puncture site. Emergency US showed findings compatible with a partially thrombosed pseudoaneurysm in the right common femoral artery. We punctured the pseudoaneurysm under US guidance and injected thrombin while compressing the right femoral artery cephalad to the neck of the pseudoaneurysm to reduce the flow inside it. Follow-up US demonstrated complete thrombosis.

Comments

The risk of major complications after vascular access is very low (generally less than 2%), although it depends on the approach, the radiologist's experience, and other factors like anticoagulant treatment or the type of intervention. The most common complication of the arterial approach is mild bleeding or hematoma (6–10%), followed by pseudoaneurysms (1–6%). The risk of major complications like bleeding that requires transfusion, arterial dissection, arterial occlusion, arteriovenous fistula, or distal embolism is much lower (all below 1%).

The incidence of iatrogenic pseudoaneurysms has increased considerably in recent years owing to a large increase in the number of catheterizations performed. Pseudoaneurysms measuring less than 2 cm normally thrombose spontaneously and do not require treatment. Pseudoaneurysms larger than 2 cm or smaller ones that do not resolve spontaneously require treatment. US-guided thrombin injection is the treatment of choice in most cases and is successful in more than 90% of cases. Complications are very rare, although some cases of distal embolism and even thrombosis of the artery distal to the pseudoaneurysm have been reported. Thrombosis can be avoided by thorough compression proximal to the neck of the aneurysm to reduce the flow within it while thrombin is injected.

Procedure Steps

1. Use US to locate the pseudoaneurysm and distinguish its neck.
2. Choose the puncture site and infiltrate local anesthetic.
3. Compress the artery proximal to the neck of the pseudoaneurysm to confirm that flow inside the pseudoaneurysm stops.
4. Puncture the pseudoaneurysm, positioning the needle as far as possible from the neck.
5. Compress the femoral artery proximal to the pseudoaneurysm.
6. Inject thrombin under US guidance and wait 30–60 s while maintaining compression.
7. Withdraw compression slowly and progressively.
8. Check the thrombosis of the pseudoaneurysm and the patency of the femoral artery.

Equipment List

1. 10 and 20 mL syringes.
2. 21½G intramuscular needle, 2% injectable lidocaine, and 8.4% sodium bicarbonate
3. US device with a linear probe and color Doppler capabilities.
4. Sterile US probe cover.
5. 20G needle.
6. Bovine thrombin (1,000 U/mL).

Case 1.6

The Thoracic Aorta. Obtaining a Thoracic Aortogram

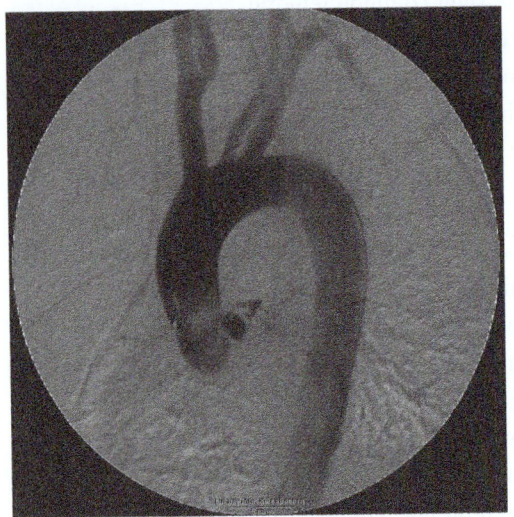

Fig. 1.6.1

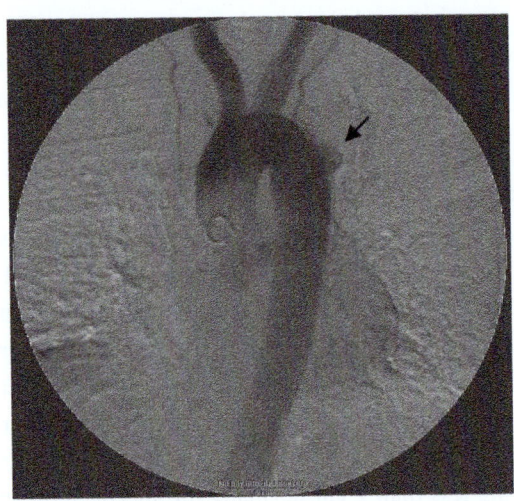

Fig. 1.6.2

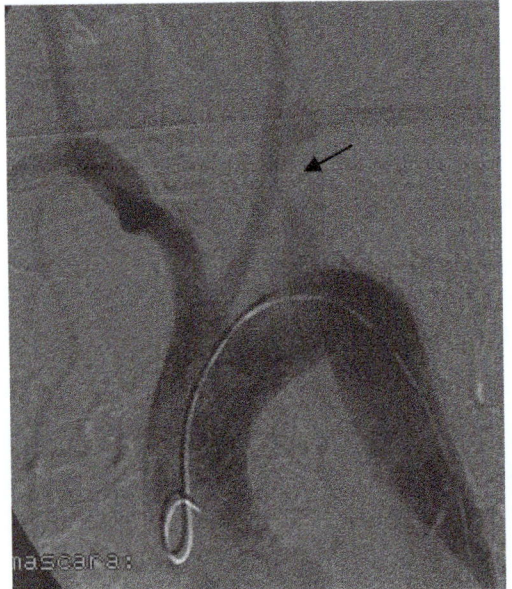

Fig. 1.6.3

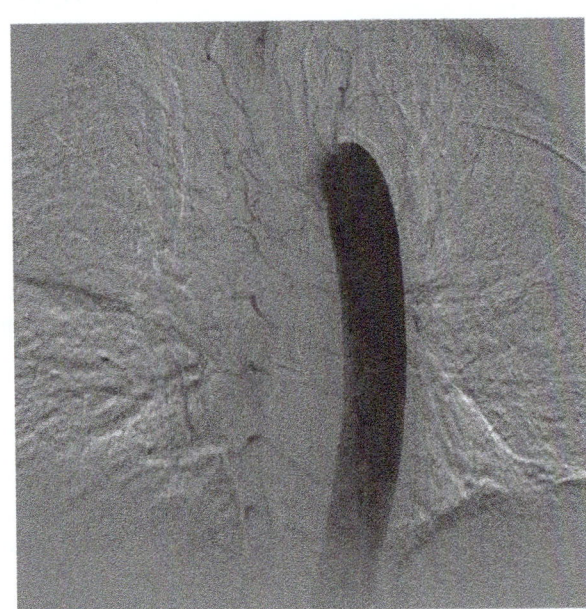

Fig. 1.6.4

Figure 1.6.1 Normal thoracic aortogram obtained using the standard right posterior oblique projection

Figure 1.6.2 Anteroposterior aortogram of the patient in Figure 1.6.1: a pseudoaneurysm (*arrow*) not appreciated in the standard projection can be seen at the beginning of the descending aorta

Figure 1.6.3 Right posterior oblique thoracic aortogram shows joint outflow from the brachiocephalic trunk and left carotid (bovine arch) as well as as a severe eccentric stenosis at the root of the left subclavian (*arrow*)

Figure 1.6.4 Arteriogram of the descending aorta: in this case, the catheter is placed at the level of the beginning of the descending aorta to obtain a better depiction of the intercostal arteries

Comments

The thoracic aorta is usually studied using femoral access; a pigtail or similar type catheter is inserted up through the abdominal aorta, thoracic aorta, and aortic arch so that the tip of the catheter is positioned approximately 2 cm above the aortic valve. The study can also be done with brachial access; the right brachial artery should be used if dissection is suspected and femoral pulses are weak.

Large volumes (30–40 mL) of contrast material must be injected at a flow of 15–20 mL/s with a high trigger speed to reduce motion artifacts due to the beating of the heart.

The standard projection for the evaluation of the aortic arch is the right posterior oblique projection, because it enables the entire length of the aortic arch and the outlets of the supraaortic trunks to be imaged. From left to right, the brachiocephalic trunk, the left carotid artery, and the left subclavian artery leave from the superior wall of the aortic arch. In adults, the normal diameters of the aortic arch and descending thoracic artery are 35 and 25 mm, respectively.

Anomalies of the aorta, the pulmonary arteries, and the supraaortic trunks sometimes form vascular rings, which may be associated to cardiac alterations.

Conjoined branching of the brachiocephalic trunk and left carotid (bovine arch) and aberrant right subclavian artery are the most common abnormalities.

Procedure Steps

1. Obtain access through the right femoral artery using the Seldinger technique.
2. Introduce the guidewire until the ascending thoracic aorta.
3. Ascend the pigtail catheter over the guidewire to the ascending aorta.
4. Withdraw the guidewire and check for correct arrangement of the distal tip of the pigtail catheter.
5. Position the catheter about 2 cm above the aortic valve.
6. Connect the catheter to the injection pump and flush the connecting systems.
7. Obtain the images.

Equipment List

1. 10 and 20 mL syringes.
2. 21½G intramuscular needle, 2% injectable lidocaine, and 8.4% sodium bicarbonate.
3. 16G Abbocath, 0.035 in. introducer sheath guidewire, and valved introducer sheath.
4. 0.035 in. conventional guidewire.
5. 5F pigtail catheter.
6. Stopcock and connections.
7. Injection pump and iodinated contrast.

Case 1.7

■

The Abdominal Aorta. Obtaining an Aortogram

Figure 1.7.1 Normal PA abdominal aortogram

Figure 1.7.2 PA abdominal aortogram in a 57-year-old male patient studied for lower limb claudication. Two right and one left polar arteries can be seen (*arrows*). Delayed perfusion of the parenchyma of the *right lower pole* defines the area fed by the polar artery

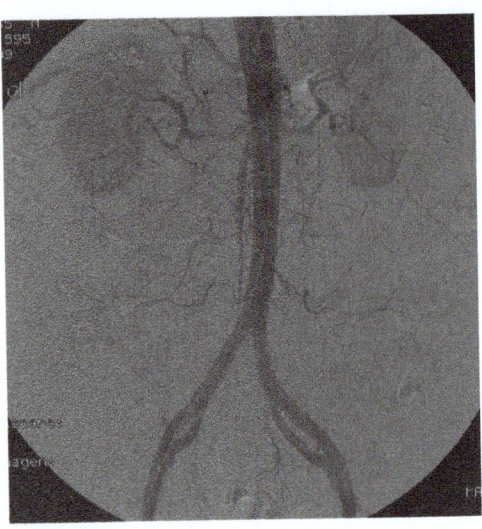

Fig. 1.7.1

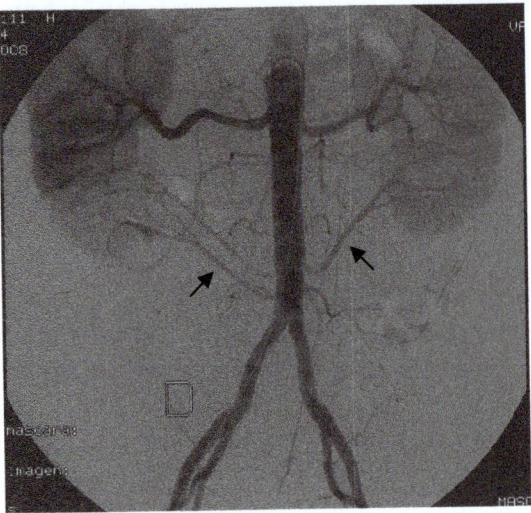

Fig. 1.7.2

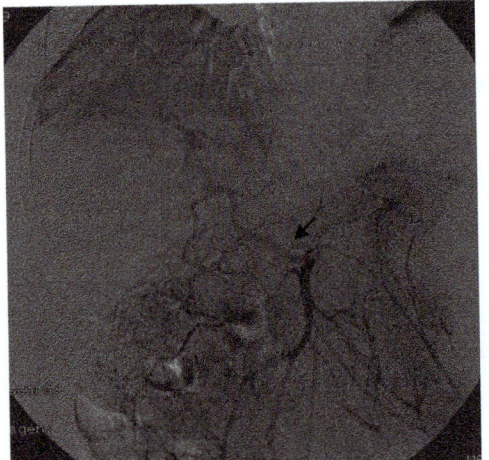

Fig. 1.7.3

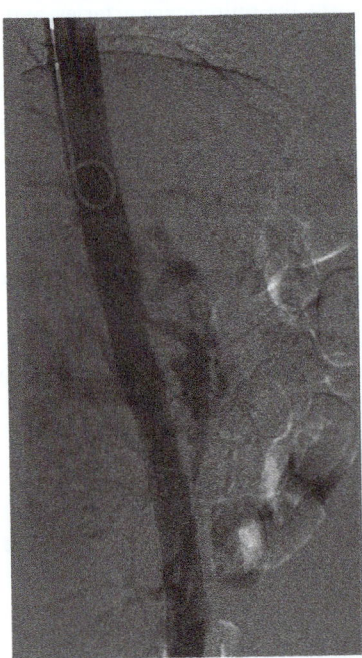

Fig. 1.7.4

Figure 1.7.3 Selective arteriogram of the superior mesenteric artery shows the existence of a right hepatic artery (*arrow*) with an independent outlet from the superior mesenteric artery
Figure 1.7.4 Lateral abdominal aortogram obtained through left brachial access shows significant stenoses of the celiac trunk and the superior mesenteric artery. The lateral projection is necessary to evaluate the ostia

Comments

Angiography of the abdominal aorta should be performed using a 4–5F straight, pigtail, or similar catheter with a multiperforated tip to enable high-flow injection. An injector should be used to administer 15–30 mL contrast material at a rate of 10–15 mL/s. Correct evaluation of the renal arteries requires the distal tip of the catheter to be placed approximately at the level of L1, and if the trunk of the celiac and mesenteric arteries is to be evaluated, the distal tip should be placed at the level of T11–T12. Although the standard projection for the evaluation of the abdominal aorta is the PA, lateral projections should be performed to evaluate the ostia of the visceral trunks, the anterior and posterior walls of the aorta, when measurements need to be taken, etc. Extreme caution is warranted during catheterization of the abdominal aorta in patients with known aneurysms and in those with severe atheromatosis to prevent detachment of the mural thrombus or atheromatous plaques.

The normal diameter of the aorta at the level of the renal arteries is 15–20 mm in a 30-year-old. From cephalad to caudal, the major branches of the abdominal aorta are the celiac trunk at the level of T12–L1, the superior mesenteric artery at the level of L1–L2, the renal arteries at the level of the superior mesenteric artery or just below it, and the inferior mesenteric at the level of L3–L4, typically from the left anterolateral aspect.

Anatomical variants of the abdominal aorta are rare; however, variants of its visceral branches are very common. Very common variants include right hepatic artery origin in the superior mesenteric artery and independent origin of the three branches of the celiac trunk. Multiple renal arteries are present in up to 25–30% of the population.

Procedure Steps

1. Approach from the femoral artery using the Seldinger technique.
2. Introduce the guidewire until the thoracic artery.
3. Advance the pigtail catheter over the guidewire to the abdominal aorta.
4. Withdraw the guidewire and check for appropriate orientation of the distal tip of the pigtail catheter.
5. Position the catheter at the level of T12–L1.
6. Connect the catheter to the injection pump and flush the connecting systems.
7. Obtain the images.

Equipment List

1. 10 and 20 mL syringes.
2. 21½G intramuscular needle, 2% injectable lidocaine, and 8.4% sodium bicarbonate.
3. 16G Abbocath, 0.035 in. introducer sheath guidewire, and valved introducer sheath.
4. 0.035 in. conventional guidewire.
5. 5F pigtail catheter.
6. Stopcock and connections.
7. Injection pump and iodinated contrast.

Case 1.8

The Pelvis. Angiographic Study

Figure 1.8.1 Arteriogram of the normal pelvis showing the common iliac artery (*black arrow*), internal iliac artery (*white arrow*), and external iliac artery (*arrowhead*)

Figure 1.8.2 Oblique arteriogram of the pelvis shows the internal iliac arteries and the femoral bifurcation better than in the PA projection

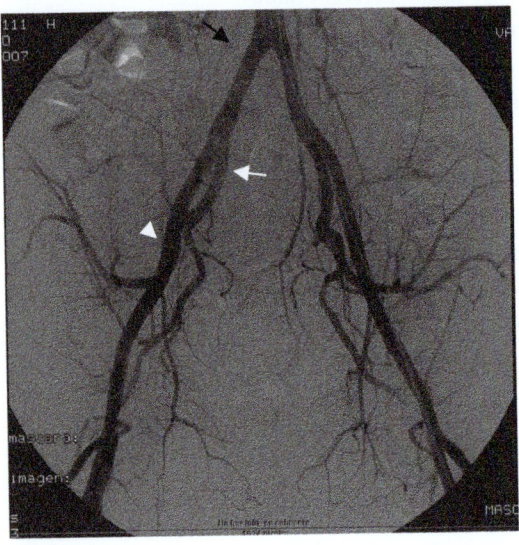

Fig. 1.8.1

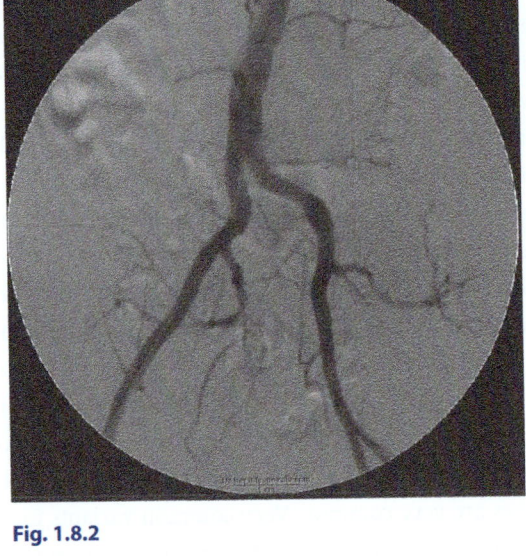

Fig. 1.8.2

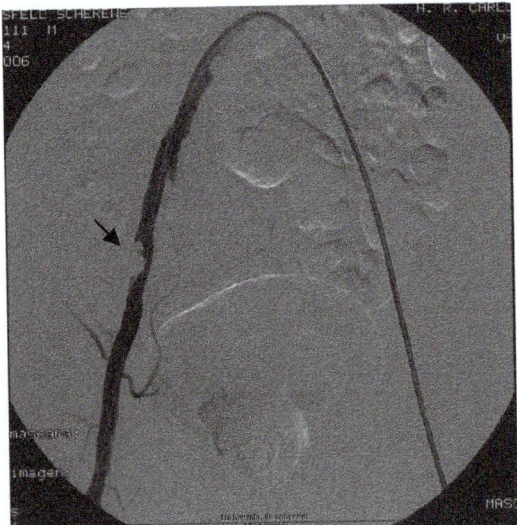

Fig. 1.8.3

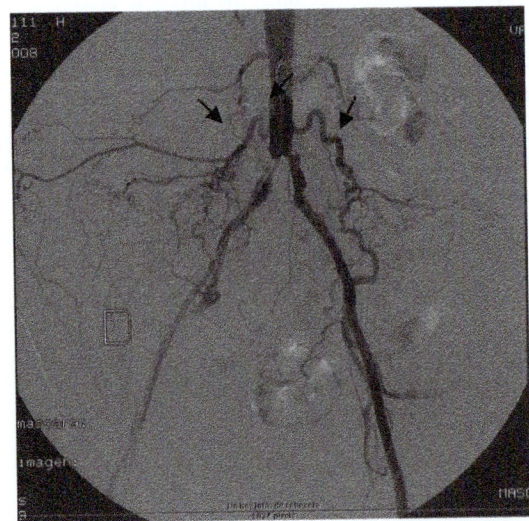

Fig. 1.8.4

Figure 1.8.3 Selective study of the right iliac artery through left femoral access (contralateral approach). Eccentric stenosis (*arrow*) due to an atheromatous plaque is seen at the level of the external iliac artery

Figure 1.8.4 Arteriogram of the pelvis showing significant stenosis of both common iliac arteries due to severe atheromatosis. Collateral vessels, in this case lumbar arteries (*arrows*), are markedly hypertrophied to compensate lack of flow from stenosed common iliac arteries

Comments

Angiographic study of the pelvis, like that of the abdominal aorta, is usually performed with vascular access through the femoral artery by placing a high-flow multiperforated catheter at the level of the aortic bifurcation; the volume and flow rate of contrast material are similar to those used to study the abdominal aorta. When the iliac arteries are severely affected and the pulses are weak or absent, US-guided arterial puncture and hydrophilic guidewires may be necessary. When this approach is very difficult, the study can be carried out using brachial access.

If the iliac arteries are occluded or severely stenosed, the catheter must be placed at the level of the renal arteries because the iliac arteries will be filled through the ipsilateral lumbar arteries. Oblique (25–30°) projections are necessary to evaluate peripheral vascular disease and for adequate depiction of the iliac and femoral bifurcations. The right posterior oblique projection will show the left iliac artery and the right femoral bifurcation, and the left posterior oblique projection will show the right iliac artery and the left femoral bifurcation.

If only one iliac artery needs to be evaluated, the study is usually done using retrograde access through the contralateral femoral artery with posterior catheterization of the iliac to be studied with a Neff, Simmons, or similar catheter. The internal iliac arteries and their branches can generally be studied in the same way, given the better angle of entry from the contralateral femoral artery.

Procedure Steps

1. Approach through the right femoral artery using the Seldinger technique.
2. Introduce the guidewire to the abdominal aorta.
3. Advance the pigtail catheter to a position above the aortic bifurcation.
4. Withdraw the guidewire and check for appropriate orientation of the distal tip of the pigtail catheter.
5. Position the catheter just above the aortic bifurcation.
6. Connect the catheter to the injection pump and flush the connecting systems.
7. Obtain the images.

Equipment List

1. 10 and 20 mL syringes.
2. 21½G intramuscular needle, 2% injectable lidocaine, and 8.4% sodium bicarbonate.
3. 16G Abbocath, 0.035 in. introducer sheath guidewire, and valved introducer sheath.
4. 0.035 in. conventional guidewire.
5. 5F pigtail catheter.
6. Stopcock and connections.
7. Injection pump and iodinated contrast.

Case 1.9
■
Lower Limbs. Angiographic Study

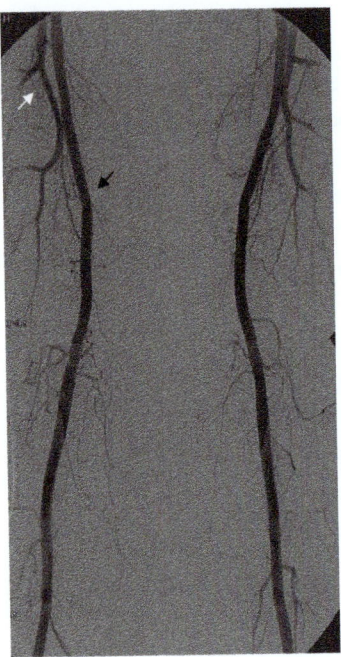

Fig. 1.9.1

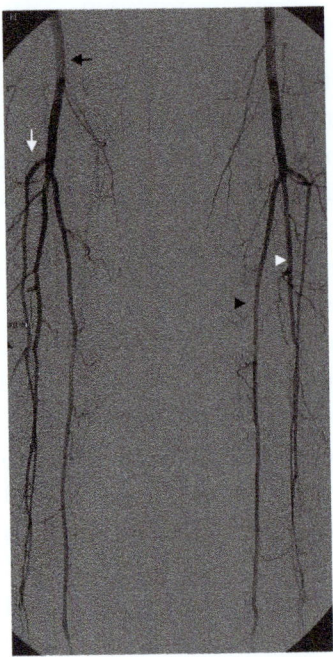

Fig. 1.9.2

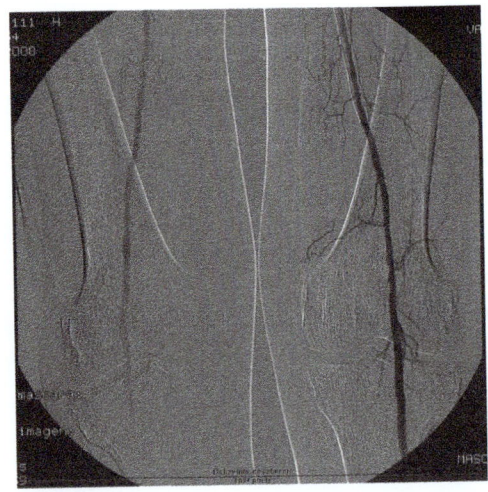

Fig. 1.9.3

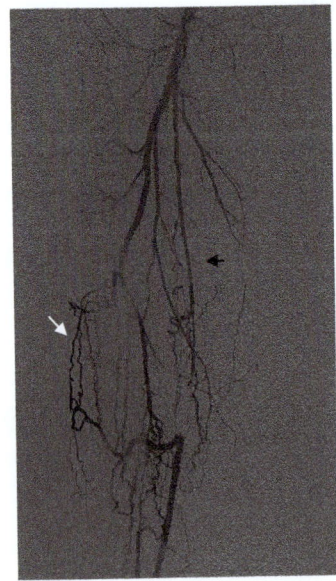

Fig. 1.9.4

Figure 1.9.1 Normal arteriogram of the lower limbs. Deep femoral artery (*white arrow*); superficial femoral artery (*black arrow*)

Figure 1.9.2 Normal arteriogram of the lower limbs at the level of the popliteal sector and distal trunks. Popliteal artery (*black arrow*), anterior tibial artery (*white arrow*), peroneal artery (*white arrowhead*), and posterior tibial artery (*black arrowhead*)

Figure 1.9.3 Arteriogram of the lower limbs at the level of the femoropopliteal sector showing markedly delayed hemodynamics of the right lower limb

Figure 1.9.4 Threadlike superficial femoral artery from its origin (*black arrow*) with filling of the distal third of the distal superficial femoral arteries through collateral branches of the deep femoral artery (*white arrow*)

Comments

For the angiographic study of both lower limbs, the catheter will remain in the iliac bifurcation, and we will inject and shoot in the different stations from the thighs to the feet; it is also possible to follow a bolus of contrast material fluoroscopically. If only one limb needs to be evaluated, a retrograde approach through the contralateral artery is usually used, with posterior catheterization of the opposite iliac artery the same as in pelvic studies, descending then to the common femoral artery and superficial femoral artery, if necessary. A single limb can also be studied using antegrade access to the ipsilateral femoral artery if iliac study is not necessary and if endovascular treatment will be carried out in the distal trunks. If the distal trunks are not clearly contrasted in the initial studies, the position of the injecting catheter in the superficial femoral artery or popliteal artery should be checked; vasodilators like glyceryl trinitrate or nitroglycerine can be administered to facilitate assessment.

With respect to the collateral circulation, if the superficial femoral artery is obstructed, the branches of the lateral circumflex artery and the perforating arteries will supply the most distal segment of the superficial femoral and popliteal arteries. If the popliteal artery is obstructed, the sural and genicular arteries at the level of the knee and proximal end of the lower leg will provide collateral supply.

Procedure Steps

1. Approach through the right femoral artery using the Seldinger technique.
2. Introduce the guidewire to the abdominal aorta.
3. Advance the pigtail catheter to a position above the aortic bifurcation.
4. Withdraw the guidewire and check for appropriate orientation of the distal tip of the pigtail catheter.
5. Position the catheter just above the aortic bifurcation.
6. Connect the catheter to the injection pump and flush the connecting systems.
7. Obtain the images.

Equipment List

1. 10 and 20 mL syringes.
2. 21½G intramuscular needle, 2% injectable lidocaine, and 8.4% sodium bicarbonate.
3. 16G Abbocath, 0.035 in. introducer sheath guidewire, and valved introducer sheath.
4. 0.035 in. conventional guidewire.
5. 5F pigtail catheter.
6. Stopcock and connections.
7. Injection pump and iodinated contrast.

Figure 1.10.1 Selective arteriogram of the right subclavian artery through a vertebral catheter. From proximal to distal, we can see the exit of the vertebral artery (*black arrow*), internal mammary artery (*white arrow*), thyrocervical trunk (*white arrowhead*), and costocervical trunk (*black arrowhead*)

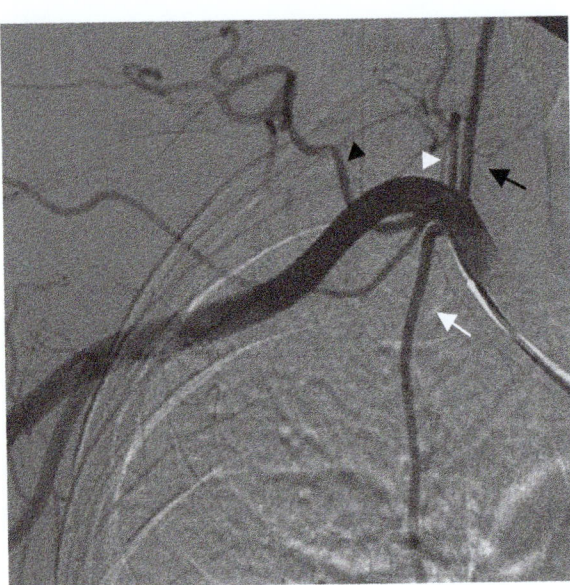

Fig. 1.10.1

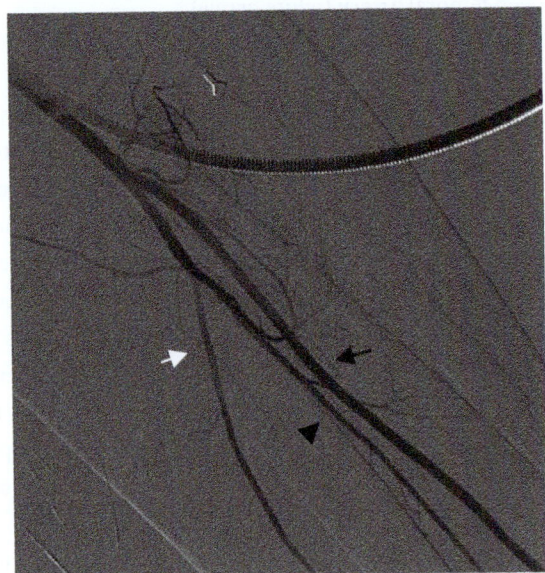

Fig. 1.10.2

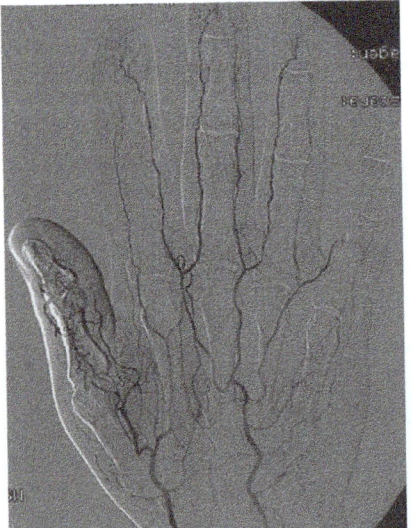

Fig. 1.10.3

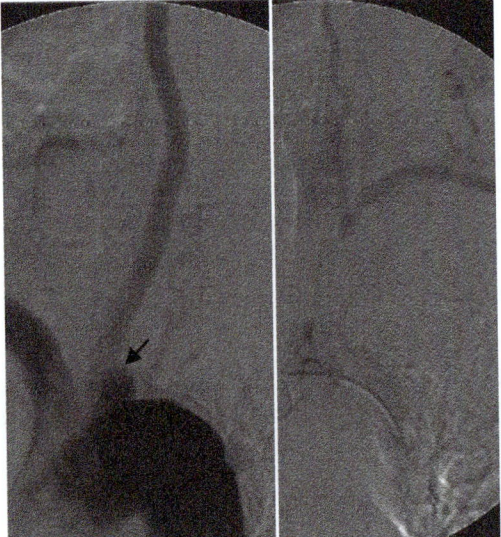

Fig. 1.10.4

Figure 1.10.2 Brachial arteriogram acquired using retrograde access through the ipsilateral brachial artery shows the normal bifurcations of the brachial artery (*black arrow*) into the radial artery (*black arrow*), cubital or ulnar artery (*white arrow*), and interosseous artery (*black arrowhead*)

Figure 1.10.3 DSA of the hand. Delayed hemodynamics of the fifth finger

Figure 1.10.4 Aortograms of the aortic arch: the image on the left shows the complete occlusion of the initial portion of the left subclavian artery (*black arrow*); the image on the *right* shows the filling of the left subclavian artery from the ipsilateral vertebral artery, which is consistent with subclavian steal syndrome

Catheterization of the brachiocephalic trunk, the left carotid artery, and the right subclavian artery can be accomplished with a 4 or 5F vertebral catheter. The simplest way is to advance the distal tip of the catheter to the ascending aorta, point the tip at the cephalad wall of the aorta, and withdraw the catheter progressively until it is introduced in the different ostia. In older patients with elongated supraaortic trunks, selective catheterization may require the use of catheters with curved tips that advance distally as they are pulled through the ostium (Simmons, Neff...). Extreme caution is necessary during the catheterization of older patients with severe atheromatosis to minimize the risk of cerebral or peripheral embolisms.

To evaluate the hand, it might be useful to dilute the contrast material with saline solution and/or administer glyceryl trinitrate and nitroglycerine to reduce pain and vasospasm of the small distal arterioles.

Obstruction of the subclavian artery at a proximal level will lead to collateral supply from the vertebrobasilar system, inverting flow at the level of the vertebral artery ipsilateral to the obstruction. When the occlusion is distal to the exit of the vertebral artery, collateral vascularization will take place through the branches of the thyrocervical, costocervical, or lateral thoracic arteries.

Comments

1. Approach through the right femoral artery using the Seldinger technique.
2. Introduce the guidewire to the thoracic aorta.
3. Advance the vertebral catheter to the thoracic aorta.
4. Withdraw the guidewire and point the tip of the catheter toward the cephalad wall of the aorta.
5. Slowly withdraw the catheter until the tip enters the different ostia and advance it with the guidewire.
6. Check the position of the catheter by injecting contrast material under fluoroscopic guidance.
7. Obtain the images.

Procedure Steps

1. 10 and 20 mL syringes.
2. 21½G intramuscular needle, 2% injectable lidocaine, and 8.4% sodium bicarbonate.
3. 16G Abbocath, 0.035 in. introducer sheath guidewire, and valved introducer sheath.
4. 0.035 in. curved-tip hydrophilic guidewire.
5. 5F vertebral catheter.
6. Stopcock and connections.

Equipment List

Further Reading

Bancroft JW, Benenati JF, Becker GJ, Katzen BT, Zemel G. Neutralized lidocaine: use in pain reduction in local anesthesia. J Vasc Interv Radiol JVIR 1992;3(1):107-109.

Carey D, Martin JR, Moore CA, Valentine MC, Nygaard TW. Complications of femoral artery closure devices. Catheter Cardio Vasc Interv 2001;52:3.

Grier D, Hartnell G. Percutaneous femoral artery puncture: practice and anatomy. Br J Cardiol 1990;63:602-604.

Hoffer EK, Bloch RD. Percutaneous arterial closure devices. J Vasc Interv Radiol 2003;14:865-886.

Jaques PF, Mauro MA, Keefe B. US guidance for vascular access. Technical note. J Vase Interv Radiol 1992;3:427-430.

Krueger K, Zaehringer M, Strohe D, Stuetzer H, Boecker J, Lackner K. Postcatheterization pseudoaneurysm: results of US-guided percutaneous thrombin injection in 240 patients. Radiology 2005;236:1104-1110.

Narins CR. Access strategies for peripheral arterial intervention. Cardiol J 2009;16(1):88-97. Review.

Sheiman RG, Brophy DP. Treatment of iatrogenic femoral pseudoaneurysms with percutaneous thrombin injection: experience in 54 patients. Radiology 2001;219(1):123-127.

Spijkerboer AM, Scholten FG, Mali WPTM, van Schaik JPJ. Antegrade puncture of the femoral artery: morphology study. Radiology 1990;176:57-60.

Noninvasive Vascular and Nonvascular Diagnosis

2

Carlos Alonso, José R. Fortuño, Joan Falcó, Lydia Alcalá, Antonio Luna, and Ramón Ribes

J.J. Muñoz and R. Ribes, *Learning Vascular and Interventional Radiology*, Learning Imaging,
DOI: 10.1007/978-3-540-87997-8_2, © Springer-Verlag Berlin Heidelberg 2010

Case 2.1
■
Coronary Artery Stenosis

Figure 2.1.1 Volume-rendered image showing focal stenosis (*arrow*) of the proximal LAD

Figures 2.1.2 and 2.1.3 Analysis of the proximal LAD at the level of the stenosis shows a hypodense focal lipoatheromatous plaque (*arrows*) measuring less than 1 cm

Figure 2.1.4 Coronariography of the LAD stenosis (*arrow*)

A 61-year-old woman presented with nonspecific chest pain. Findings at blood tests and ECG were normal; stress test was inconclusive. CT study of the coronary arteries was performed to rule out disease.

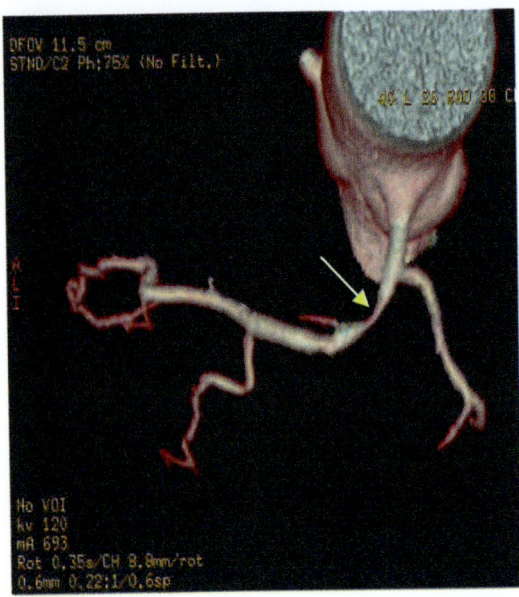

Fig. 2.1.1

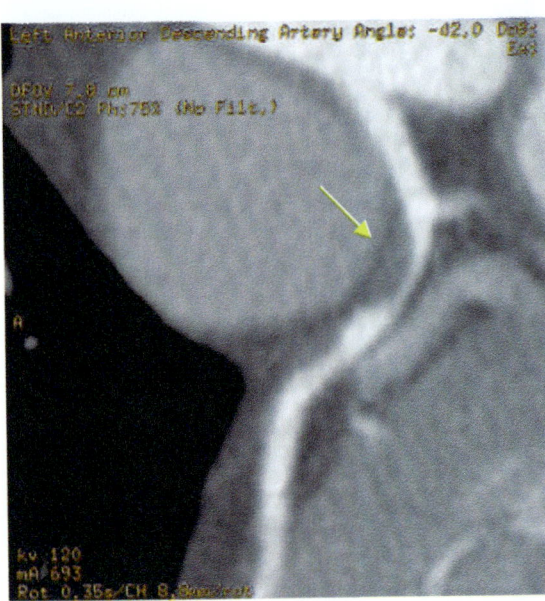

Fig. 2.1.2

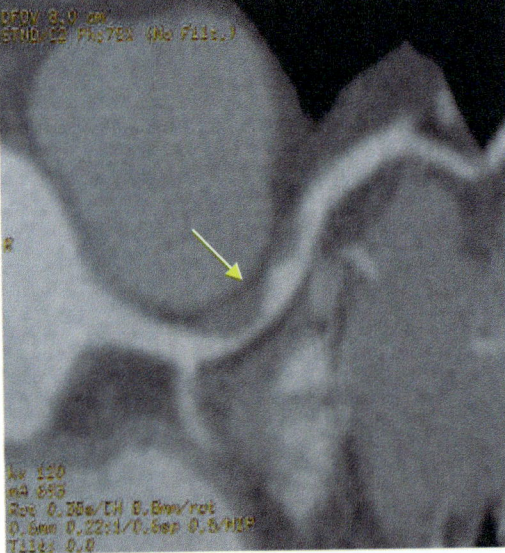

Fig. 2.1.3

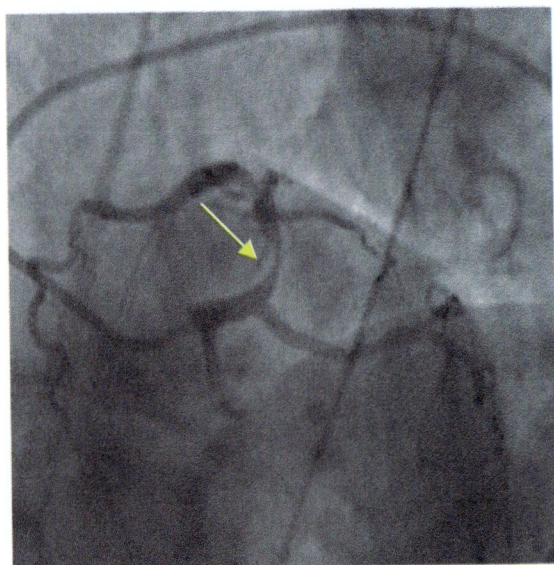

Fig. 2.1.4

Two coronary arteries arise from the heart: the *right* coronary artery and the *left* coronary artery, which branches into the left anterior descending artery (LAD) and the left circumflex artery (LCx).

The LAD runs toward the apex of the heart, with septal and diagonal branches on both sides. The LCx descends through the coronary sulcus and gives rise to one or more left marginal arteries.

The right coronary artery bifurcates into the posterolateral artery and the posterior descending artery (PDA), which runs through the posterior interventricular sulcus; the origin of the PDA determines cardiac dominance (right in 85% of cases).

CT of the coronary arteries makes it possible to evaluate these vessels; with a negative predictive value of 99–100%, this technique is very useful for ruling out disease. Its sensitivity and specificity range from 80 to 95% and depend on the number of detectors in the scanner, the caliber of the vessel evaluated, and the type of patient.

The current indications for CT of the coronary arteries include atypical chest pain with normal ECG and enzyme levels, clinically or electrically inconclusive stress tests, bypass follow-up, stent follow-up, congenital anomalies, and even triple rule-out (i.e., triple evaluation of coronary arteries, pulmonary arteries, and aortic disease).

Comments

Greet the patient and fill out the form (reason for the examination, fundamental heart disease, medication). If the patient is on beta-blockers, do not administer any medication; if not, administer 50 g metoprolol 1–1.5 h before the examination.

Use an 18G trocar to insert a cannula for vascular access.

Have the patient lie down and attach the ECG electrodes.

Administer sublingual nitroglycerine if blood pressure is normal.

Explain the procedure and practice breath-holding.

Load contrast material and saline solution in the two compartments of the injector.

Imaging protocol: inject 70–80cc contrast material at a rate of 5 mL/s + 40 mL saline solution at a rate of 3.5 mL/s.

120 Kv 700 mAs.

Tube modulation (greater radiation at end-diastole).

Center the study on the area from the tracheal carina to the apex of the heart.

Start the study performed with smart prep by placing the ROI at the root of the aorta; begin image acquisition when the density surpasses 150 HU.

Choose the reconstruction protocol: below 70 bpm, use segment mode (beat information), reconstructing by default 75% of the R-R cycle (end-diastolic phase), which is the reconstruction with the least heart movement. Above 70 bpm, use the Bursa mode, which analyzes the information from several beats.

Reconstruct each vessel at the workstation using dedicated programs (volume rendering, MIP, RMP, lumen, curve, etc.).

Complete the report, analyzing the number of stenoses, their location, degree (significant >50%), state of the remaining vessels, etc.

Procedure

Case 2.2
■
Evaluating a Coronary Bypass with MDCT

Figure 2.2.1 Volume-rendered image shows the root of the aorta with an aortic graft to supply the distal portion of the right coronary artery

Figure 2.2.2 Volume-rendered image shows two other aortic grafts to supply the diagonal and oblique marginal branches; the native arteries are severely calcified

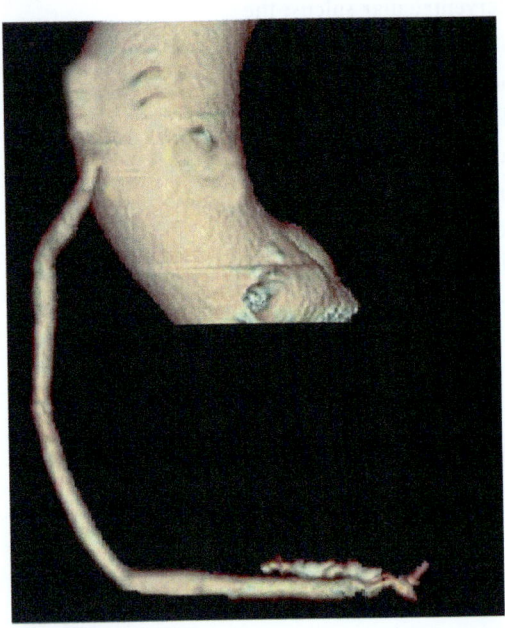

Fig. 2.2.1

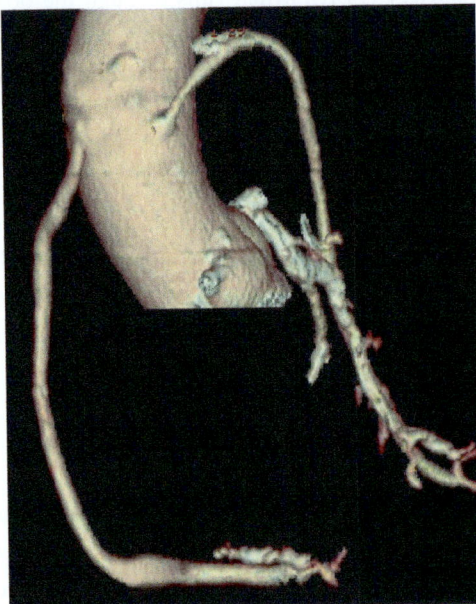

Fig. 2.2.2

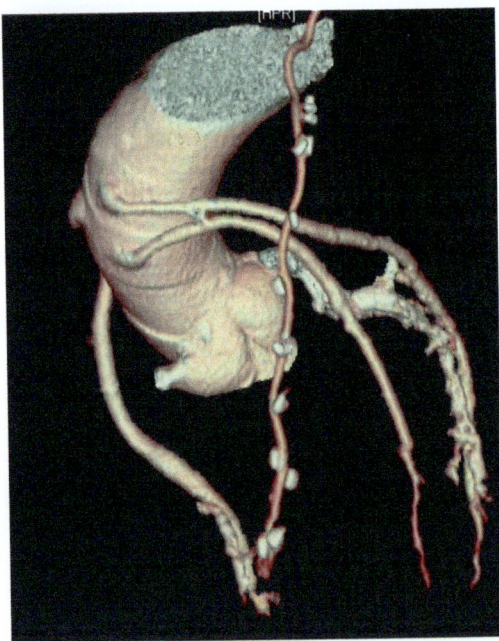

Fig. 2.2.3

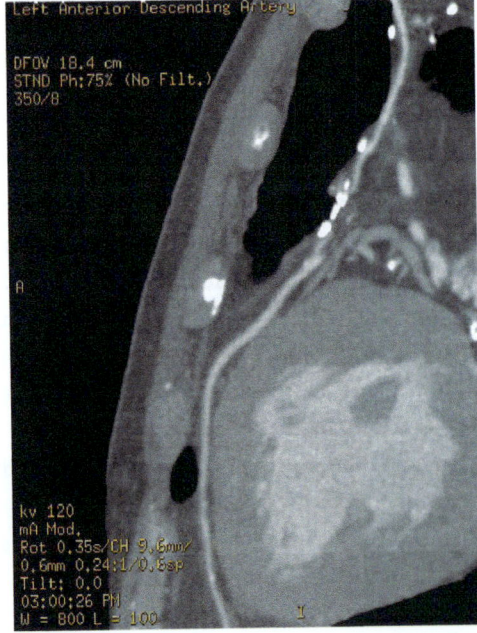

Fig. 2.2.4

Figure 2.2.3 Volume-rendered image shows a mammary graft supplying the LAD
Figure 2.2.4 Curved multiplanar reconstruction following the axis of the internal mammary graft to evaluate its lumen and rule out disease

A 64-year-old man presented with chest complaints and mild dyspnea. He had a history of ischemic heart disease treated 4 years before with quadruple bypass. We performed CT of the coronary arteries to evaluate the bypasses and rule out bypass occlusion.

Comments

Ischemic heart disease can be treated surgically or percutaneously.

When only one or two vessels are involved, ischemic heart disease is treated by heart catheterization through the diseased vessel followed by the dilation of the stenosis and stenting.

When three or more vessels are involved, ischemic heart disease is treated by the surgical placement of grafts from the aorta using donor arteries or veins or by using the internal mammary artery to reestablish flow to stenosed vessels. Surgical treatment is only possible when the distal beds of the different coronary arteries are patent.

Before the advent of MDCT, the patency of bypasses and stents could only be studied by repeated heart catheterization, which, although relatively safe, is not without risk.

Today, the assessment of stents or bypasses is one of the indications for the CT examination of the coronary arteries.

Procedure

Greet the patient and fill out the form (reason for the examination, fundamental heart disease, medication). If the patient is on beta-blockers, do not administer any medication; if not, administer 50 g metoprolol 1–1.5 h before the examination.

Use an 18G trocar to insert a cannula for vascular access.

Have the patient lie down and attach the ECG electrodes.

Administer sublingual nitroglycerine if blood pressure is normal.

Explain the procedure and practice breath-holding.

Load contrast material and saline solution in the two compartments of the injector.

Imaging protocol: inject 70–80cc contrast material at a rate of 5 mL/s + 40 mL saline solution at a rate of 3.5 mL/s.

120 Kv 700 mAs.

Tube modulation (greater radiation at end-diastole).

Center the study on the area from the supraaortic trunks to the apex of the heart.

Start the study performed with smart prep by placing the ROI at the root of the aorta; begin image acquisition when the density surpasses 150 HU.

Choose the reconstruction protocol: below 70 bpm, use segment mode (beat information), reconstructing by default 75% of the R-R cycle (end-diastolic phase), which is the reconstruction with the least heart movement. Above 70 bpm, use the Bursa mode, which analyzes the information from several beats.

Reconstruct each vessel at the workstation using dedicated programs (volume rendering, MIP, RMP, lumen, curve, etc.).

Complete the report, analyzing the number of stenoses, their location, degree (significant >50%), state of the remaining vessels, etc.

Case 2.3

■

Congenital Anomaly of the Coronary Vessels

Figures 2.3.1 and 2.3.2 Volume-rendered images of the aortic root with anterior and superior views of the right and left coronary arteries show that the right coronary artery originates from the left common trunk

Figure 2.3.3 Volume-rendered image of the heart shows the path of the right coronary artery passing through the aortic root and the trunk of the pulmonary artery

Figure 2.3.4 Curved multiplanar reconstruction of the right coronary artery shows its path between the aortic root and the pulmonary trunk

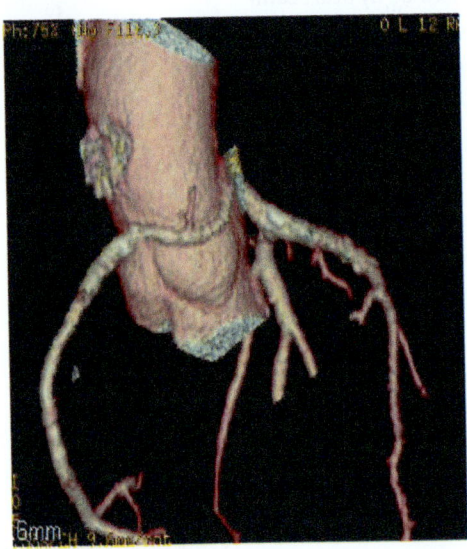

Fig. 2.3.1

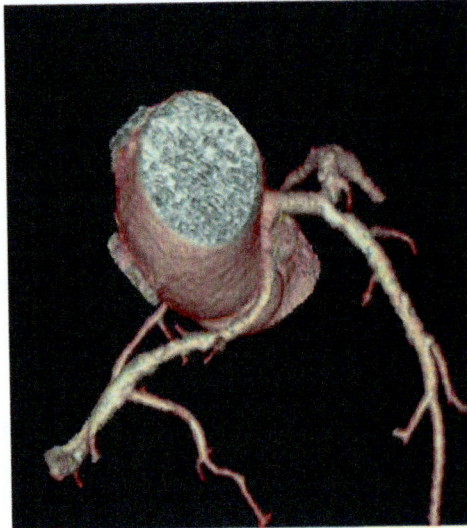

Fig. 2.3.2

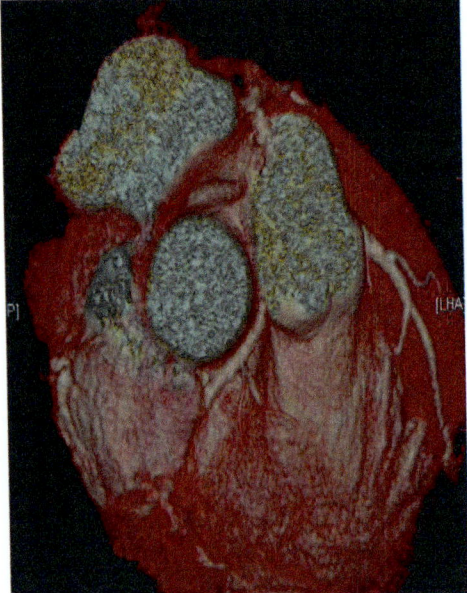

Fig. 2.3.3

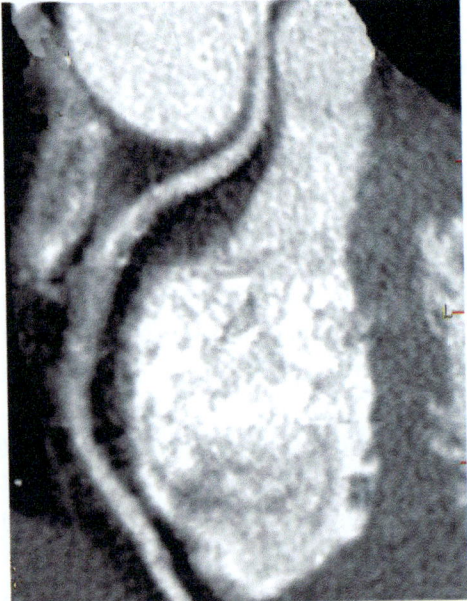

Fig. 2.3.4

A 36-year-old man presented with chest discomfort that increased with physical exercise. Findings at ECG and echocardiography were normal.

CT study of the coronary arteries is a simple, noninvasive way to evaluate congenital disease.

Congenital anomalies of the coronary arteries are found in 1% of all patients undergoing heart catheterization. There are three types: ectopia originating in the coronary sinus, absence of the artery, and ectopia originating in the main pulmonary artery (associated to fistulas). The first two types are the most common.

The origin of the right coronary artery in the left common trunk with a path between the aortic root and the trunk of the pulmonary artery seen in this case is one of the malignant congenital anomalies; it is associated to arrhythmias, syncope, and sudden death due to compression of the right coronary artery between the two large arterial trunks.

Greet the patient and fill out the form (reason for the examination, fundamental heart disease, medication). If the patient is on beta-blockers, do not administer any medication; if not, administer 50 g metoprolol 1–1.5 h before the examination.

Insert a cannula for vascular access.

Have the patient lie down and attach the ECG electrodes.

Administer sublingual nitroglycerine if blood pressure is normal.

Explain the procedure and practice breath-holding.

Load contrast material and saline solution in the two compartments of the injector.

Imaging protocol: inject 70–80cc contrast material at a rate of 5 mL/s + 40 mL saline solution at a rate of 3.5 mL/s.

120 Kv 700 mAs.

Tube modulation (greater radiation at end-diastole).

Center the study on the area from the tracheal carina to the apex of the heart.

Start the study performed with smart prep by placing the ROI at the root of the aorta; begin image acquisition when the density surpasses 150 HU.

Choose the reconstruction protocol: below 70 bpm, use segment mode (beat information), reconstructing by default 75% of the R-R cycle (end-diastolic phase), which is the reconstruction with the least heart movement. Above 70 bpm, use the Bursa mode, which analyzes the information from several beats.

Reconstruct each vessel at the workstation using dedicated programs (volume rendering, MIP, RMP, lumen, curve, etc.).

Complete the report, analyzing the number of stenoses, their location, degree (significant >50%), state of the remaining vessels, etc.

A 64-detector MDCT is best, although the examination can be performed with fewer detectors with longer periods of breath-holding; use the ECG to synchronize the study.

Double-head injector.

Iodinated contrast material.

18G trocar.

Beta-blockers.

Administer sublingual nitroglycerine a few minutes before the study.

Comments

Procedure

Equipment Required

Case 2.4
Stenosis in a Carotid Stent due to Intimal Hyperplasia

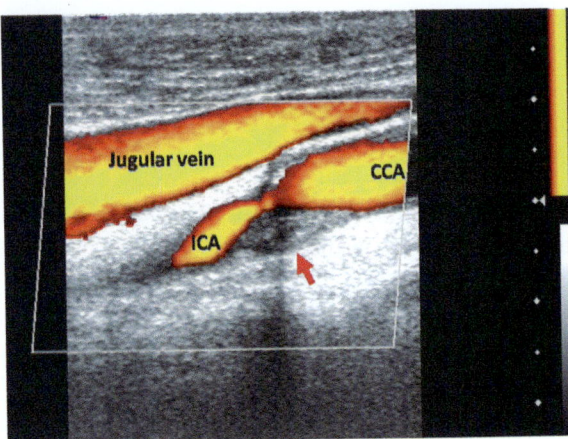

Fig. 2.4.1

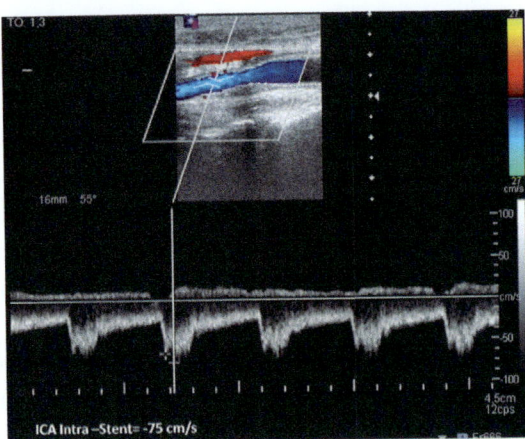

Fig. 2.4.2

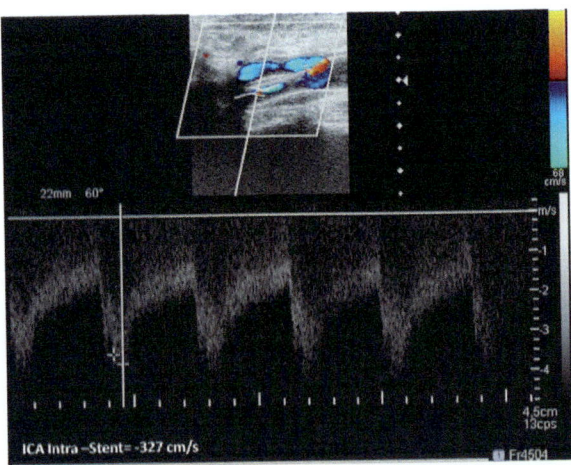

Fig. 2.4.3

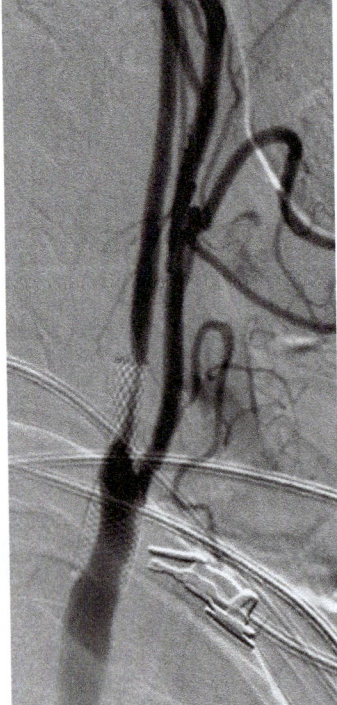

Fig. 2.4.4

Figure 2.4.1 Power-Doppler US shows significant stenosis in the left internal carotid artery caused by a predominantly hypoechoic plaque (*arrow*)

Figure 2.4.2 Follow-up pulsed Doppler US 30 days after stent placement shows the absence of pathological findings distal to the stent

Figure 2.4.3 Follow-up pulsed Doppler US 6 months after stent placement shows narrowing of the lumen, turbulent flow, and a considerable increase in the systolic peak in the area distal to the stent, compatible with significant stenosis within the stent

Figure 2.4.4 Selective arteriogram of the left carotid arteries corroborates the stenosis within the stent due to intimal hyperplasia

A 54-year-old man with multiple cardiovascular risk factors presented after a transitory ischemic attack manifesting as amaurosis fugax in his left eye. Doppler US showed significant (>70%) stenosis of the left internal carotid artery, and a carotid stent was percutaneously placed in the context of a randomized clinical trial.

Comments

Carotid stenting is an efficacious alternative to endarterectomy for symptomatic stenosis of the carotid arteries. However, due to the possibility of stenosis within the stent, strict Doppler US follow-up is necessary after stenting.

Although numerous recommendations have been published, there is no consensus regarding the Doppler criteria for restenosis. However, it seems clear that a baseline study should be performed to enable comparison with follow-up US examinations. Turbulent flow within the stent, increases of 80% over the baseline peak systolic blood flow (Vps), or Vps >200 cm/s are highly suggestive of hemodynamically significant restenosis greater than 80%, although each imaging center should validate its US findings.

In our case, the findings were normal in the baseline and 30-day follow-up Doppler US examinations but highly pathological in the 6-month follow-up, coinciding with a recurrence of symptoms. As the treatment of choice for symptomatic restenosis was angioplasty, we were able to corroborate the US findings by angiography prior to balloon dilation.

Case 2.5

Significant Stenosis in the Middle Portion of the Cephalic Vein

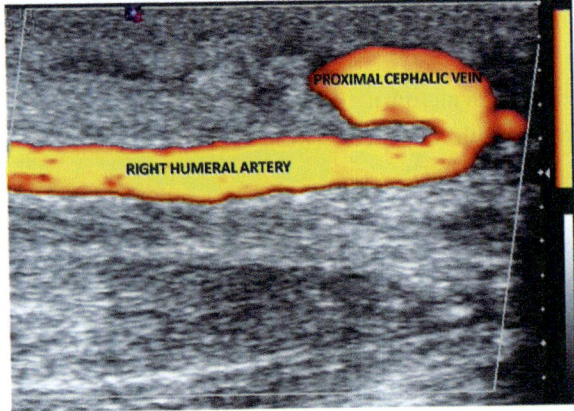

Fig. 2.5.1

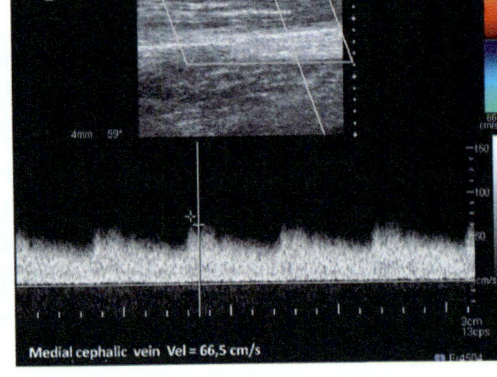

Fig. 2.5.2

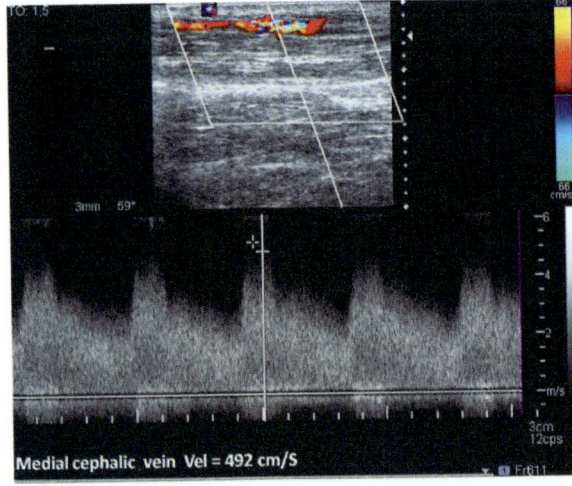

Fig. 2.5.3

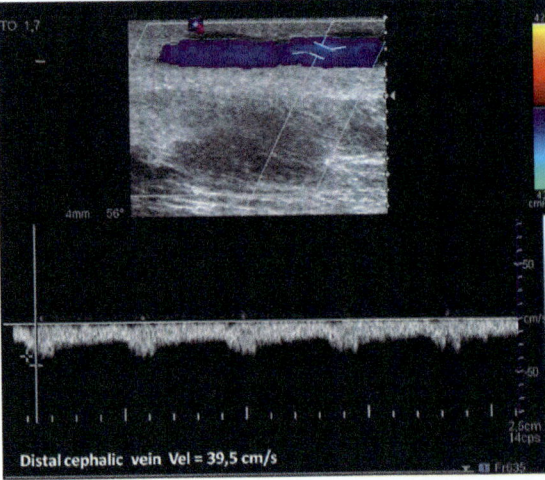

Fig. 2.5.4

Figure 2.5.1 Power Doppler US of the humeral artery shows an arteriovenous anastomosis and a patent proximal cephalic vein

Figure 2.5.2 Pulsed Doppler in the middle portion of the cephalic vein proximal to the stenotic area shows a peak systolic blood flow of 66 cm/s

Figure 2.5.3 Pulsed Doppler in the area of maximum turbulent flow in the cephalic vein stenosis reveals a peak systolic flow of 492 cm/s

Figure 2.5.4 Pulsed Doppler in the poststenotic segment of the cephalic vein shows a peak systolic flow of 39.5 cm/s

A 45-year-old man with terminal kidney failure secondary to glomerulonephritis was undergoing hemodialysis by means of an arteriovenous fistula between the right humeral artery and the right cephalic vein. Dialysis had become difficult in recent weeks, with problematic puncture and considerably increased venous pressures, so he was referred for Doppler US evaluation prior to treatment.

Comments

Doppler US is a first-line technique for the evaluation of hemodialysis fistula dysfunction. If performed by duly trained personnel using 10–15 MHz probes, it makes it possible to detect changes in the morphology of arteries, veins, or the anastomosis that cause dysfunction as well as to decide on the best treatment and best approach if treatment is to be percutaneous.

The problem usually originates in the return vein, where significant stenoses that deteriorate the quality of dialysis can appear and ultimately cause thrombosis and loss of vascular access.

The diagnostic criteria for stenosis are the same as those used in other vascular territories, i.e., significant narrowing of the vascular lumen, turbulent flow, increased peak systolic flow, and increased peak systolic flow ratio between the pre- and post-stenotic segments. In the present case, we observed a significant stenosis in the cephalic vein, with peak systolic flow of nearly 50 m/s and a ratio between the pre and poststenotic segments >7.

Case 2.6
Fibromuscular Dysplasia of the Right Renal Artery

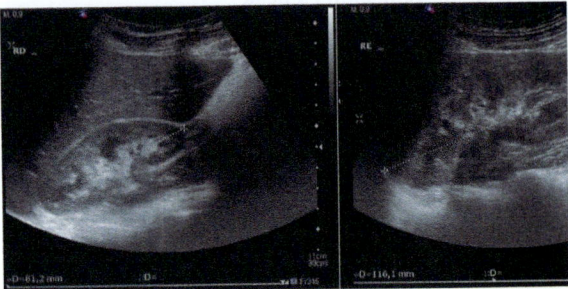

Fig. 2.6.1

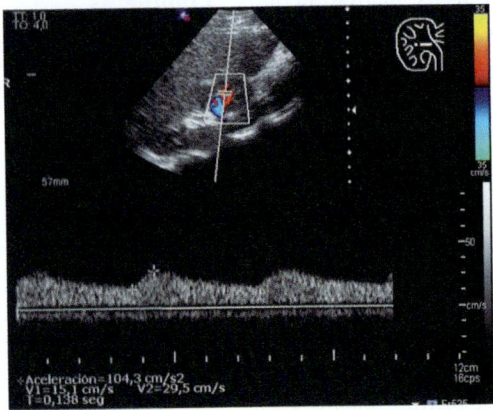

Fig. 2.6.2

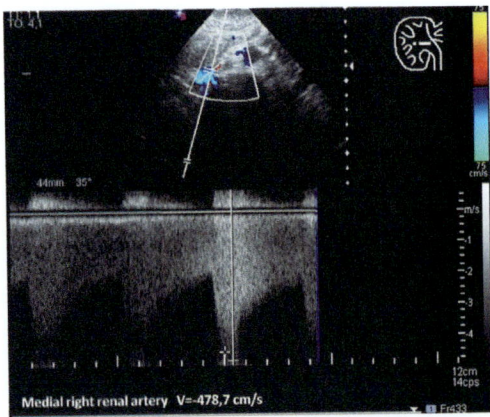

Fig. 2.6.3

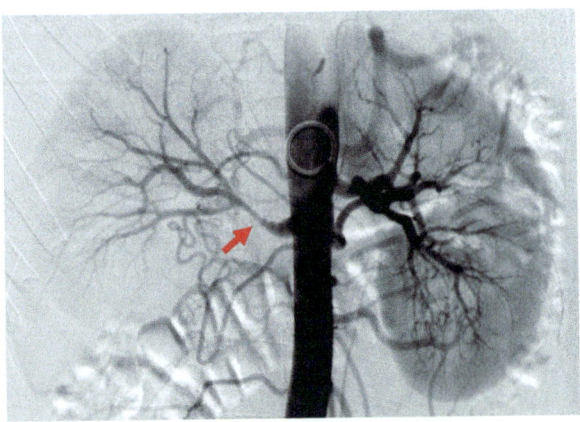

Fig. 2.6.4

Figure 2.6.1 B mode US shows atrophy of the right kidney compared to the left, without alterations in corticomedullary differentiation or in the excretory system

Figure 2.6.2 Intrarenal pulsed Doppler US shows a parvus-tardus spectral waveform image

Figure 2.6.3 Pulsed Doppler US in the middle portion of the right renal artery shows a peak systolic flow of 478 cm/s

Figure 2.6.4 Nonselective aortorenal arteriogram shows asymmetric uptake in the renal parenchyma and the characteristic string-of-pearls angiographic image (*arrow*) in the middle portion of the right renal artery

A 22-year-old woman with no relevant history or other symptoms presented with arterial hypertension of recent appearance that responded poorly to drug treatment. Doppler US was performed to rule out a vascular origin of the hypertension.

Comments

Although arterial hypertension is usually idiopathic, its recent onset with poor response to drug therapy in a young person requires Doppler US investigation of possible renal vascular disease.

Doppler US shows severe renal asymmetry, stenosis of the middle portion of the renal artery with peak systolic flow >4 m/s and parvus-tardus spectral waveform image with a peak systolic acceleration time >0.1 s. Although Doppler US is not specific, these imaging findings taken together with the epidemiological data strongly suggest that, in a young woman without atheromatosis, the cause is fibromuscular dysplasia involving the renal artery. Fibromuscular dysplasia is a noninflammatory vasculitis that affects large vessels; its cause is unknown. Although only the renal artery is involved in 75% of cases, bilateral involvement occurs occasionally, and extension to the carotid-vertebral vascular segment is not uncommon. More rarely, fibromuscular dysplasia can affect the splanchnic artery territory or the lower limbs.

The most characteristic angiographic finding is the string-of-pearls appearance of the artery caused by multiple concentric focal stenoses in the middle or distal portions of the renal artery, which can also have a more linear appearance.

Although the natural history of the disease is unpredictable in patients with poor blood pressure control, percutaneous angioplasty is recommended and resolves hypertension in more than 70% of cases.

Case 2.7
Vesical Carcinoma with Extension to the Right Ureter

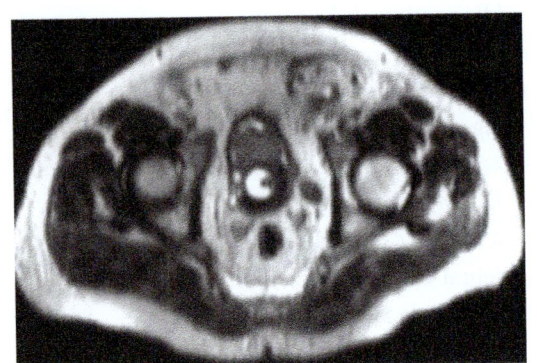

Fig. 2.7.1

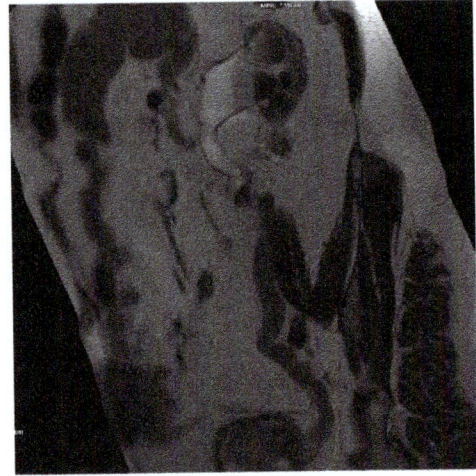

Fig. 2.7.2

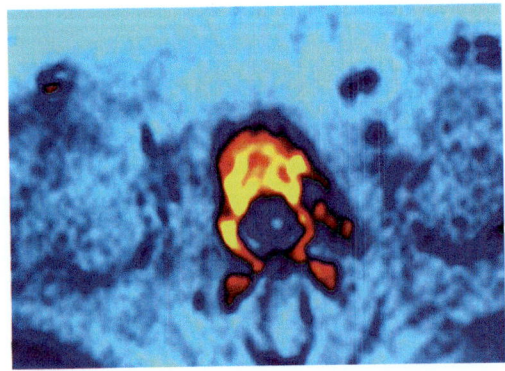

Fig. 2.7.3

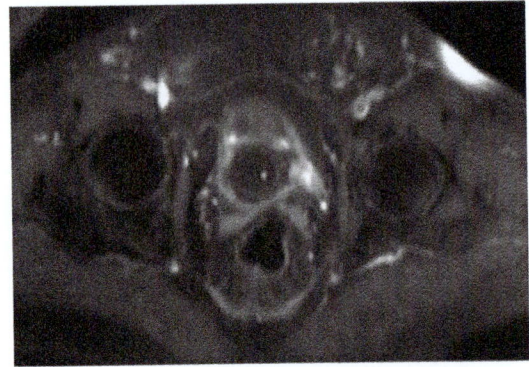

Fig. 2.7.4

Figure 2.7.1 Axial T2-weighted MRI shows a large solid mass inside a barely-filled bladder

Figure 2.7.2 Multiplanar reconstruction of a T2-weighted MR image shows the mass extending to the left ureter, obstructing the pyeloureteral junction and causing hydronephrosis, with fluid levels in the calyces, probably due to detritus deposits

Figure 2.7.3 Fusion of T2-weighted and diffusion-weighted ($b = 800$) image shows marked restriction of diffusion in the vesical mass and its extension to the most distal portion of the left ureter

Figure 2.7.4 Contrast-enhanced fat-suppressed T1-WI MR shows heterogeneous gadolinium uptake

An 82-year-old man with bladder cancer treated with transurethral resection presented anuria due to bladder distension and gross hematuria after urinary catheter placement.

Comments

The prevalence of primary bladder tumors ranges from 2 to 6%, making them the fourth most common tumor. Bladder tumors are normally malignant and have a high rate of recurrence. The most common histological type is the urothelial tumor (90%), followed by squamous cell tumors (2–15%) and adenocarcinoma (2%). It is most common among men between 50 and 70 years old. Active tobacco use is a significant risk factor. Other risk factors include contact with certain chemical substances (beta-naphthylamines) and the presence of vesical diverticula, kidney stones, and urinary infections or irritations.

Gross hematuria, hypogastric pain, and dysuria are present in 80% of patients with vesical carcinoma.

In the early stages, most vesical carcinomas are focal, low grade, and less than 2.5 cm in diameter; however, urothelial carcinomas are multicentric in 30–40% of cases and may occur synchronically with a carcinoma in the upper urinary tract.

Screening for vesical carcinoma should be carried out with US, confirmed with cystoscopy and biopsy, and staged with unenhanced and enhanced MRI.

Case 2.8
■ Cholangiocarcinoma

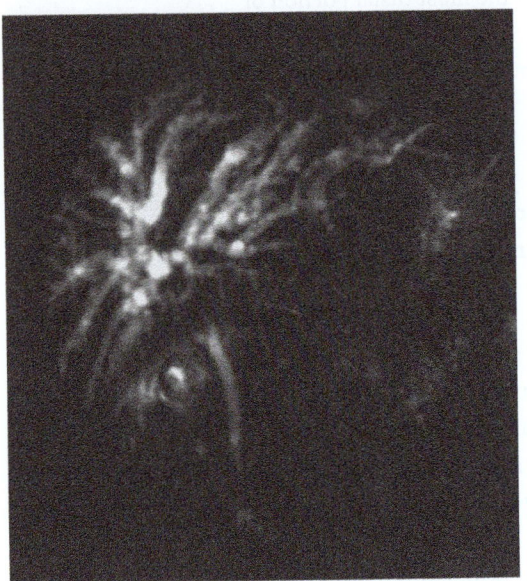

Fig. 2.8.1

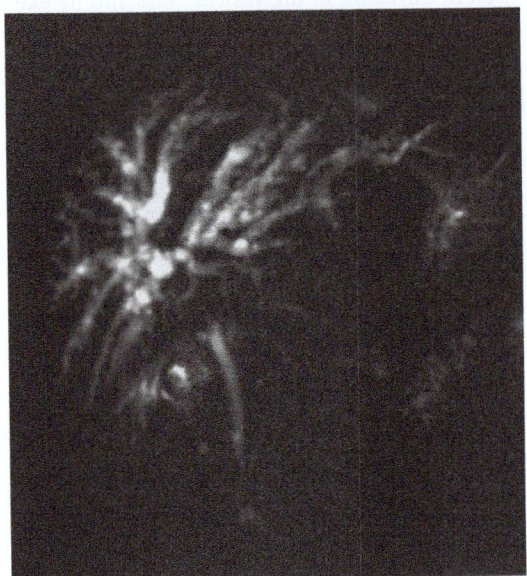

Fig. 2.8.2

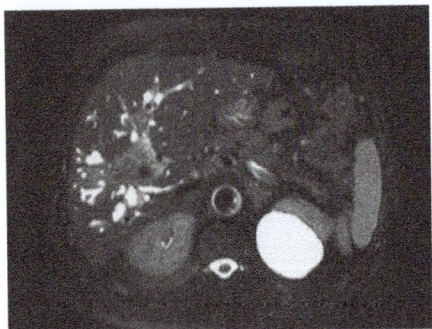

Fig. 2.8.3

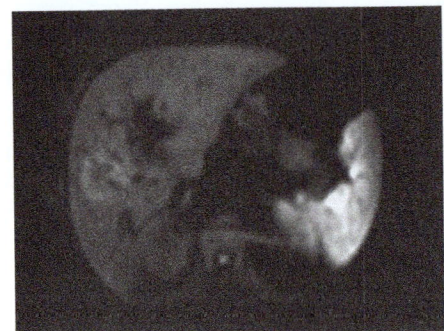

Fig. 2.8.4

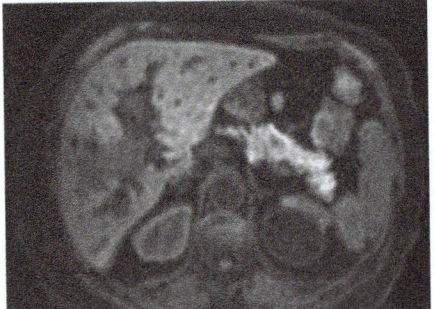

Fig. 2.8.5

Figure 2.8.1 MR cholangiography shows marked dilation of the intrahepatic biliary duct with abrupt interruption of the hepatic hilum; the caliber of the common bile duct is normal

Figure 2.8.2 T2-weighted MR images show that the above-mentioned interruption is accompanied by a moderately hyperintense solid lesion with ill-defined margins that is infiltrating liver segment V

Figure 2.8.3 Restricted diffusion in the most peripheral portion with b values = 1,000 indicates peripheral hypercellularity and central fibrosis

Figure 2.8.4 The lesion is hypointense on unenhanced fat-suppressed T1-weighted sequences

Figure 2.8.5 The lesion shows late enhancement after the administration of gadolinium

A 79-year-old woman presented obstructive jaundice, abdominal pain, asthenia, anorexia, and weight loss. Laboratory test results were nonspecific, showing only a pattern suggestive of cholestasis.

Comments

Klatskin's tumor is an uncommon tumor of the intrahepatic bile duct that usually occurs at the confluence of the right and left hepatic ducts. It accounts for about 85% of bile duct tumors and 1% of all malignant tumors. Nearly all (95%) Klatskin tumors are adenocarcinomas and some secrete mucin; they are classified by their type of presentation into exophytic, infiltrating, polypoid, and mixed.

Klatskin tumors occur predominantly in women older than 70 years of age. Predisposing factors include ulcerative colitis, sclerosing cholangitis, Caroli's disease, choledochal cyst, hepatic parasitic infestations, and exposure to chemicals (Thorotrast).

The differential diagnosis should include lithiasis without a posterior acoustic shadow, sclerosing cholangitis, gallbladder carcinoma, and metastases from breast cancer, colon cancer, or melanoma.

Treatment depends on the extent of the tumor: if there is vascular invasion or the tumor is unresectable, interventional techniques are used for biliary decompression, although the use of chemotherapy is also under study.

Case 2.9
■
Choledocolithiasis and Caroli's Disease

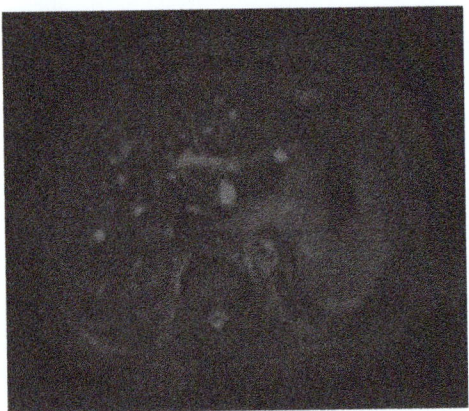

Fig. 2.9.1

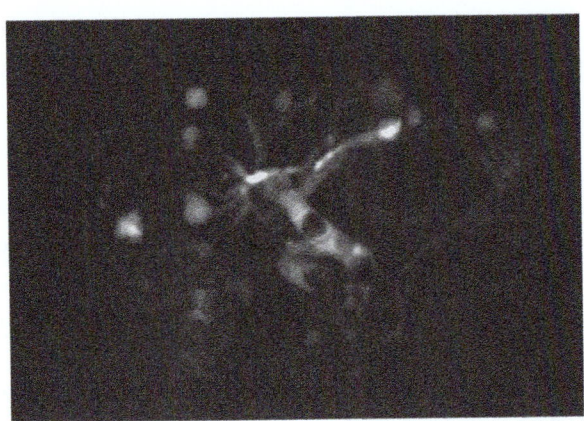

Fig. 2.9.2

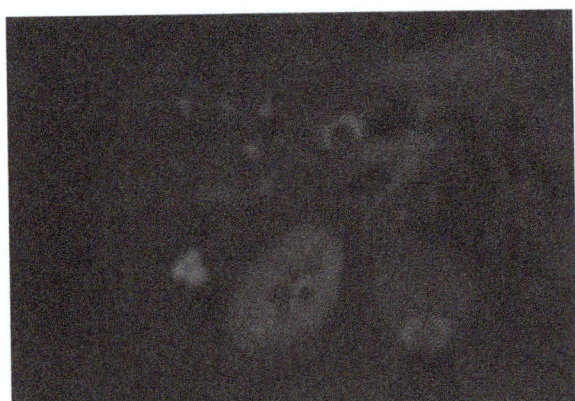

Fig. 2.9.3

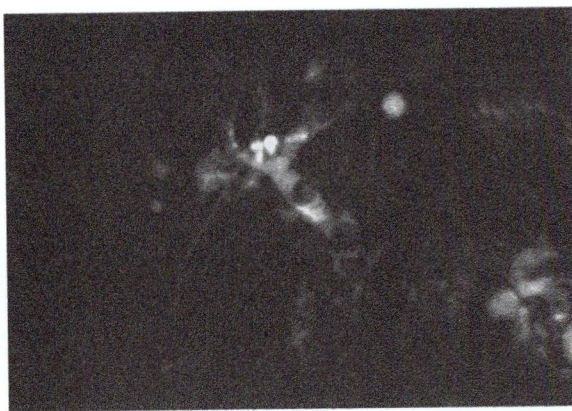

Fig. 2.9.4

Figure 2.9.1 Multiple well-defined intrahepatic lesions that are hyperintense on this fat-suppressed T2-weighted sequences

Figure 2.9.2 MR cholangiography. The lesions were connected to the biliary tree

Figure 2.9.3 Fat-suppressed T2-WI MR. The central dot sign is seen in some of the cysts

Figure 2.9.4 MR cholangiography. The intra and extrahepatic bile ducts are greatly dilated with multiple filling defects in the common bile duct compatible with obstructive choledo-cholithiasis in a patient with prior cholecystectomy

An 85-year-old man presented with right hypochondrial pain of 2 days' evolution and jaundice in the previous hours with elevated liver enzymes. He had no fever or leukocytosis.

Caroli's disease is a congenital disease with autosomal recessive transmission, which causes an alteration in the embryological formation of the walls of the biliary tract. It is classified as a fibrocystic liver disease.

Comments

Caroli's disease causes multifocal dilation of the intrahepatic biliary tract without affecting the extrahepatic ducts. It is associated with cholangiocarcinoma in 7% of cases.

It is essential to demonstrate that the cysts communicate with the biliary tree to differentiate it from polycystic disease, hamartomas, or multiple liver abscesses. Cysts in Caroli's disease can measure up to 5 cm, unlike hamartomas, which tend to be smaller (7–15 mm). Caroli's disease results in a characteristic appearance of alternating stenosis and dilation in the biliary tract. The central dot sign, consisting of a fibrovascular bundle situated at the center of the dilated biliary radical containing a dilated portal radical which has enhanced after the administration of contrast material, is also very characteristic of Caroli's disease. MR cholangiography has supplanted ERCP as the technique of choice to characterize Caroli's disease.

Case 2.10
■ Renal Lithiasis and Nonobstructive Ureterolithiasis

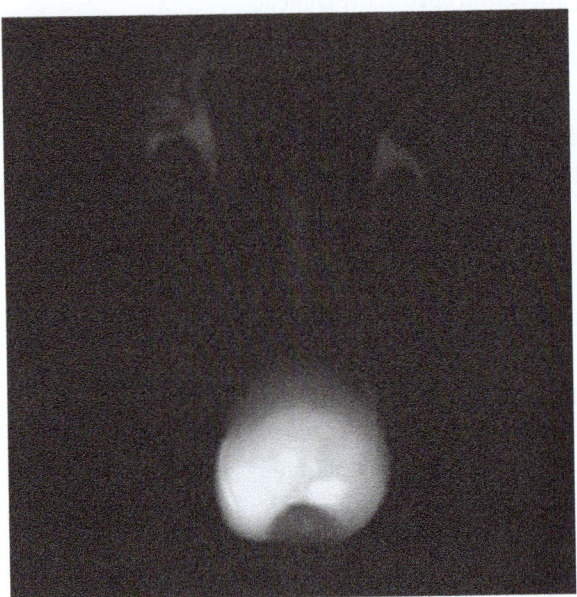

Fig. 2.10.1

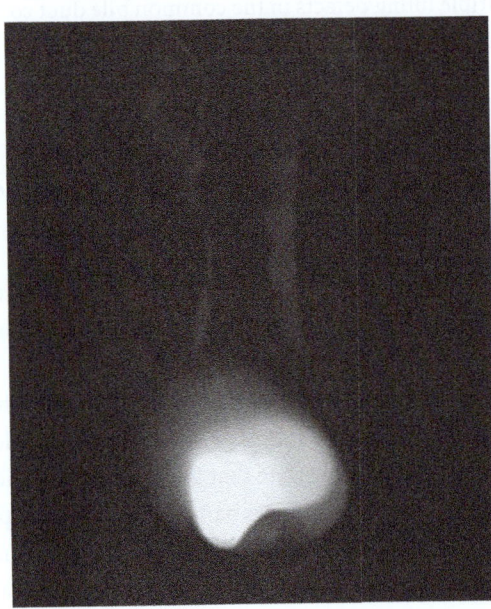

Fig. 2.10.2

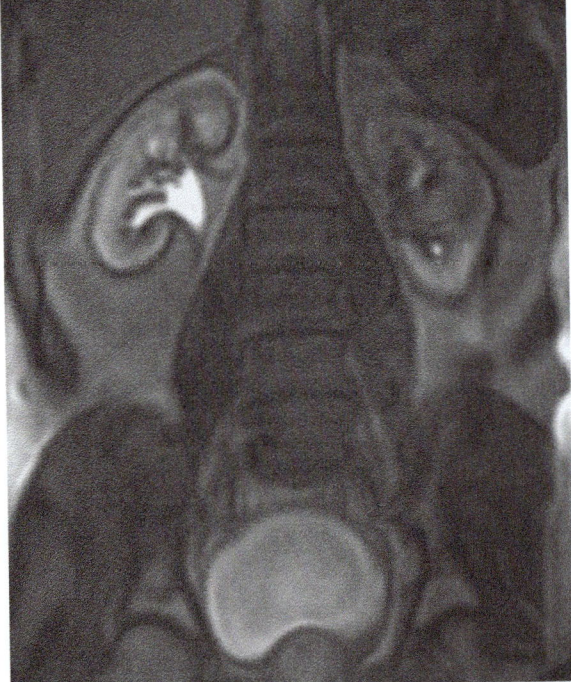

Fig. 2.10.3

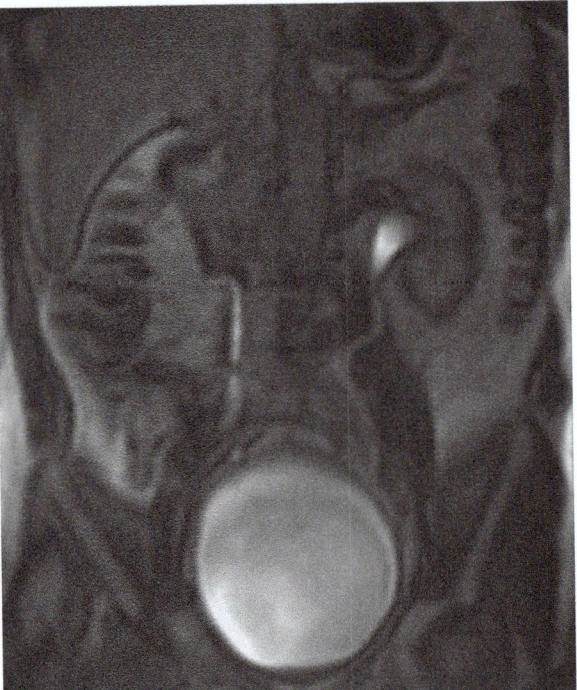

Fig. 2.10.4

Figure 2.10.1 MR urography filling defect in the right middle calyceal group extending from the ipsilateral renal pelvis

Figure 2.10.2 MR urography shows a second filling defect in the right lumbar ureter that does not cause proximal hydronephrosis

Figures 2.10.3 and 2.10.4 Gadolinium-enhanced MRI demonstrates good, symmetrical excretion by both kidneys. The lack of enhancement in the filling defects and good flow of contrast confirm that the right lithiasis is not obstructive

A 64-year-old man with right renal fossa pain of abrupt onset radiating to the genitals presented with hematuria.

Nephrolithiasis is a disease consisting of calculi in the urinary tract.

It affects 10% of the general population and is especially predominant in sedentary men or those exposed to heat.

Calculi are classified according to their composition as calcium oxalate, calcium phosphate, uric acid (which are radiotransparent), struvite (magnesium, ammonium, and phosphate), and cystine (which appear in childhood).

The clinical presentation ranges from typical colic pain in the renal fossa that radiates to the genitals to continuous low back pain or to painless hematuria or urine infections.

The imaging differential diagnosis is mainly with ureteral tumors, which do not normally calcify, have restricted diffusion, and enhance after the administration of contrast agents.

The importance of MRI in the diagnosis rests on two pillars: first, it is a noninvasive examination that enables visualization of the entire urinary system and surrounding tissues; thus, we can see an extrarenal mass causing hydronephrosis by compressing a ureter. Second, in patients with kidney failure or allergies to contrast agents, we can study the entire excretory system with great spatial resolution without administering gadolinium. Moreover, the patient is spared the radiation inherent in other imaging studies.

Comments

Further Reading

Abou-El-Ghar ME, El-Assmy A, Refaie HF, El-Diasty T. Bladder cancer: diagnosis with diffusion-weighted MR imaging in patients with gross hematuria. Radiology 2009; 251:415–421; published online before print as 10.1148/radiol.2503080723.

Achenbach S, Moselewski F, Ropers D, et al. Detection of calcified and noncalcified coronary atherosclerotic plaque by contrast-enhanced, submillimeter multidetector spiral computed tomography: a segment-based comparison with intravascular ultrasound. Circulation 2004; 109:14–17.

Bloom CM, Langer B, Wilson SR. Role of US in the detection, characterization, and staging of cholangiocarcinoma. Radiographics 1999; 19:1199.

Brancatelli G, Federle MP, Vilgrain V, Vullierme M-P, Marin D, Lagalla R. Fibropolycystic liver disease: CT and MR imaging findings. Radiographics 2005; 25:659–670.

Bruzzi JF, Rémy-Jardin M, Delhaye D, Teisseire A, Khalil Ch, Rémy J. When, why and how to examine the heart during thoracic ct: Part 1, basic principles. AJR Am J Roentgenol 2006; 186:324–332.

Bruzzi JF, Rémy-Jardin M, Delhaye D, Teisseire A, Khalil Ch, Rémy J. When, why and how to examine the heart during thoracic ct: Part 2, clinical applications. AJR Am J Roentgenol 2006; 186(2):333–341.

Datta J, White Ch, Gilkeson R, Meyer C, Kansal S, Jani M, Arildsen R, Read K. Anomalous coronary arteries in adults: depiction at multi-detector row CT angiography. Radiology 2005; 235:812–818.

Deserno WM, Harisinghani MG, Taupitz M, Jager GJ, Witjes JA, Mulders PF, Hulsbergen van de Kaa CA, Kaufmann D, Barentsz JO. Urinary bladder cancer: preoperative nodal staging with ferumoxtran-10-enhanced MR imaging. Radiology 2004; 233:449–456; published online before print as 10.1148/radiol.2332031111.

Frazier A, Qureshi F, Read K, Gilkeson R, Poston R, White Ch. Coronary artery bypass grafts: assessment with multidetector CT in the early and late postoperative settings. Radiographics 2005; 25:881–896.

Han JK, Choi BI, Kim AY, An SK, et al. Cholangiocarcinoma: pictorial essay of CT and cholangiographic findings. Radiographics 2002; 22:173.

Heimbach JK, Gores GJ, Haddock MG, Alberts SR, Pedersen R, Kremers W, Nyberg SL, Ishitani MB, Rosen CB. Predictors of disease recurrence following neoadjuvant chemoradiotherapy and liver transplantation for unresectable perihilar cholangiocarcinoma. Transplantation 2006; 82(12):1703–1707.

Heuschmid M, Kuettner A, Schroeder S, Trabold T, Feyer A, Seemann MD, Kuzo R, Claussen CD, Kopp AF. ECG-gated 16-MDCT of the coronary arteries: assessment of image quality and accuracy in detecting stenoses. AJR Am J Roentgenol 2005; 184:1413–1419.

Hoffmann MH, Shi H, Manzke R, et al. Noninvasive coronary angiography with 16-detector row CT: effect of heart rate. Radiology 2005; 234:86–97.

Hoffmann U, Pena A, Moselewski F, Ferencik M, Abbara S, Cury R, Chae CU, Nagurney JT. MDCT in early triage of patients with acute chest pain. AJR Am J Roentgenol 2006; 187:1240–1247.

Kim M-J, Mitchell DG, Ito K, Outwater EK. Biliary dilatation: differentiation of benign from malignant causes-value of adding conventional MR imaging to MR cholangiopancreatography. Radiology 2000; 214:173.

Kuettner A, Kopp AF, Schroeder S, et al. Diagnostic accuracy of multidetector computed tomography coronary angiography in patients with angiographically proven coronary artery disease. J Am Coll Cardiol 2004; 43:831–839.

Lawyer L, Pannu HK, Fichman EK. MDCT evaluation of the coronary arteries: how we do it; data acquisition, postprocessing, display, and interpretation. AJR Am J Roentgenol 2005; 184:1402–1412.

Lee WJ, Lim HK, Jang KM, Kim SH, et al. Radiologic spectrum of cholangiocarcinoma: emphasis on unusual manifestations and differential diagnoses. Radiographics 2001; 21:97.

Leschka S, Alkadhi H, Plass A, et al. Accuracy of MSCT coronary angiography with 64-slice technology: first experience. Eur Heart J 2005; 26:1482–1487.

Levy AD, Rohrmann CA Jr, Murakata LA, Lonergan GJ. Caroli's disease: radiologic spectrum with pathologic correlation. AJR Am J Roentgenol 2002; 179:1053–1057.

Leyendecker JR, Barnes CE, Zagoria RJ. MR urography: techniques and clinical applications. Radiographics 2008; 28:23–46.

Mahnken A, Mühlenbruch G, Günther RW, et al. Cardiac CT: coronary arteries and beyond. J Eur Radiol 2007; 17:994–1008.

Morteleé KJ, Ros PR. Cystic focal liver lesions in the adult: differential CT and MR imaging features. Radiographics 2001; 21:895–910.

Nakanishi T, Kayashima Y, Inoue R, Sumii K, Gomyo Y. Pitfalls in 16-detector row CT of the coronary arteries. Radiographics 2005; 25:425–438.

Nieman K, Cademartiri F, Lemos PA, Raaijmakers R, Pattynama PM, de Feyter PJ. Reliable non-invasive coronary angiography with fast submillimeter multislice spiral computed tomography. Circulation 2002; 106:2051–2054.

Nieman K, Oudkerk M, Rensing BJ, et al. Coronary angiography with multi-slice computed tomography. Lancet 2001; 357:599–603.

Nikolau C, Knez A, Rist C, et al. Accuracy of 64-MDCT in the diagnosis of ischemic heart disease. AJR Am J Roentgenol 2006; 187:111–117.

Pannu HK, et al. Coronary CT angiography with 64 MDCT: assessment of vessel visibility. AJR Am J Roentgenol 2006; 187:119–126.

Pannu HK, et al. β-blockers for cardiac CT: a primer for the radiologist. AJR Am J Roentgenol 2006; 186:S341–S345.

Pannu HK, Flohr TG, Corl FM, Fishman EK. Current concepts in multi-detector row CT evaluation of the coronary arteries: principles, techniques, and anatomy. Radiographics 2003; 23:S111–S125.

Pannu HK, Jacobs J, Lai S, Fishman EK. Coronary CT angiography with 64-MDCT: assessment of vessel visibility. AJR Am J Roentgenol 2006; 187:119–126.

Pavone P, Laghi A, Catalano C, Passariello R. Caroli's disease: evaluation with MR cholangiography. AJR Am J Roentgenol 1996; 166:216–217.

Pugliese F, Cademartiri F, et al. Multidetector CT for visualization of coronary stents. Radiographics 2006; 26:887–904.

Rothpearl A, Frager D, Subramanian A, Bashist B, Baer J, Kay C, Cooke K, Raia C. MR urography: technique and application. Radiology 1995; 194:125.

Schoenhagen P, Halliburton S, Stillman AE, Kuzmiak SA, Nissen SE, Tuzcu EM, White RD. Noninvasive imaging of coronary arteries: current and future role of multi-detector row CT. Radiology 2004; 232:7–17.

Schoepf UJ, Becker CR, Ohnesorge BM, Yucel EK. CT of coronary artery disease. Radiology 2004; 232:18–37.

Schroeder S, Kopp AF, Baumbach A, et al. Noninvasive detection and evaluation of atherosclerotic coronary plaques with multislice computed tomography. J Am Coll Cardiol 2001; 37:1430–1435.

Silverman SG, Leyendecker JR, Amis ES Jr. What is the current role of CT urography and MR urography in the evaluation of the urinary tract? Radiology 2009; 250:309–323.

Sudah M, Vanninen RL, Partanen K, Kainulainen S, Malinen A, Heino A, Ala-Opas M. Patients with acute flank pain: comparison of MR urography with unenhanced helical CT. Radiology 2002; 223:98–105; published online before print as 10.1148/radiol.2231010341.

Takeuchi M, Sasaki S, Ito M, Okada S, Takahashi S, Kawai T, Suzuki K, Oshima H, Hara M, Shibamoto Y. Urinary bladder cancer: diffusion-weighted MR imaging – accuracy for diagnosing T stage and estimating histologic grade. Radiology 2009; 251:112–121.

Vitellas KM, Keogan MT, Freed KS, Enns RA, et al. Radiologic manifestations of sclerosing cholangitis with emphasis on MR cholangiopancreatography. Radiographics 2000; 20:959.

Wong JT, Wasserman NF, Padurean AM. Bladder squamous cell carcinoma. Radiographics 2004; 24:855–860.

Wong-You-Cheong JJ, Woodward PJ, Manning MA, Sesterhenn IA. From the archives of the AFIP: neoplasms of the urinary bladder: radiologic-pathologic correlation. Radiographics 2006; 26:553–580.

Zenooz NA, Reza Habibi R, Mammen L, Finn JP, Gilkeson RC. Coronary artery fistulas: CT findings. Radiographics 2009; 29:781–789.

Fundamentals of Vascular Interventions

3

Esther Boullosa

J.J. Muñoz and R. Ribes, *Learning Vascular and Interventional Radiology*, Learning Imaging,
DOI: 10.1007/978-3-540-87997-8_3, © Springer-Verlag Berlin Heidelberg 2010

Case 3.1
■
Renal Artery Fibrodysplasia. Treatment with Angioplasty

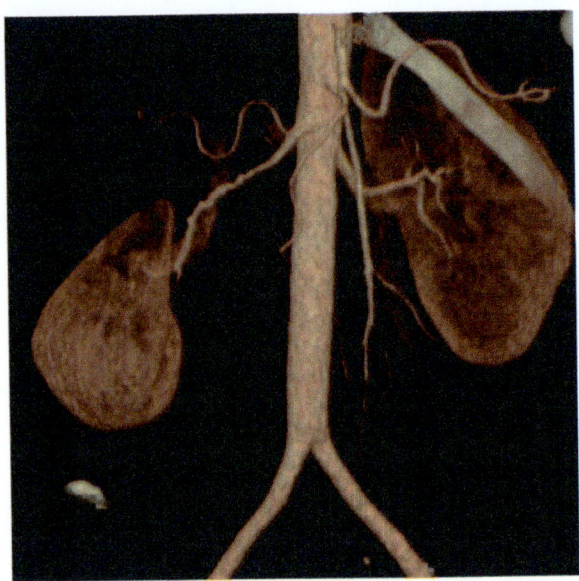

Fig. 3.1.1

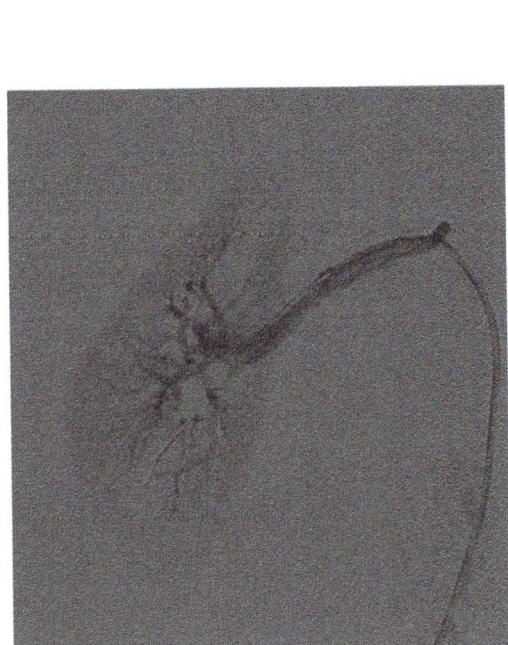

Fig. 3.1.2

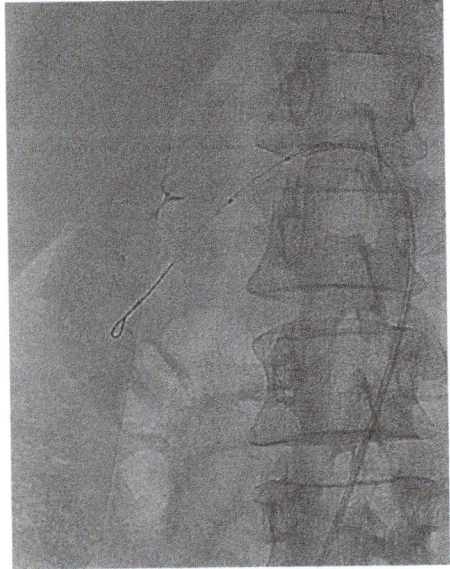

Fig. 3.1.3

Fig. 2.1.4

Figure 3.1.1 3D reconstruction of a CT angiogram of the renal arteries (volume rendering) shows the corkscrew shape of the right renal artery

Figure 3.1.2 Selective renal arteriogram obtained via selective catheterization with a 4F visceral catheter confirms the findings at CT angiography, showing diffuse stenoses and the characteristic string-of-pearls appearance of the renal artery, which are compatible with fibrodysplasia of the right renal artery

Figure 3.1.3 Catheterization of the renal artery stenosis: after placing a guidewire in the ostium of the renal artery, a balloon catheter (6 mm in diameter and 20 mm long) is advanced over the guidewire (radiopaque marks show the length of the balloon)

Figure 3.1.4 Selective renal arteriogram after percutaneous transluminal angioplasty: the rupture of fibrous bands confirms the good outcome

A 46-year-old woman presented with an 8-year history of poorly controlled hypertension treated with two drugs and diastolic heart dysfunction as the only sign of visceral repercussions. Renal function tests showed hyperaldosteronism and hyperreninemia but no microalbuminuria.

Renal CT angiography performed for suspected renal vascular disease showed that the right renal artery had a corkscrew shape suggestive of renal dysplasia.

These findings were confirmed at selective arteriography and the lesions were treated with angioplasty. Angiography confirmed the success of the procedure and the patient's hypertension resolved.

Comments

Secondary hypertension accounts for less than 5% of all cases of hypertension. Renovascular hypertension is one type of secondary hypertension. Its most common cause is atherosclerosis; however, in 10–30% of cases, it is caused by fibromuscular dysplasia.

The first case of fibromuscular disease was reported by Leadbetter and Burkland in 1938. In 1971, researchers at the Mayo Clinic and at the Cleveland Clinic established uniform terminology for nonarteriosclerotic fibromuscular lesions of the renal artery based on the arterial layer affected. Thus, there are three main types of dysplasia, depending on whether it affects the intima, medial layer, or the adventitia.

Medial fibroplasia is the most common cause of fibromuscular dysplasia, accounting for 70% of all cases. It usually occurs in women between 25 and 50 years of age and often involves both the renal arteries. The lesion characteristically affects the two distal thirds of the main renal artery and can extend to its main branches. It is often detected in other vascular territories, such as the carotid, mesenteric, or iliac. Arteriography shows the typical string-of-pearls appearance of the main renal artery or its main branches.

Percutaneous transluminal balloon angioplasty is the treatment of choice for symptomatic arterial stenosis secondary to fibromuscular dysplasia. Clinical outcome and patency after balloon angioplasty are at least as good as after surgery, but with the additional advantage of less morbidity and mortality. The immediate results and clinical outcome are good in about 94% of cases, and patency at 5 years is greater than 90%. The rate of restenosis is about 10%, and restenosis is very easy to treat with another percutaneous transluminal angioplasty.

In summary, fibromuscular dysplasia is a potentially curable type of secondary hypertension. Fibromuscular dysplasia should be suspected in cases involving young women and/or patients who rapidly develop severe hypertension. In these cases, Doppler US of the renal arteries seems to be the best screening technique. In positive cases, arteriography will reach the definitive diagnosis and will also enable treatment when percutaneous transluminal angioplasty is possible.

Procedure Steps

1. Apply a transdermal patch of 5 mg nitroglycerine.
2. Use a retrograde approach through the right common femoral artery.
3. Perform selective renal arteriography with a 4F visceral catheter.
4. Recanalize the stenosis with a 0.14 guidewire.
5. Introduce a 6F guiding catheter in the ostium of the renal artery; this will enable angiograms to be performed throughout the procedure.
6. Introduce a balloon catheter (6 mm in diameter and 20 mm long) over the guidewire and perform angioplasty while controlling the pressure with a manometer.
7. Obtain a follow-up angiogram through the introducer sheath. Prescribe acetylsalicylic acid for 6 months.

Equipment List

1. 150 cm long 0.035 in. angled hydrophilic guidewire. Terumo Radiofocus
2. 4F visceral catheter.
3. 65 cm long 4F SHK 1.0® catheter. Cordis
4. 180 cm long 0.014 in. miraclebros® 12 metallic guidewire. Abbott
5. 50 cm long 6F Veripath® peripheral guiding catheter. Abbott
6. Viatrac 14 plus® monorail peripheral balloon angioplasty catheter (6 mm in diameter and 20 mm long), 135 cm long guiding catheter. 0.014 in. guidewire. Abbott
7. 20cc disposable manometer. Biometrix B.V.

Case 3.2
■
Tibiofibular Angioplasty

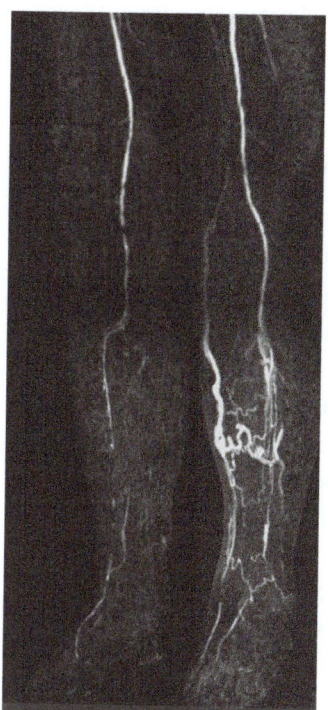

Fig. 3.2.1

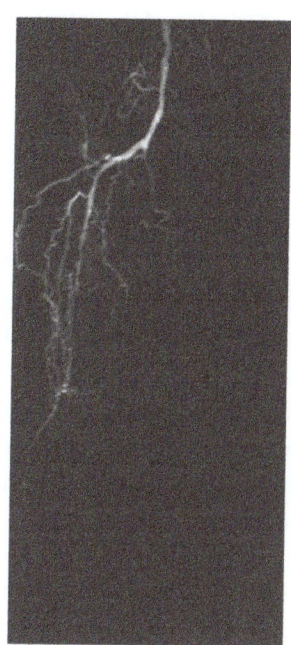

Fig. 3.2.2

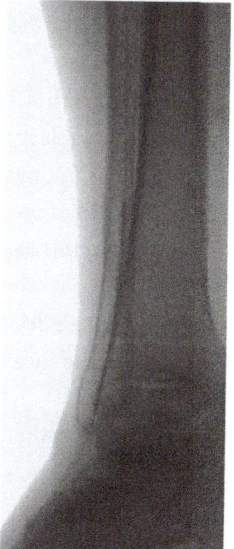

Fig. 3.2.3

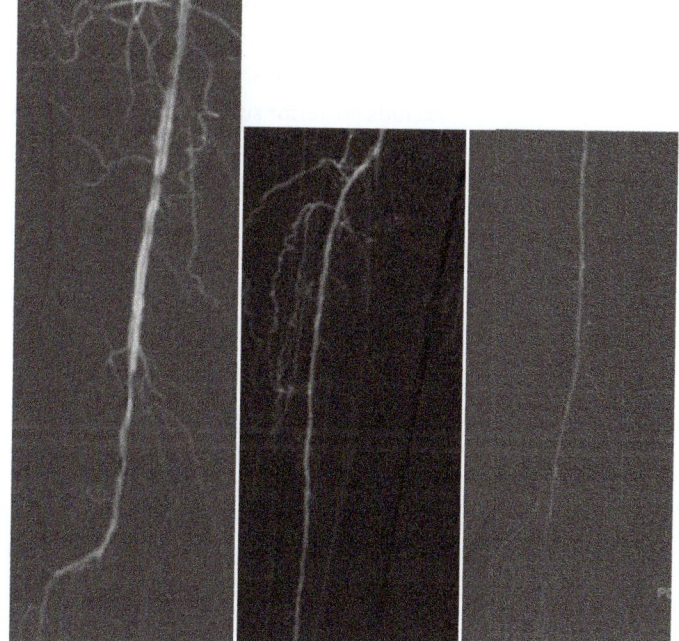

Fig. 3.2.4

Figure 3.2.1 Arterial MR angiogram of the lower limbs: In the right lower limb, a short occlusion is seen in the second portion of the popliteal artery and in the middle and lower thirds of the anterior tibial artery (the only vessel with outflow, which is revascularized distal to the pedal artery)

Figure 3.2.2 Selective antegrade arteriogram prior to treatment. Antegrade approach through the ipsilateral common femoral artery confirms the findings at MR angiography; the image shows occlusion of the anterior tibial artery approximately 6 cm from its origin

Figure 3.2.3 Balloon angioplasty in the anterior tibial artery to the pedal artery with a balloon catheter measuring 2 mm in diameter and 120 mm long

Figure 3.2.4 Antegrade selective arteriogram after percutaneous transluminal angioplasty: the results after angioplasty of the popliteal and anterior tibial arteries are acceptable

A 79-year-old woman was admitted for trophic lesions in her right lower limb of 1 month's evolution and a 15-day history of pain at rest.

She was being followed on an outpatient basis by a vascular surgeon for her atherosclerotic disease.

She had a history of insulin-dependent diabetes mellitus, hypertension, hypertensive heart disease, and hypercholesterolemia.

Faced with critical ischemia in a woman with multiple risk factors for surgical revascularization, we unblocked the occlusions in the popliteal and anterior tibial arteries and performed angioplasty with balloon catheters (5 mm by 40 mm long and 3 mm and 2 mm by 120 mm long, respectively). At the end of the procedure, she had recovered her pedal pulse. At discharge, she remained asymptomatic and her wounds were healing correctly.

Comments The BASIL (bypass versus angioplasty in severe ischemia of the leg) trial showed that endovascular treatment and surgery were comparable in the treatment of critical ischemia in the lower limbs, but percutaneous transluminal angioplasty is cheaper and does not exclude posterior surgical treatment. Percutaneous transluminal angioplasty should be the treatment of choice in patients with a life expectancy of less than 2 years.

The treatment of infrapopliteal lesions has usually been reserved for cases of critical ischemia, because it is technically difficult to use conventional peripheral angioplasty material in small caliber vessels. Recent publications show that percutaneous transluminal angioplasty in distal vessels can be very efficacious, with a success rate of 80% for tibiofibular angioplasty. Using material for coronary angioplasty has improved the results of infrapopliteal endovascular interventions.

The optimum treatment of infrapopliteal arterial lesions requires the appropriate selection of patients and lesions; the success rate is higher in patients with less than five focal stenoses with separations between them.

The aim of treatment is to eliminate pain at rest, cure the ulcers, and save the limb, rather than to achieve long-term patency of the vessel. The basic principle for curing ulcers is based on increasing the supply of oxygenated blood to maintain tissue integrity. Recent clinical trials suggest that percutaneous treatment saves limbs in the long-term in 80% of patients and can be considered the treatment of choice in patients with critical ischemia threatening the preservation of the limb.

1. Use an antegrade approach through the right common femoral artery.
2. Recanalize the occlusion in the popliteal artery using a straight hydrophilic guidewire and 4F multipurpose catheter.
3. Administer 3,000–5,000 IU sodium heparin and 100–200 µg nitroglycerine intraarterially.
4. Perform angioplasty with a balloon catheter measuring 5 mm in diameter and 40 mm in length.
5. Exchange the balloon catheter over the guidewire for a multipurpose catheter.
6. Use a 0.014 in. guidewire to recanalize the tibial artery until the pedal artery.
7. Advance a balloon catheter (2 mm in diameter and 120 mm long) over the guidewire and perform the angioplasty.
8. Replace the balloon catheter with another of greater diameter and equal length and perform angioplasty in the proximal anterior tibial artery.
9. Perform angiography through the introducer sheath to check the results.
10. Prescribe lifelong antiplatelet therapy with 80–100 mg acetylsalicylic acid every 24 h.

1. Two-piece 19G metallic needle for the Seldinger approach. Boston Scientific
2. 180 cm long 0.035 in. stiff straight-tipped THSF Amplatz guidewire. Cook
3. 10 cm long 5F vascular introducer sheath with a hemostatic valve. Introducer II®. Terumo Radiofocus
4. 80 cm long 4F multipurpose angiographic catheter A2®. Cordis
5. 150 cm long angled 0.035 in. hydrophilic guidewire. Terumo Radiofocus
6. Ultrathin SDS angioplasty balloon catheter (5 mm in diameter and 40 mm long), 90 cm long delivery catheter. 0.035 in. guidewire. Boston Scientific
7. 300 cm long 0.014 in. skipper deep® metallic STF guidewire. Invatec
8. Amphirion deep® balloon angioplasty catheter (3 mm in diameter and 80 mm long). Invatec
9. Amphirion deep® balloon angioplasty catheter (2 mm in diameter and 120 mm long). Invatec
10. 20cc disposable manometer Biometrix B.V.

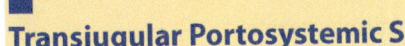

Case 3.3

Transjugular Portosystemic Shunt

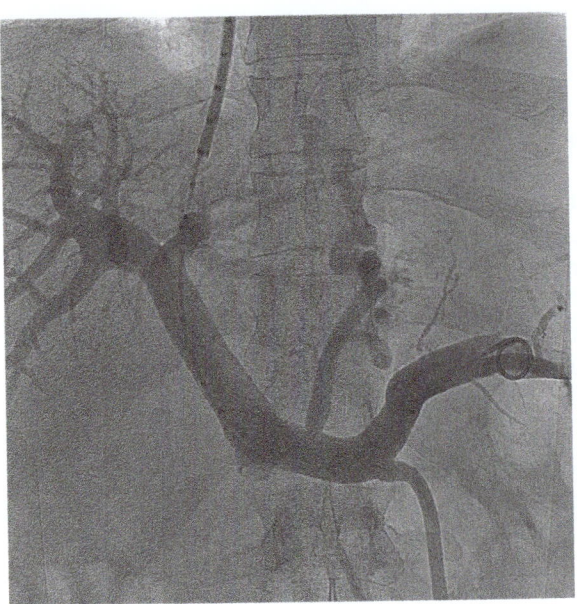

Fig. 3.3.1

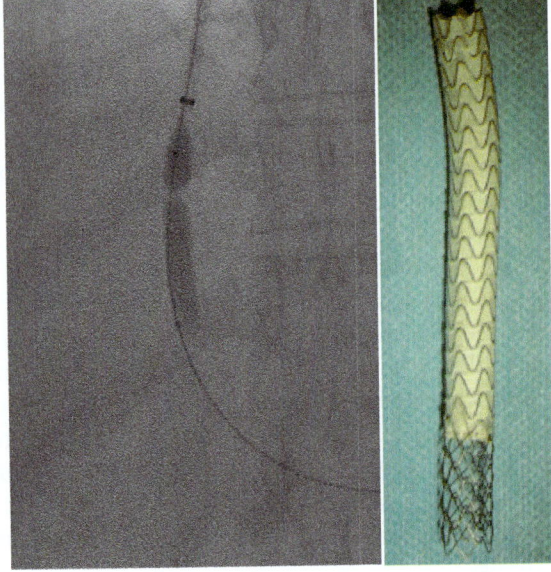

Fig. 3.3.2

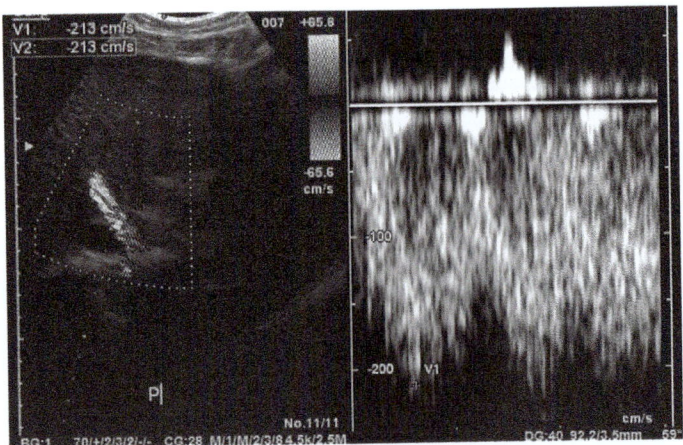

Fig. 3.3.3

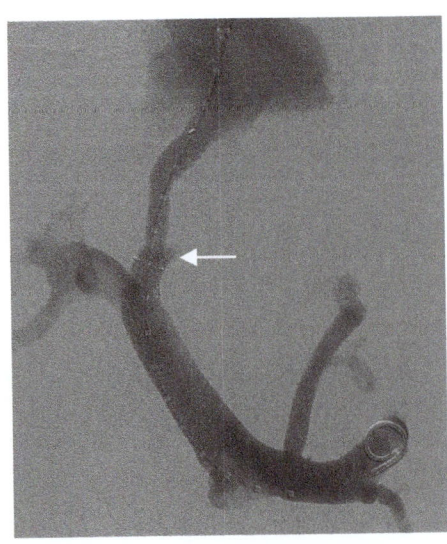

Fig. 3.3.4

Figure 3.3.1 Direct portography performed with a calibrated 5F pigtail catheter shows varicose dilation of the left gastric artery

Figure 3.3.2 Dilatation of the hepatic tract: the notch in the balloon shows the pressure applied at the entry to the hepatic vein. The image on the right shows a partially coated Viatorr stent-graft

Figure 3.3.3 Portogram after stenting, uncoated segment inside the stent (*arrow*), patent portosystemic shunt, and decreased size of the varices

Figure 3.3.4 Follow-up US 1 month after transjugular intrahepatic portosystemic shunt (TIPS) confirms the patency of the stent with color Doppler and duplex US; the velocity of blood flow in the stent was 200 cm/s

A 45-year-old man was admitted to the reanimation unit with hypovolemic shock after bleeding due to fundal varices. During hospitalization, he was diagnosed with chronic liver disease and portal hypertension due to alcoholism. After sclerotherapy of the varices proved ineffective, he was successfully treated with transjugular intrahepatic portosystemic shunt (TIPS) (pre-TIPS portosystemic gradient: 15 mmHg, post-TIPS gradient: 10 mmHg). He presented no signs of rebleeding during hospitalization. At discharge, he was asymptomatic and able to eat and had no problems with hemodynamics or encephalopathy.

Comments

TIPS consists of creating an intrahepatic communication between the portal vein and a hepatic vein with the aim of reducing portal pressure. TIPS is absolutely indicated in variceal bleeding in the following cases: (1) hemorrhage that cannot be controlled endoscopically, and (2) in recurrent hemorrhage in cases of failed medical and endoscopic treatment.

Other indications for TIPS are refractory ascites, hepatic hydrothorax (both due to reduced hydrostatic pressure in the portal vein), veno-occlusive liver disease, Budd–Chiari syndrome, hypertensive gastropathy, hepatorenal syndrome, and hepatopulmonary syndrome.

Procedure Steps

1. Most patients require general anesthesia.
2. US-guided access through the right internal jugular vein.
3. Use a multipurpose 4F catheter to catheterize a hepatic vein.
4. Measure the free and wedged hepatic vein pressure and calculate the pressure gradient.
5. Introduce a stiff Amplatz guidewire and exchange the multipurpose catheter for a 10F introducer sheath.
6. Introduce the Colapinto needle over the guidewire, withdraw the guidewire, and insert the trocar. Turn the entire set anteromedially inside the hepatic vein. Advance the trocar 4–5 cm toward the portal vein, then carefully withdraw the metallic part of the trocar, aspirating with a contrast-filled syringe. When blood is aspirated, inject the contrast agent; if puncture of the portal branch is confirmed, advance a hydrophilic guidewire to the portal vein and finally place it in the splenic vein or in the superior mesenteric vein. Immediately advance the trocar catheter and replace the hydrophilic guidewire with a stiff Amplatz guidewire.

7. Insert a calibrated pigtail catheter over the guidewire. Measure the portal pressures and perform portography, simultaneously injecting contrast material in the introducer sheath placed in the hepatic vein to evaluate the portal anatomy, varices, and size of the intrahepatic tract (to choose the prosthesis). Replace the pigtail catheter with an 8 or 10 mm angioplasty balloon and dilate the intrahepatic tract; the two notches that appear on the balloon are the entrances to the portal vein and hepatic vein.

8. Advance the introducer sheath to the portal vein and introduce the prosthesis, placing the 2 cm uncoated part inside the portal vein and the coated part in the intrahepatic tract and hepatic vein to the inferior vena cava.

9. Measure the gradient between invasive portal pressure and hepatic vein pressure and obtain a portogram to confirm the results of the procedure.

Equipment List

1. TIPS Procedure pack. Tipss-200®. Cook. 035 in. Extra stiff Amplatz guidewire, modified 16G Ross Colapinto needle, 10.0F Flexor® Check-Flo® introducer sheath, 12.0F dilator , 5.0F multipurpose catheter, angioplasty balloon catheter (8 and 10 mm in diameter), 70 cm long Aurous® 5F calibrated pigtail catheter.
2. 80 cm long 4F A2® multipurpose angiographic catheter. Cordis
3. 150 cm long 0.035 in. straight hydrophilic guidewire. Terumo Radiofocus
4. 180 cm long 0.035 in. straight-tipped stiff Amplatz guidewire. Cook
5. 260 cm long angled 0.035 in. hydrophilic guidewire. Terumo Radiofocus
6. 20cc disposable manometer. Biometrix B.V.
7. Partially coated Viatorr® prosthesis (10 mm in diameter and 70 + 20 mm long). Gore

Case 3.4
Digestive Visceral Artery Stenting

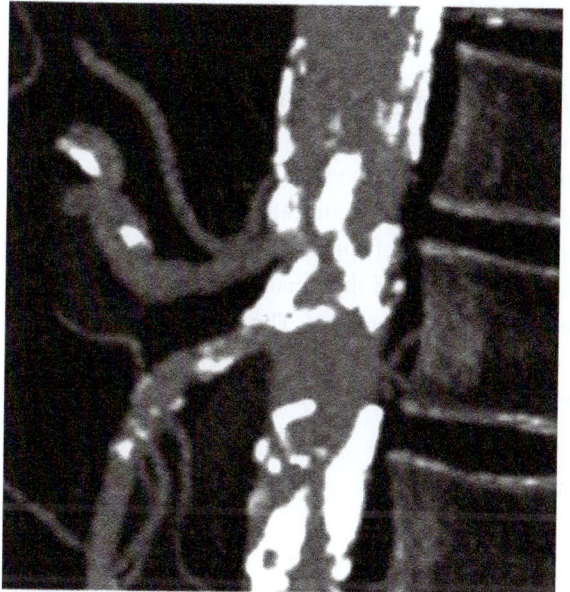

Fig. 3.4.1

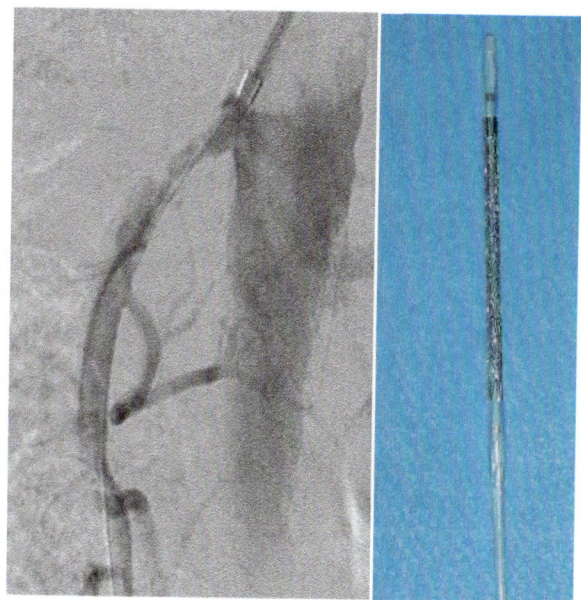

Fig. 3.4.2

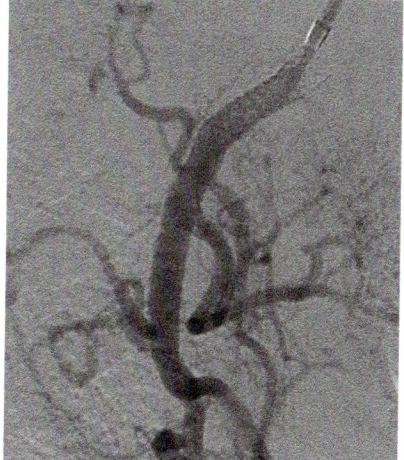

Fig. 3.4.3

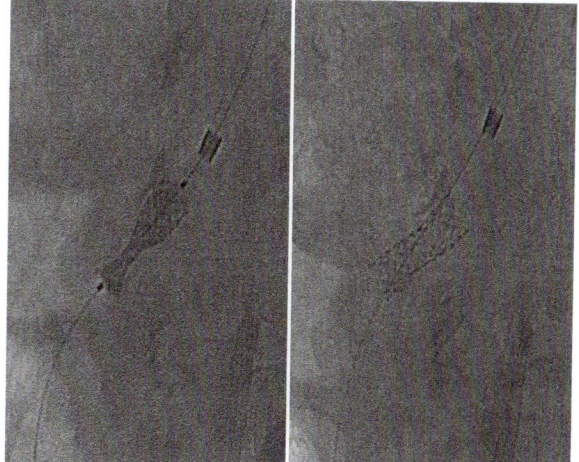

Fig. 3.4.4

Figure 3.4.1 CT angiogram. MIP reconstruction of the aorta and digestive trunks shows aortic atheromatosis with significant stenosis at the origin of the superior mesenteric artery (SMA); the caliber of the celiac trunk is normal

Figure 3.4.2 Selective arteriogram of the SMA through a 6F introducer sheath (approach through the left axillary artery) confirms the findings at CT angiography. The image on the right shows the stent in the delivery catheter: radiopaque marks on its tips indicate the extremes of the balloon

Figure 3.4.3 Implantation of the expandable balloon prosthesis: the extremes of the balloon begin to dilate before the center; the final diameter of the stent depends on the pressure applied with the balloon

Figure 3.4.4 Arteriogram after the procedure shows the good angiographic outcome. The patient's symptoms improved within hours and he was able to resume oral feeding

A 69-year-old man with a history of hypertension, type II diabetes mellitus that was poorly controlled with oral antidiabetics, hypercholesterolemia being treated with statins, ischemic heart disease, and smoking until 3 months was referred for a 6-month history of symptoms and signs of chronic intestinal ischemia (significant postprandial pain and weight loss (8 kg)). CT angiography showed stenosis of approximately 90% in the origin of the superior mesenteric artery (SMA). We recanalized the stenosis, approaching through the axillary artery and placing an expandable balloon stent. The angiographic outcome was good and the patient reported alleviation of symptoms on resuming eating 4 h after the procedure. He has remained symptom free throughout 2 years follow-up.

Comments   The term intestinal ischemia covers three distinct clinical conditions: acute intestinal ischemia, chronic intestinal ischemia, and ischemic colitis.

Chronic mesenteric ischemia nearly always occurs in patients with significant, diffuse atheromatous disease who often have a prior history of atheromatous disease in other territories. Atherosclerotic disease accounts for 90% of the cases of chronic mesenteric ischemia.

In the pretreatment workup of stenosis of the celiac trunk and SMA, multidetector CT enables treatment planning and determination of the best point of vascular access. In cases of suspected celiac trunk involvement, it is essential to perform the differential diagnosis with extrinsic compression of the arcuate ligament.

Classical surgical treatment includes endarterectomy and aortomesenteric or aortoceliac bypass; these procedures have high rates of perioperative mortality (17%) and major complications (15–35%). With improvements in materials and techniques, endovascular treatment, comprising percutaneous angioplasty with or without stent placement in one or more mesenteric arteries, achieves technical success in 90–100% of cases, with lower rates of periprocedural mortality (0–13%) and complications (0–25%). Because atherosclerotic ostial lesions are the most common cause of mesenteric stenosis or occlusions, expandable balloon stents are preferred over self-expanding balloon stents.

Alleviation of symptoms is reported in 95% of patients, and stenting of the mesenteric arteries is considered a safe and efficacious alternative to surgery in patients with chronic mesenteric ischemia.

1. Approach through the left axillary artery (because the patient had significant calcified stenosis in the SMA and absent femoral pulses due to atheromatous disease in both iliac axes).
2. Introduce a pigtail catheter using a hydrophilic guidewire and perform lateral arteriography of the abdomen to evaluate the ostium of the digestive visceral arteries. Without moving the position of the angiographic arch, replace the pigtail catheter with a multipurpose catheter. Catheterize the SMA with a 0.014 in. guidewire and a multipurpose catheter.
3. Administer 3,000 IU sodium heparin and 100 μg nitroglycerine intraarterially.
4. Introduce an expandable balloon stent (7 mm in diameter and 18 mm long).
5. Through the introducer sheath, obtain as many angiograms as necessary to know precisely the appropriate positioning of the stent for placement.
6. Open the expandable balloon stent, controlling the pressure with a manometer. Check the results by arteriography. The patient can be discharged after 24 h and will need 80–100 mg acetylsalicylic acid for at least 6 months after the procedure.

1. 45 cm long 6F contralateral introducer sheath. Destination®. Terumo Radiofocus
2. 150 cm long angled 0.035 in. hydrophilic guidewire. Terumo radiofocus
3. 100 cm long 5F pigtail angiographic catheter. Cordis
4. 80 cm long 4F A2® multipurpose angiographic catheter. Cordis
5. 180 cm long 0.014 in. miraclebros® 12 metallic guidewire. Abbott
6. Rx Herculink elite® expandable balloon stent (7 mm in diameter and 18 mm long). Abbott
7. 20cc disposable manometer. Biometrix B.V.

Figure 3.5.1 Arterial phase contrast-enhanced liver CT shows a hypodense collection in segment II of the left liver lobe

Figure 3.5.2 Selective left hepatic arteriogram shows extravasation of contrast material from an artery in segment II of the left liver lobe

Figure 3.5.3 Hepatic arteriogram after embolization with microcoils: no extravasation of contrast material is seen in this subtracted image. The unsubtracted image in the *right lower corner* shows details of the microcoils in place

Figure 3.5.4 Follow-up abdominal CT 1 month after embolization shows that the intra-parenchymal collection has disappeared and there is no evidence of active bleeding. The microcoils cause a metallic artifact

A 22-year-old man admitted for penetrating abdominal trauma (a knife wound in the epigastric region). CT angiography showed hepatic laceration with active bleeding in segment II–IV. As the patient presented hypotension and tachycardia and clinical worsening was foreseen,

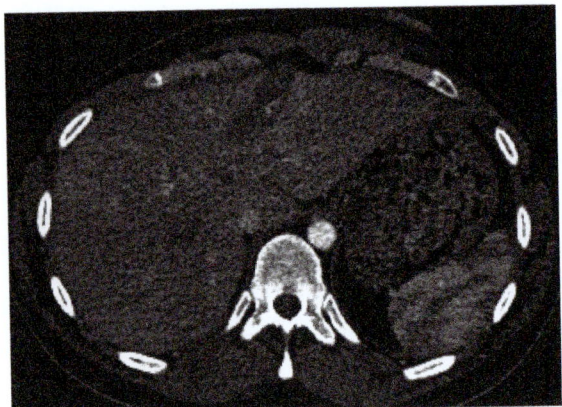

Fig. 3.5.1

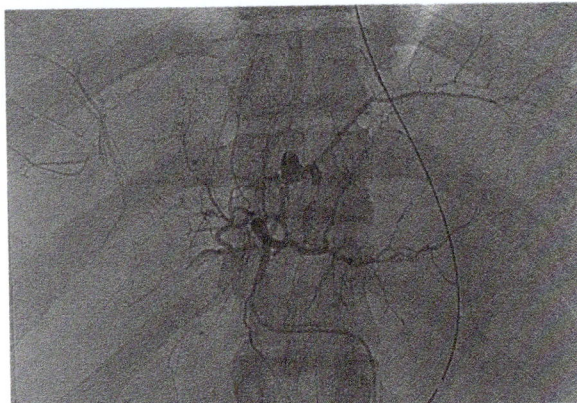

Fig. 3.5.2

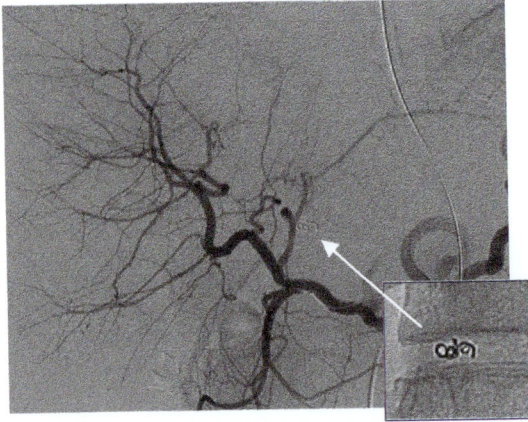

Fig. 3.5.3

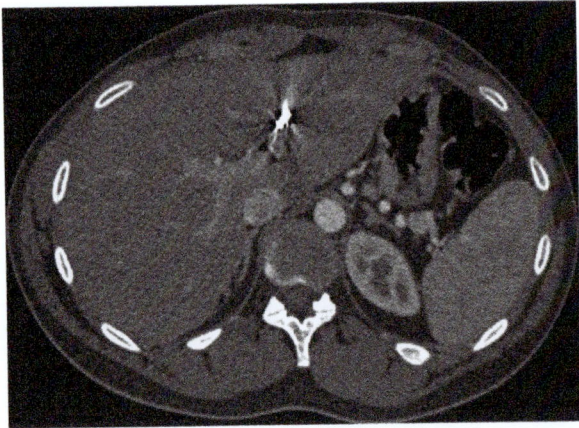

Fig. 3.5.4

selective hepatic arteriography was performed to confirm active bleeding in the left liver lobe.

We selectively catheterized the segmental artery and embolized it with microcoils measuring 3 mm in diameter and 3 cm in length until the iodinated contrast material stopped flowing and no extravasation of contrast material could be appreciated on subtracted angiograms.

The patient evolved favorably and was discharged from the hospital without consequences 10 days after the trauma.

Comments

Before the advent of arterial embolization, the only treatment available for abdominal trauma with liver lesions and active bleeding was surgery. Nowadays, with the development of endovascular techniques, only a small percentage of these patients undergo surgery. It is easy to identify the bleeding vessel, and occluding it is highly effective.

In cases of liver trauma, if the patient is stable and no lesions that justify exploratory laparotomy are seen at CT, the treatment is conservative.

If signs of active bleeding are seen at CT and the patient is hemodynamically unstable, if time permits, a liver arteriogram should be performed to locate the point of bleeding to be embolized. Embolization immediately stops the bleeding, and signs of clinical improvement are often evident as soon as the procedure has been completed.

Embolization should be as selective as possible (either resorbable materials like gelfoam or nonresorbable microcoils can be used). The advantage of hepatic embolization is that the liver has double circulation (20% through the hepatic artery and 80% through the portal vein), so arterial occlusion is well tolerated and can be achieved using nonresorbable materials: note that in the case described above, there are no areas of ischemia in the liver in the 1-month follow-up CT examination.

Procedure Steps

1. Approach through the right common femoral artery.
2. Selectively catheterize the hepatic artery with a 4F SHK catheter.
3. Perform hepatic arteriography with an injector. In this case, angiographic signs of active bleeding (pseudoaneurysms) were seen in segments II and IV of the left liver lobe.
4. Introduce a 2.4F microcatheter and a 0.16 in. hydrophilic microguidewire through the 4F catheter for superselective catheterization of the segmental arteries of the left liver lobe.
5. Once the damaged artery is embolized through the microcatheter with 0.018 microcoils (3 mm in diameter and 3 cm long), push the coils with 2 mL saline solution.
6. Perform subtracted arteriography of the liver to ensure that there is no extravasation of iodinated contrast material.

Equipment List

1. 10 cm long 5F vascular introducer sheath with a hemostatic valve. Introducer II®. Terumo Radiofocus
2. 150 cm long 0.035 in. hydrophilic guidewire. Terumo Radiofocus guide wire M.
3. 65 cm long 4F 1.0 SHK catheter. Cordis
4. 130 cm long 2.4F microcatheter. Terumo Progreat
5. 200 cm long 0.016 in. 45-degree angled hydrophilic guidewire. Terumo Radiofocus GT with gold coil.
6. 0.018 in. multiple-curled soft platinum TM Microcoils (3 mm in diameter and 3 cm long). Cook MWCE-18S-3.0-3-HILAL

Case 3.6
Embolization of Hepatocellular Carcinoma

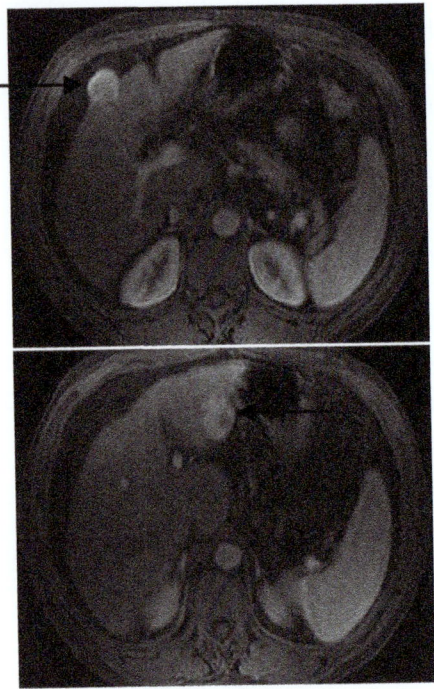

Fig. 3.6.1

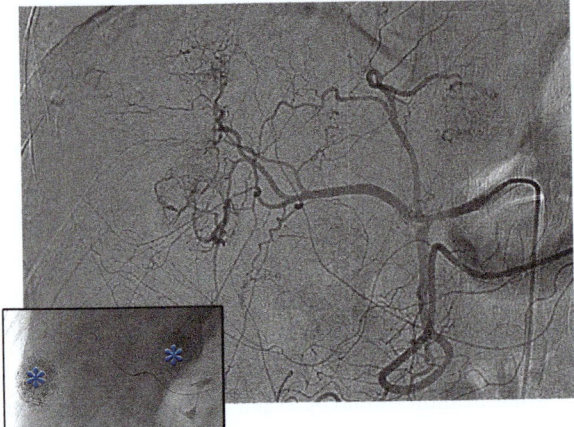

Fig. 3.6.2

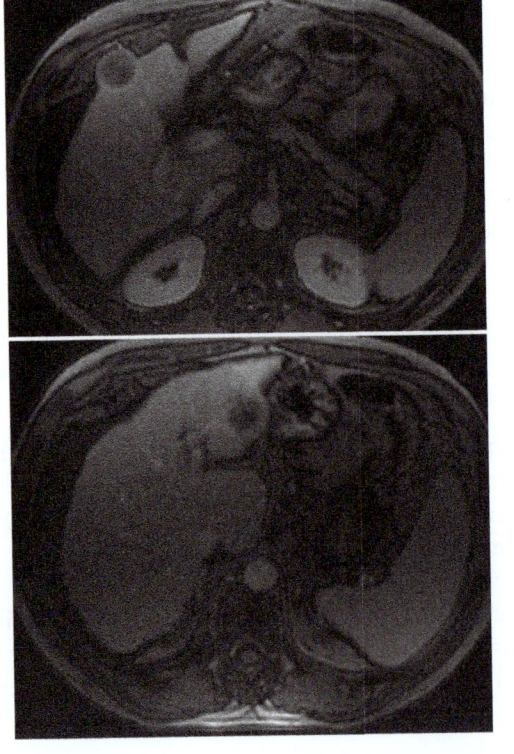

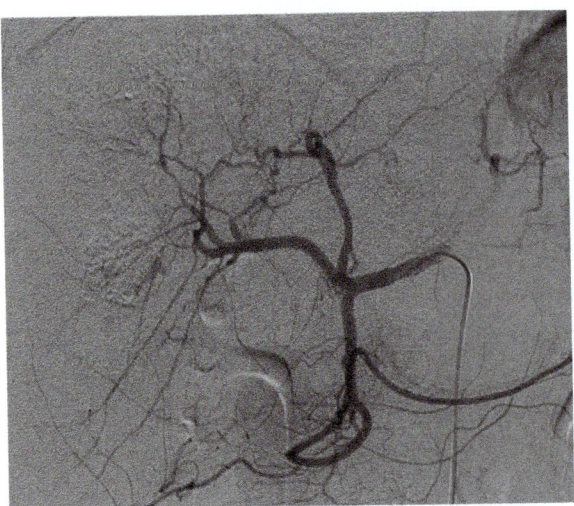

Fig. 3.6.3

Fig. 3.6.4

Figure 3.6.1 T1-weighted MR image, dynamic study: after gadolinium administration, two of the three masses visualized are shown in segments III and IV of the left liver lobe. The behavior of the masses is suggestive of hepatocellular carcinoma: the masses are hypervascular in the arterial phase (*arrows*)

Figure 3.6.2 Hepatic arteriogram confirms the two dominant hypervascular masses in the left liver lobe; another mass measuring 10 mm and two others measuring less than 1 cm are seen in the right liver lobe. The detailed image at the lower left shows lipiodol uptake in larger masses (marked with *asterisks*)

Figure. 3.6.3 Subtracted arteriogram of the liver after embolization: no hypervascular masses are seen

Figure 3.6.4 Gadolinium-enhanced MR image, dynamic study 1 month after treatment: in the arterial phase, due to necrosis in response to endovascular treatment, the hypervascular masses seen before embolization show no uptake

A 48-year-old man was admitted for hematemesis after NSAID ingestion; during hospitalization, he was diagnosed with chronic liver disease due to hepatitis C virus and alcohol abuse, as well as multifocal hepatocellular carcinoma. At least three focal lesions measuring 32, 26, and 10 mm were seen in segments III and IV of the left liver lobe and in segment VIII of the right liver lobe. His functional stage was Child B7. Because at least three lesions were found in two different lobes and the larger lesions were very exophytic (one was in contact with the lesser curvature of the stomach), we decided to treat the patient with chemical embolization and evaluate the response. The patient was discharged from the hospital 24 h after the procedure. In the 1-month follow-up MRI, we observed necrosis of the larger masses and no evidence of focal lesions with strong uptake.

Comments

Hepatocellular carcinoma is the most common malignant neoplasm of the liver. The incidence of hepatocellular carcinoma has increased in recent years, and it is now the fifth most common tumor in the world; it occurs in patients with cirrhosis of the liver and is the main cause of death in these patients.

According to the treatment algorithm for hepatocellular carcinoma in the Barcelona classification, patients in the early stage (A) (i.e., a single tumor ≤5 cm or up to three nodules <3 cm) are candidates for curative treatment; options include liver transplantation, resection, and percutaneous treatments. Patients in the intermediate stage (B) (i.e., tumor >5 cm or multifocal) or in the advanced stage (C) (i.e., extrahepatic dissemination or vascular invasion) have a 3-year survival rate of 10–50% and are candidates for locoregional or palliative treatments. The best palliative treatment is arterial chemoembolization.

Procedure Steps

1. Approach through the right common femoral artery and insert a 5F arterial introducer sheath.
2. Introduce a 4F cobra catheter over the guidewire and catheterize the common hepatic artery. Perform selective arteriography to detect hypervascular masses. In this case, three hypervascular masses and other small foci of hypervascularization were detected.

3. Introduce the 0.016 in. Terumo Progreat microcatheter and microguidewire through the 4F hydrophilic catheter and superselectively catheterize the branches that supply the largest tumors.
4. Superselectively embolize the arteries supplying the tumors using an emulsion of 5 mL lipiodol and 50 mg adriamycin.
5. Perform arteriography to confirm the absence of arterial supply to the liver tumors.
6. Prescribe 8 mg/8 h oral ondansetron hydrochloride (Zofran Zydis®) for 2 days and a single 30 mg dose of prednisone (Dacortín®) every 24 h for 3 days to alleviate postembolization syndrome.

Equipment List

1. 10 cm long 5F vascular introducer sheath with a hemostatic valve. Introducer II®. Terumo Radiofocus
2. 150 cm long 0.035 in. angled hydrophilic guidewire. Terumo Radiofocus guide wire M.
3. 80 cm long 4F cobra C3 hydrophilic angiographic catheter. Terumo Radiofocus Glidecath
4. 130 cm long 2.4F microcatheter. Terumo Progreat
5. 200 cm long 0.016 in. 45-degree angled hydrophilic guidewire. Terumo Radiofocus GT with gold coil.
6. Iodinated contrast oil: lipiodol
7. Adriamycin 50 mg
8. 500–700 µm calibrated microspheres. Embosphere Microspheres®. Biosphere Medical

Case 3.7

■
**Breakage of a
Central Venous
Catheter from a
Reservoir**

Figure 3.7.1 Anteroposterior chest X-ray shows a venous catheter tunneled from the left hemithorax to the ipsilateral subclavian vein; there seems to be an interruption in the catheter as it runs adjacent to the clavicle. A metallic artifact related to the needle projects onto the opacity of the reservoir

Figure 3.7.2 CT slice (*upper image*) and fluoroscopy (*lower image*) show extravasation of contrast material in the segment of the catheter adjacent to the entrance to the vein, in contact with the clavicle, and reflux of contrast material toward the subcutaneous pouch that harbors the unicameral reservoir

Figure 3.7.3 Approaching from the right common femoral vein, we trap the free tip of the catheter with a gooseneck snare while releasing the catheter from the reservoir to pull it toward the inferior vena cava. Different sizes of Amplatz gooseneck snares

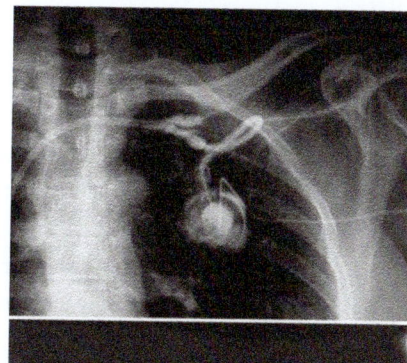
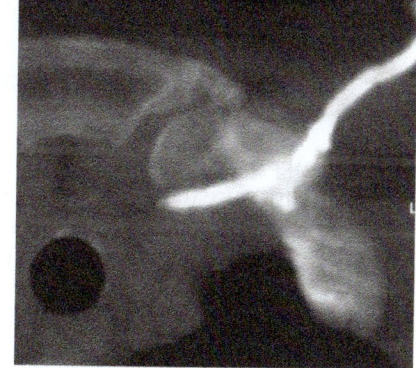

Fig. 3.7.2

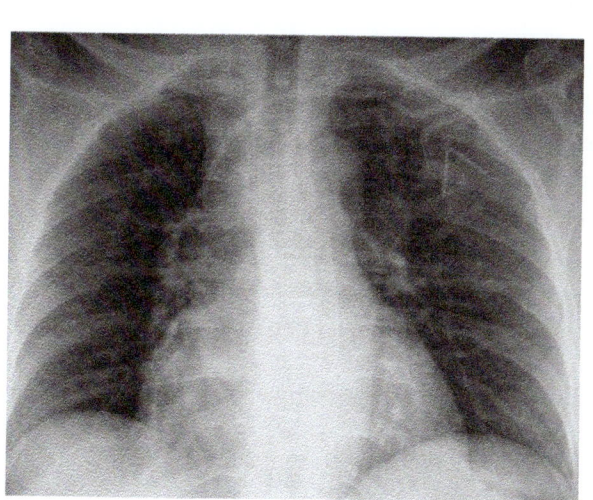

Fig. 3.7.1

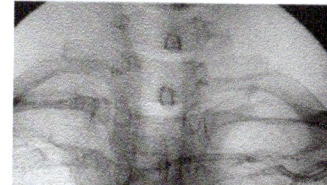
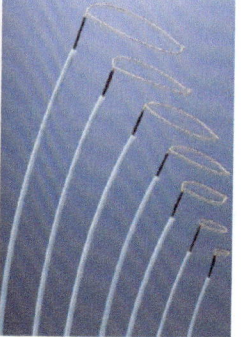

Fig. 3.7.3

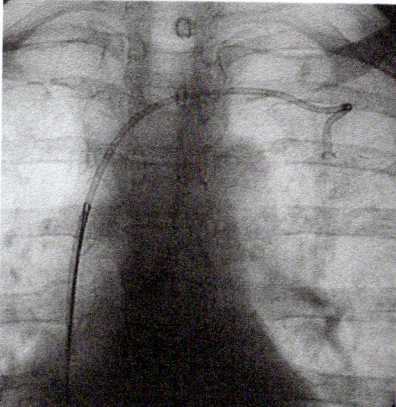

Fig. 3.7.4

Figure 3.7.4 Once the free portion was introduced into the inferior vena cava, the snare was placed in a segment of the catheter closer to the rupture to enable it to be pulled better. The broken catheter was then removed through the common femoral vein

A 49-year-old woman with a subcutaneous reservoir placed 3 years earlier in her left hemithorax with a catheter tunneled to the ipsilateral subclavian vein to administer chemotherapy for ovarian cancer presented for routine radiologic follow-up of her disease. We observed discontinuity and elbowing of the catheter in the left hemithorax and when we tried to heparinize it, the patient experienced pain adjacent to the clavicle.

After confirming the incomplete break in the catheter, we approached through the right common femoral vein and trapped the catheter with a gooseneck snare, disconnecting it from the subcutaneous reservoir. The patient was sent home after the catheter was removed and 6 h rest was recommended for the punctured limb.

Comments

The percutaneous removal of intravascular foreign bodies avoids major surgery in many cases.

In the present case, detecting the partial break in the catheter avoided its migration and made its removal easier.

Diverse techniques for the percutaneous removal of foreign bodies have been reported. However, the most widely used technique is the simple and efficacious one described here.

Intravascular fragments are successfully removed in 95% of cases, and thus thoracotomy or venotomy are avoided. Complications during percutaneous extraction are rare; these include cardiac arrhythmias, fragmentation of the foreign body, lesions to the vein, and embolization.

Procedure Steps

1. Approach through the right common femoral artery.
2. Introduce the curry snare through the delivery catheter until the free segment of the endovenous catheter is reached.
3. Withdraw the catheter that delivers the snare a few centimeters so that the 25 mm snare opens.
4. Maneuver the snare under fluoroscopic guidance to grasp the free tip of the foreign body with the metallic snare.
5. Withdraw everything toward the inferior vena cava.
6. Without releasing the catheter from the snare, disconnect the catheter from the reservoir in the subcutaneous pouch.
7. Once the catheter is disconnected, advance the snare toward a segment that is closer to the break to achieve greater traction strength and pull the catheter with greater security.
8. Remove everything through the common femoral vein.
9. Instruct the patient to rest the punctured member for 6 h.

Equipment List

1. 10 cm long 7F vascular introducer sheath with hemostatic valve. Introducer II®. Terumo Radiofocus
2. 150 cm long 0.035 in. angled hydrophilic guidewire. Terumo Radiofocus
3. 120 cm long 6F nitinol curry snare with a 24 mm loop. Hooker® MedItalia
4. Wound care kit (to remove the subcutaneous reservoir).

Case 3.8

Breakage of a Venous Catheter in the Left Pulmonary Artery

Figure 3.8.1 Anteroposterior chest X-ray (detail from a lateral projection) shows a unicameral metallic reservoir in the right hemithorax; the radiopaque tubular structure superimposed on the cardiac silhouette is an endovenous catheter that has migrated to the left pulmonary artery

Figure 3.8.2 The catheter that has migrated to the left pulmonary artery is caught with a 5F pigtail catheter and pulled to a position where it will be easier to grab its free tip with the snare

Figure 3.8.3 Once the catheter has been withdrawn from the right atrium, its free tip is trapped with the snare and removed through the common femoral artery

Figure 3.8.4 Chest X-ray after the removal of the subcutaneous reservoir following the removal of the catheter

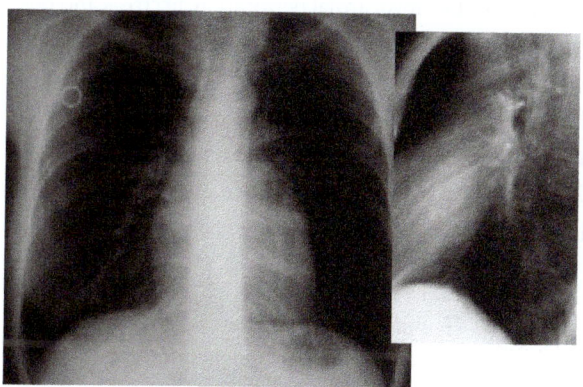
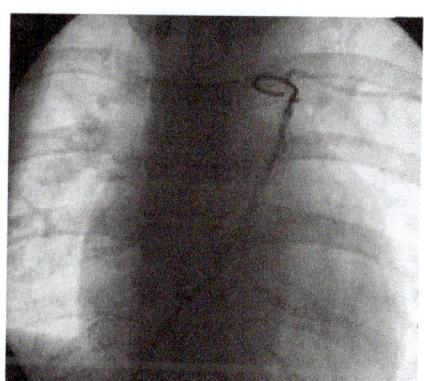

Fig. 3.8.1

Fig. 3.8.2

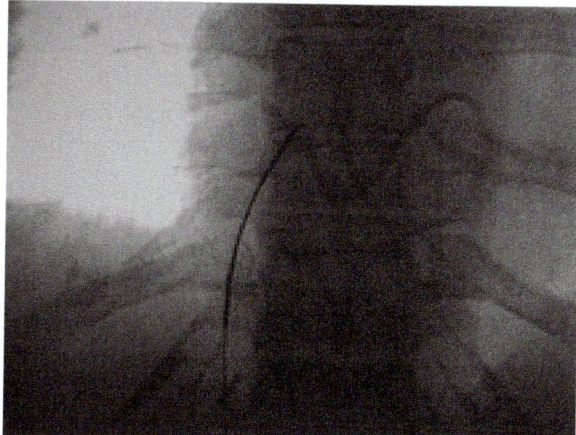
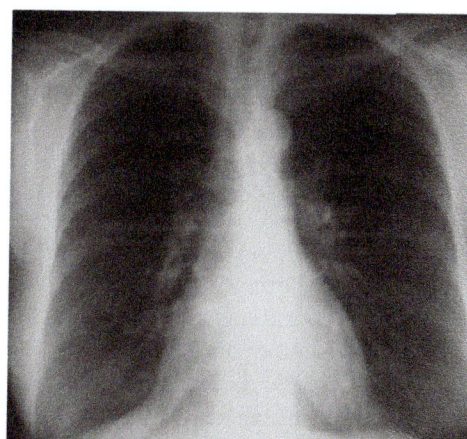

Fig. 3.8.3

Fig. 3.8.4

A 39-year-old woman with a history of left mastectomy for inflammatory breast cancer who had a subcutaneous reservoir placed in her right hemithorax with a tunneled catheter to the ipsilateral subclavian vein 6 months earlier underwent routine chest X-ray examination for her disease. The tunneled catheter had become disconnected from the reservoir and migrated to the left pulmonary artery, and the patient referred chest pain and palpitations in the previous month.

We trapped the catheter with a gooseneck snare and removed it through the common femoral vein. Then we removed the subcutaneous reservoir from the right hemithorax and sent the patient home to rest the punctured limb.

Comments

Implantable devices for venous access eliminate the need for repeated puncture in patients who require prolonged intravenous treatment. These devices consist of a reservoir connected to a catheter whose distal tip is placed in the superior vena cava or right atrium. Catheter breakage and intravascular migration are rare complications. In the present case, the catheter became disconnected from the reservoir and migrated to the pulmonary artery. Centrally embolized foreign bodies can lead to serious complications like myocardial perforation, necrosis and posterior tamponade, myocardial infarction, valve perforation, pulmonary embolism, and infectious complications like endocarditis or septic embolisms. The mortality depends on the time the embolized catheter remains in the vessels and the place where it is lodged (complications associated to lodging in the right heart are more serious, those arising from lodging in the inferior vena cava are less serious, and those due to lodging in the pulmonary artery are even less serious). In any case, the foreign body should be removed as soon as possible to avoid death.

Procedure Steps

1. Approach through the right common femoral vein.
2. Catheterize the pulmonary artery with a 4F multipurpose catheter.
3. While maneuvering through the chambers of the heart, be especially careful to avoid causing runs of extrasystoles.
4. Exchange the multipurpose catheter for a 5F pigtail catheter over the Amplatz guidewire.
5. Wrap the pigtail catheter around the migrated catheter and pull it so that the free tip of the broken catheter comes into a position where it is easy to catch with the snare.
6. The broken catheter is moved to the right atrium or to the inferior vena cava, where it is easier to snare, and the snare is advanced in its delivery catheter to the migrated catheter.
7. The delivery catheter is withdrawn a few centimeters and the snare is turned under fluoroscopic guidance until the free tip of the foreign body is inside the loop.
8. The deliver catheter is advanced until it closes the snare around the foreign body.
9. Everything is withdrawn through the right common femoral vein and the patient is advised to rest the punctured limb for 6 h.

Equipment List

1. 10 cm long 7F vascular introducer sheath with hemostatic valve. Introducer II®. Terumo Radiofocus
2. 150 cm long 0.035 in. angled hydrophilic guidewire. Terumo Radiofocus
3. 80 cm long 4F multipurpose A2® angiographic catheter. Cordis
4. 180 cm long 0.035 in. extrastiff straight-tipped Amplatz THSF guidewire. Cook
5. 65 cm long 5F pigtail angiographic catheter. Cordis
6. 120 cm long 6F nitinol curry snare with a 24 mm loop. Hooker® MedItalia
7. Wound care kit (to remove the subcutaneous reservoir).

Case 3.9

Aortobifemoral Graft Thrombolysis

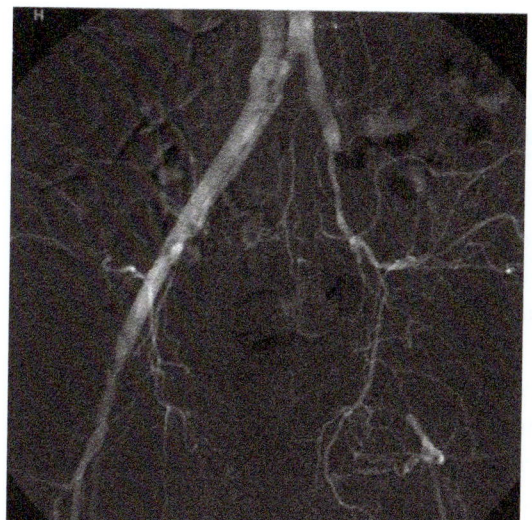

Fig. 3.9.1

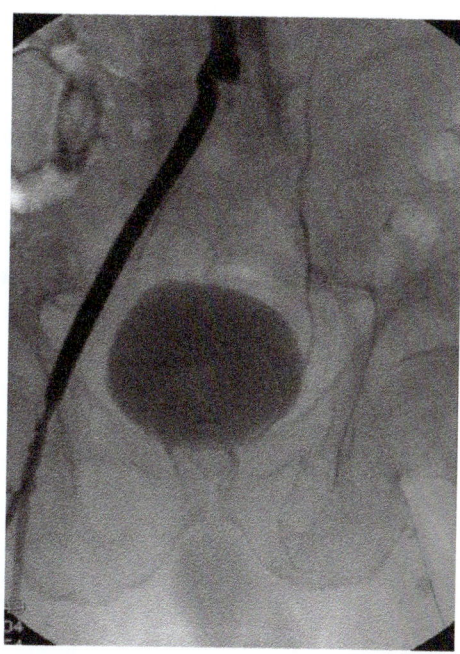

Fig. 3.9.2

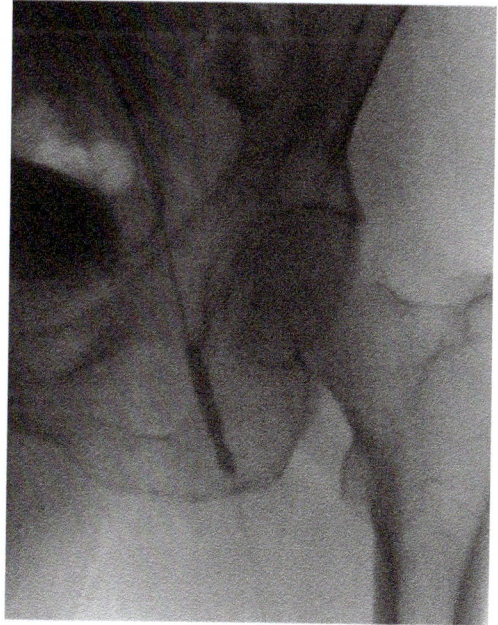

Fig. 3.9.3

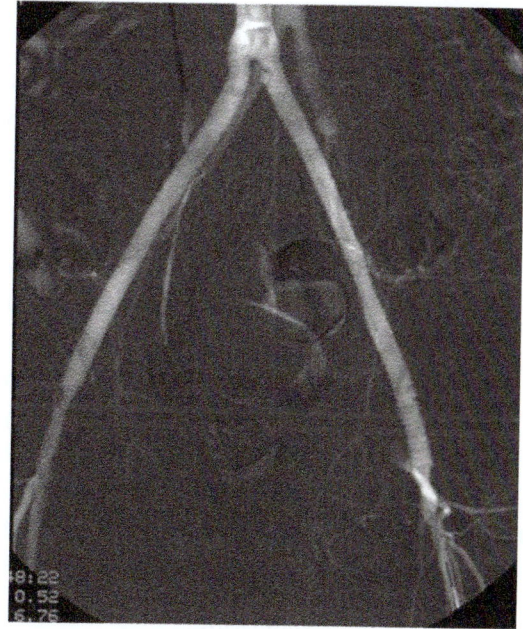

Fig. 3.9.4

Figure 3.9.1 Pelvic arteriogram performed using a pigtail catheter in the infrarenal aorta shows occlusion of the left branch of the aortobifemoral bypass that is revascularized through the deep femoral artery. The aortic cone and native iliac arteries are also filled

Figure 3.9.2 Pelvic arteriogram after recanalization of the occluded branch using a multi-perforated catheter prior to in situ thrombolysis. Note the radiopaque markings on the microcatheter, which indicate the segment of the multiperforated catheter

Figure 3.9.3 Dilatation of the distal anastomosis of the bypass with a balloon catheter measuring 7 mm in diameter and 40 mm in length after significant stenosis was observed in the arteriogram obtained 18 h after starting thrombolytic treatment

Figure 3.9.4 Pelvic arteriogram showing the final outcome: patency has been restored to the occluded branch of the bypass, and the stenosis of the distal anastomosis has been dilated

A 74-year-old man presented at the emergency department with a 1-week history of left foot pain at rest. He was diagnosed with acute arterial ischemia of the left leg secondary to occlusion of the left branch of the aortobifemoral bypass performed 14 years earlier to treat Leriche syndrome.

At physical examination, pulses were absent in the left leg and its skin was cold and pale with delayed venous filling but motility and sensitivity were preserved. After confirming the diagnosis, we performed endovascular treatment of the occluded branch of the bypass consisting of thrombolysis within the prosthesis and angioplasty of the distal anastomosis.

The patient was discharged from the hospital 48 h after endovascular treatment was initiated; his left femoral pulse was normal and his symptoms had disappeared.

Comments

Acute occlusion of a prosthetic vascular graft causes sudden limb pain. As the condition progresses, the pain is followed by paresthesias, functional impotence, and eventually tissue necrosis.

The speed of progression of the symptoms depends on the length of the thrombosed segment and whether collateral vessels are present. Acute ischemia of the limbs threatens both the viability of the limb and the patient's life. Acute ischemia (<14 days' evolution) responds better to intraarterial thrombolytic treatment than to surgery, which is the treatment of choice in patients with chronic symptoms (>14 days). Furthermore, thrombolytic treatment is the first line approach for thrombosis of prosthetic grafts. The age of the graft is also an important prognostic factor: grafts less than 1-year-old have a worse prognosis, because a graft that develops early thrombosis indicates an inadequate caliber, poor quality distal bed, etc., and these problems are difficult to solve. In this case of a patient with acute ischemia (IIA) of less than 14 days' evolution due to thrombosis of a vascular graft in place for more than 1 year, the treatment of choice is in situ intraarterial thrombolysis.

Procedure Steps

1. Approach through the left axillary artery. Confirm the occlusion of the left branch of the bypass with diagnostic arteriography.
2. Recanalize the occlusion with a multipurpose catheter and stiff hydrophilic guidewire.

3. Pass a 0.014 in. guidewire through the multipurpose catheter and replace the multipurpose catheter with a multiperforated microcatheter, which has two radiopaque marks that indicate the length of the multiperforated segment, leaving the distal radiopaque mark in the patent artery.

4. Administer a 300,000 IU bolus of urokinase for thrombolysis; because the multiperforated segment of the catheter does not cover the entire thrombosed segment, withdraw the catheter slightly after 20–30 min to ensure that the thrombolytic drug is administered evenly throughout the thrombosed segment.

5. Place the distal tip of a catheter (e.g., the same microcatheter) in the proximal end of the thrombosis and continuously perfuse the thrombolytic drug (100,000 IU urokinase/h) until the following day.

6. Perform a blood test 4 and 12 h after initiating thrombolysis. Administer analgesics through continuous endovenous perfusion throughout the treatment. Prescribe antacids, a soft diet, and vigilance of the arterial access and possible bleeding points. Suspend subcutaneous and intramuscular medication.

7. Obtain an arteriogram the following day; in this case, stenosis of the distal anastomosis was seen.

8. After introducing a thin guidewire, replace the microcatheter with a 4F multipurpose catheter to catheterize the native artery.

9. Once in the native artery, introduce an Amplatz-type exchange guidewire, withdraw the multipurpose catheter, and introduce a balloon catheter measuring 7 mm in diameter and 40 mm in length.

10. Perform angioplasty controlled with a manometer and check the results with an arteriogram obtained with a 5F pigtail catheter.

Equipment List

1. 45 cm long 6F contralateral shapeable introducer sheath. Destination®. Terumo Radiofocus
2. 65 cm long 4F pigtail angiographic catheter. Cordis
3. 80 cm long 4F multipurpose angiographic catheter A2®. Cordis
4. 260 cm 0.035 in. straight stiff hydrophilic guidewire. Terumo Radiofocus
5. 300 cm long 0.014 in. miraclebros® 12 metallic guidewire. Abbott
6. 135 cm long 3F Pulse spray Pro® multiperforated infusion catheter with a 20 cm perforated section. Angiodynamics
7. 0.035 in. exchange guidewire.
8. 135 cm long delivery catheter and Ultrathin SDS® balloon angioplasty catheter (7 mm in diameter and 40 mm long). Boston Scientific
9. 20cc disposable manometer. Biometrix B.V.

Case 3.10
Native Artery Thrombolysis

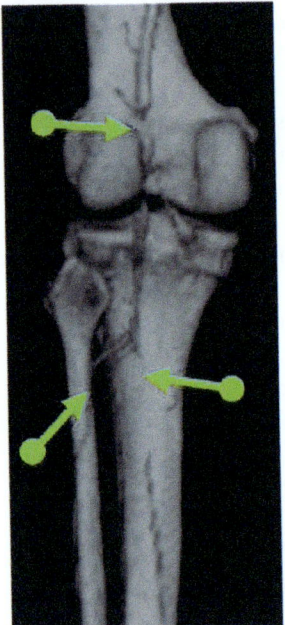

Fig. 3.10.1

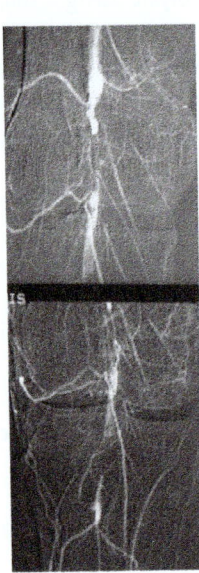

Fig. 3.10.2

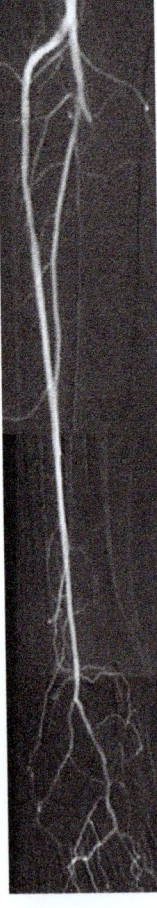

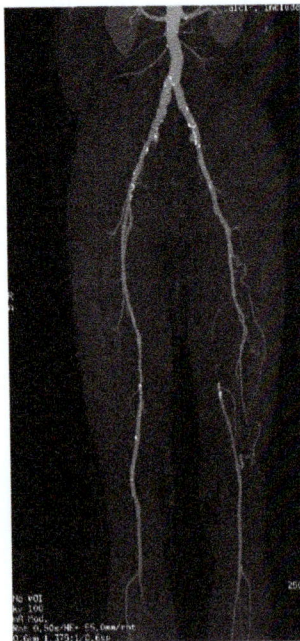

Fig. 3.10.3   **Fig. 3.10.4**

Figure 3.10.1 CT angiogram shows occlusion of the popliteal artery, anterior tibial artery, and tibioperoneal trunk (*arrows*)

Figure 3.10.2 Selective antegrade arteriogram confirms the findings

Figure 3.10.3 Antegrade arteriogram after thrombolytic treatment and angioplasty of the popliteal and distal lesions demonstrates the patency of the previously occluded arteries and the absence of residual stenoses

Figure 3.10.4 CT angiogram 4 years after thrombolytic treatment shows that the femoropopliteal trunk and the anterior tibial and peroneal arteries remain patent without significant stenoses

A 69-year-old man was admitted with a 4-day history of right foot pain at rest of abrupt onset. At physical examination, popliteal and distal pulses in the right leg were absent and the right foot was cold, pallid, and poorly perfused, although movement was preserved. Acute arterial ischemia of the right leg was diagnosed clinically and arterial thrombosis was suspected. CT angiography confirmed diffuse lesions in the superficial femoral artery, short occlusion of the popliteal artery (first–second portion), and occlusion of infrapopliteal arteries (the anterior tibial arteries a few centimeters from its origin and the tibioperoneal trunk from its origin).

Using an antegrade approach through the ipsilateral common femoral artery, we recanalized the occluded segments and performed in situ thrombolysis for 24 h followed by angioplasty of the underlying stenosing lesions.

During outpatient follow-up, the patient remained asymptomatic with positive pedal pulses. CT angiography 4 years after treatment confirmed the patency of the arteries treated.

In cases of acute arterial ischemia, the first aspect to evaluate is its clinical grade: Is the limb viable? Is it threatened? Does it require urgent treatment?

Comments

- Grade I Viable – preserved sensitivity and mobility – permits nonurgent treatment.
- Grade IIA Slight threat – minimal loss of sensitivity, preserved mobility – requires urgent treatment.
- Grade IIB Immediate threat – loss of sensitivity and mobility, intense pain at rest – requires urgent treatment.
- Grade III Irreversible – profound loss of sensation, muscular rigidity, foot clubbing – the only treatment possible is amputation.

In grades I and IIA, if symptoms have been present for less than 14 days, thrombolysis is the first line of treatment, because the risks involved are minor compared to those of surgical treatment, especially considering that, as in this case, patients tend to have many comorbidities. However, the outcome in thrombolysis of distal occlusions is worse than in iliofemoral thrombosis, and as was demonstrated in the STILE study, native artery occlusions do not respond to thrombolytic treatment as well as prosthetic shunts.

Procedure Steps

1. Use an antegrade approach through the ipsilateral common femoral artery.
2. Introduce an Amplatz guidewire using the needle and catheterize the superficial femoral artery. Introduce a 5F arterial introducer sheath over the guidewire.
3. Perform diagnostic arteriography.
4. Introduce a multipurpose catheter and then pass a hydrophilic guidewire through it to recanalize the obstruction.
5. Once the occluded segment is recanalized, introduce a 0.014 in. guidewire through the multipurpose catheter to exchange it for a perforated microcatheter; administer a bolus of 300,000 IU urokinase over 20–30 min.
6. Connect the catheter to a perfusion pump and continuously perfuse 100,000 IU urokinase/h with the catheter placed a few centimeters in the proximal extreme of the thrombosed segment.
7. Obtain blood tests 4 and 12 h after starting thrombolysis. Administer analgesics through continuous endovenous perfusion throughout the treatment. Prescribe antacids, a soft diet, and vigilance of the arterial access and possible bleeding points. Suspend subcutaneous and intramuscular medication.
8. The following day, perform angiography to check femoropopliteal patency, stenosis in the superficial femoral artery and in the anterior tibial and peroneal arteries.
9. Replace the microcatheter with a balloon catheter measuring 6 mm in diameter and 40 mm in length.
10. Check the outcome by angiography.

Equipment List

1. Two-piece 19G Seldinger-approach metallic needle. Boston Scientific
2. 180 cm long 0.035 in. extrastiff straight-tipped Amplatz THSF guidewire. Cook.
3. 10 cm long 5F vascular introducer sheath with hemostatic valve. Introducer II®. Terumo Radiofocus
4. 80 cm long 4F A2® multipurpose angiographic catheter. Cordis
5. 150 cm long 0.035 in. angled hydrophilic guidewire. Terumo Radiofocus
6. 90 cm long 3F Pulse spray Pro® multiperforated infusion with a 20 cm long perforated segment. Angiodynamics.
7. 180 cm long 0.014 in. miraclebros® 12 metallic guidewire. Abbott
8. Ultrathin SDS® balloon angioplasty catheter (6 mm in diameter and 40 mm in length), 90 cm long. Boston Scientific.
9. 20cc disposable manometer. Biometrix B.V.
10. Medication: urokinase, sodium heparin, nitroglycerine.

Further Reading

AbuRahma AF, Stone PA, Bates MC, Welch CA. Angioplasty/stenting of the superior mesenteric artery and celiac trunk: Early and late outcomes. J Endovasc Ther 2003;10:1046–1053.6.

Adam DJ, et al. Bypass versus angioplasty in severe ischaemia of the leg (BASIL): multicentre randomised controlled trial. Lancet 2005;366:1925–1934.

Airoldi F, Palatresi S, Marana I, et al. Angioplasty of atherosclerotic and fibromuscular renal artery stenosis: time course and predicting factors of the effects on renal function. Am J Hypertens 2000;13:1210–1207.

Allen RC, Martin GH, Rees CR, et al. Mesenteric angioplasty in the treatment of chronic intestinal ischemia. J Vasc Surg 1996;24:415–421; discussion 421–423.

Andrews RT, Venbrux AC, Magee CA, Bova DA. Placement of a flexible endovascular stent across the femoral joint: an in vivo study in the swine model. J Vasc Interv Radiol 1999;10:1219–1228.

Angermayr B, Cejna M, Koenig F, et al. Survival in patients undergoing transjugular intrahepatic portosystemic shunt: ePTFE-covered stentgrafts versus bare stents. Hepatology 2003;38:1043–1050.

Barjau E, Hernández E, Cairols M, Sancho C, Simeón JM. ¿Son los fibrinolíticos un tratamiento útil en las reintervenciones de bypass femoropoplíteo? Angiología 2001;53:17–27.

Barrio J, Ripoll C, Banares R, Echenagusia A, Catalina MV, Camunez F, Simo G, Santos L. Comparison of transyugular intrahepatic portosystemic shunt dysfunction in PTFE-covered stent-grafts versus bare stents. Eur J Radiol 2005;55:120–124.

Bartorelli AL, Fabbiocchi F, Montorsi P, Loaldi A, Tamborini G. Successful transcatheter management of Palmaz stent embolization after superior vena cava stenting. Cathet Cardiovasc Diagn 1995;34:162–166.

Becker GJ, Holden RW, Klatte EC. Therapeutic embolization with absolute ethanol. Semin Intervent Radiol 1984;1:118.

Bernhardt LC, Wegner GP, Mendenhall JT. Intravenous catheter embolization to the pulmonary artery. Chest 1970;57:329–332.

Bloomfield DA. The nonsurgical retrieval of intracardiac foreign bodies: an international survey. Cathet Cardiovasc Diagn 1978;4:114.

Bosch FX, Ribes J, Borras J. Epidemiology of primary liver cancer. Semin Liver Dis 1999;19:271–285.

Brawn LA, Ramsay LE. Is "improvement" real with percutaneous transluminal angioplasty in the management of renovascular hypertension? Lancet 1987;2:1313–1316.

Brooks B. The treatment of traumatic arteriovenous fistula. South Med J 1930;23:100.

Brown DJ, Schermerhorn ML, Powell RJ, et al. Mesenteric stenting for chronic mesenteric ischemia. J Vasc Sur 2005;42:268–274.

Bruix J, Sherman M, Llovet JM, Beaugrand M, Lencioni R, Christensen E, Burroughs A, et al. Clinical management on hepatocellular carcinoma. Conclusions of the Barcelona-2000 EASL Conference. J Hepatol 2001;35:421–430.

Bruix J, Sala M, Llovet JM. Chemoembolization for hepatocellular carcinoma. Gastroenterology 2004;127(5 suppl 1):S179–S188.

Bureau C, Garcia-Pagan JC, Otal P, et al. Improved clinical outcome using polytetrafluoroethylene-coated stents for TIPS: results of a randomized study. Gastroenterology 2004;126:469–475.

Burkart DJ, Borsa JJ, Anthony JP, et al. Thrombolysis of occluded peripheral arteries and veins with tenecteplase: a pilot study. J Vasc Interv Radiol 2002;13:1099–1102.

Canzanello VJ, Millan VG, Spiegel JE, et al. Percutaneous transluminal renal angioplasty in management of atherosclerotic renovascular hypertension: results in 100 patients. Hypertension 1989;13:163–172.

Castañeda ZWR, Sanchez R, Amplatz K. Experimental observations on short and long-term effects of arterial occlusion with ivalon. Radiology 1978;126:783.

Castañeda-Zuñiga WE, Yormanek A, Tadavarthy M, et al. The mechanism of ballon angioplasty. Radiology 1980;135:565–571.

Cekirge S, Weiss JP, Foster RG, Neiman HL, McLean GK. Percutaneous retrieval of foreign bodies: experience with the nitinol gooseneck snare. J Vasc Interv Radiol 1993;4:805–810.

Chuapetcharasopon C, Wright KC, Wallace S, Dobben RL, Gianturco C. Treatment of experimentally induced atherosclerosis in swine iliac arteries: a comparison of self-expanding and balloon-expanded stents. Cardiovasc Intervent Radiol 1992;15:143–150.

Cicuto KP, McLean GK, Oleaga JA, et al. Renal artery stenosis: anatomic classification for percutaneous transluminal angioplasty. AJR Am J Roentgenol 1981;137:599–601.

Cohen GS, Ball DS. Delayed Wallstent migration after a transjugular intrahepatic portosystemic shunt procedure: relocation with a loop snare. J Vasc Interv Radiol 1993;4:561–563.

Colapinto RF, McLoughlin MJ, Weisbrod GL. The routine lateral aortogram and the celiac compression syndrome. Radiology 1972;103:557.

Collier J, Sherman M. Screening for hepatocellular carcinoma. Hepatology 1998;27:273–278.

Conrad M, Shepard A, Rubinfeld I, Burke M, Nypaper T, Reddy D, et al. Long-term results of catheter-directed thrombolysis to treat infrainguinal bypass graft occlusion: the urokinase era. J Vasc Surg 2003;37:1009–1016.

Debrun G, Lacour P, Caron JP, Hurt M, Comoy J, Keravel Y. Detachable balloon and calibrated-leak balloon techniques in the treatment of cerebral vascular lesions. J Neurosurg 1978;49:635.

Di Mario C, et al. Drug-eluting bioabsorbable magnesium stent. J Interv Cardiol 2004;17:391–395.

Djindjian R, Cophignon J, Theron J, Merlan JJ, Houdart R. Superselective arteriography embolization by the femoral route in neuroradiology: study of 60 cases. Neuroradiology 1973;6:132.

Doering RB, Stemmer EA, Connolly JE. Complications of indwelling venous catheters, with particular reference to catheter embolus. Am J Surg 1967;114:259–266.

Dondeliger RF, Lepontre B, Kurdziel JC. Percutaneous vascular foreign body retrieval: experience of an 11-year period. Eur J Radiol 1991;12:4–10.

Donelli G. Vascular catheter-related infection and sepsis. Surg Infect (Larchmt) 2006;7:s25–s27.

Dorros G, et al. Below-the-knee angioplasty: tibioperoneal vessels, the acute outcome. Cathet Cardiovasc Diagn 1990;19:170–178.

Dorros G, et al. Tibioperoneal (outflow lesion) angioplasty can be used as primary treatment in 235 patients with critical limb ischemia: five-year follow-up. Circulation 2001;104:2057–2062.

Dotter CT, Judkins NIP. Transluminal treatment of arteriosclerotic obstruction. Description of a new technique and a preliminary report of its application. Circulation 1964;30: 654–670.

Dotter CT, Rosch J, Bilbao MK. Transluminal extraction of catheter and guide fragments from the heart and great vessels; 29 collected cases. Am J Roentgenol Radium Ther Nucl Med 1971;111:467–472.

Dotter CT, Rosch J, Lakin PC, Lakin RC, Pegg JE. Injectable flow-guided coaxial catheters for selective angiography and controlled vascular occlusion. Radiology 1972;104(2):421–423.

Dotter CT, Rosch J, Seaman AJ. Selective clot lysis with low-dose streptokinase. Radiology 1974;111:31–37.

Drescher P, McGuckin J, Rilling WS, Crain MR. Catheter-directed thrombolytic therapy in peripheral artery occlusions: combining reteplase and abciximab. AJR Am J Roentgenol 2003;180(5):1385–1391.

Druskin MS, Siegel PD. Bacterial contamination of indwelling intravenous polyethylene catheters. JAMA 1963;185:966–968.

Duda SH, Tepe G, Luz O, et al. Peripheral arterial occlusion: treatment with abciximab plus urokinase versus with urokinase alone – a randomized pilot trial (the PROMPT study). Radiology 2001;221:689–696.

Duda SH, et al. Drug-eluting and bare nitinol stents for the treatment of atherosclerotic lesions in the superficial femoral artery: long-term results from the SIROCCO trial. J Endovasc Ther 2006;13:701–710.

Egglin TKP, Dickey KW, Rosenblatt M, Pollak JS. Retrieval of intravascular foreign bodies: experience in 32 cases. AJR Am J Roentgenol 1995;164:1259–1264.

Fisher RG, Ferreyro R. Evaluation of current techniques for non-surgical removal of intravascular iatrogenic foreign bodies. AJR Am J Roentgenol 1978;130:541–548.

Gabelmann A, Kramer S, Gorich J. Percutaneous retrieval of lost or misplaced intravascular objects. AJR Am J Roentgenol 2001;176:1509–1513.

Gianturco C, Anderson JH, Wallace S. Mechanical devices for arterial oclusion. AJR Am J Roentgenol 1975;124:428.

Górriz E, Carreira JM, García JM, Maynar M. Diagnóstico y terapéutica endoluminal. Radiología Intervencionista. Editorial Masson. Embolización. Introducción. Capítulo 16.1 358–363.

Graor RA, Risius B, Young JR, et al. Thrombolysis of peripheral arterial bypass grafts: surgical thrombectomy compared with thrombolysis: a preliminary report. J Vasc Surg 1988;7:347–355.

Harrison EG Jr, McCormack LJ. Pathologic classifications of renal arterial disease in renovascular hypertension. Mayo Clin Proc 1971;46:161–167.

Hartnell GG, Jordan SJ. Percutaneous removal of a misplaced Palmaz stent with a coaxial snare technique. J Vasc Interv Radiol 1995;6:799–801.

Henry M, Klonaris C, Amor M, Henry I, Tzvetanov K. State of the art: which stent for which lesion in peripheral interventions? Tex Heart Inst J 2000;27:119–126.

Hirsch AT, Haskal ZJ, Hertzer NR, Bakal CW, Creager MA, Halperin JL, Hiratzka LF, Murphy WR, Olin JW, Puschett JB, Rosenfield KA, Sacks D, Stanley JC, Taylor LM Jr, White CJ, White J, White RA. ACC/AHA 2005 guidelines for the management of patients with peripheral arterial disease (lower extremity, renal, mesenteric, and abdominal aortic): a collaborative report [trunc]. Bethesda, MD: American College of Cardiology Foundation; 2005:192p.

Howell M, Krajcer Z, Diethrich EB, Motarjeme A, Bacharach M, Dolmatch B, et al. Wallgraft endoprosthesis for the percutaneous treatment of femoral and popliteal artery aneurysms. J Endovasc Ther 2002;9:76–81.

Hutto JD, Reed AB. Endovascular repair of an acute blunt popliteal artery injury. J Vasc Surg 2007;45:188–190.

Hye R, Turner C, Valji K, Wolf Y, Roberts A, Bookstein J, et al. Is thrombolysis of occluded popliteal and tibial bypass grafts worthwhile? J Vasc Surg 1994;20:588–597.

Izumi R, Shimizu K, Ii T, Yagi M, Matsui O, Nonomura A, Miyazaki I. Prognostic factors of hepatocellular carcinoma in patients undergoing hepatic resection. Gastroenterology 1994;106:720–727.

Khosla S, Jain P, Manda R, et al. Acute and long-term results after intra-arterial thrombolysis of occluded lower extremity bypass grafts using recombinant tissue plasminogen activator for acute limb-threatening ischemia. Am J Ther 2003; 10:3–6.

Klinge J, Mali WP, Puijlaert CB, et al. Percutaneous transluminal renal angioplasty: initial and long-term results. Radiology 1989;171:501–506.

Koseoglu K, Parilda M, Oran I, Memisb A. Retrieval of intravascular foreign bodies with goose neck snare. Eur J Radiol 2004;49:281–285.

Kudo T, et al. Changing pattern of surgical revascularization for critical limb ischemia over 12 years: endovascular vs. open bypass surgery. J Vasc Surg 2006;44:304–313.

Lammer J. Femoropopliteal artery obstruction: from the balloon to the stent graft. Cardiovasc Intervent Radiol 2001;24:73–83.

Lammer J, Dake MD, Bleyn J, et al.; International Trial Study Group. Peripheral arterial obstruction: prospective study of treatment with a transluminally placed self-expanding stent-graft. Radiology 2000;217:95–104.

Leadbetter WF, Burkland CF. Hypertension in unilateral renal disease. J Urol 1938;39:611–626.

Leung DA, Spinosa DJ, Hagspiel KD, Angle JF, Matsumoto AH. Selection of stents for treating iliac arterial occlusive disease. J Vasc Interv Radiol 2003;14:137–152.

Lewis AL, Gonzalez MV, Lloyd AW, Hall B, Tang Y, Willis SL, et al. DC bead: in vitro characterization of a drug-delivery device for transarterial chemoembolization. J Vasc Interv Radiol 2006;17(2 pt 1):335–342.

Libertino JA, Beckmann CF. Surgery and percutaneous angioplasty in the management of renovascular hypertension. Urol Clin North Am 1994;21:235–243.

Lipton M, Cynamon J, Bakal CW, Sprayregen S. Percutaneous retrieval of two Wallstent endoprostheses from the heart through a single jugular sheath. J Vasc Interv Radiol 1995;6: 469–472.

Llovet JM, Bru C, Bruix J. Prognosis of hepatocellular carcinoma: the BCLC staging classification. Semin Liver Dis 1999;19:329–338.

Luesenhof AJ, Spence WT. Artificial embolization of cerebral arteries: report of use in a case of arteriovenous malformation. JAMA 1960;172:1153.

Mahler F, Schneider E, Hess H; Steering Committee, Study on Local Thrombolysis. Recombinant tissue plasminogen activator versus urokinase for local thrombolysis of femoropopliteal occlusions: a prospective, randomized multicenter trial. J Endovasc Ther 2001;8:638–647.

Mangell P, Malina M, Vogt K, et al. Are self-expanding stents superior to balloon-expanded in dilating aortas? An experimental study in pigs. Eur J Vasc Endovasc Surg 1996;12:287–294.

Matsi PJ, Suhonen MT, Pirinen AE, Soimakallio S. Chronic critical lower-limb ischemia: prospective trial of angioplasty with 1-36 months of follow-up. Radiology 1993;188:381–387.

Matsumoto AH, Barth KH, Selby JB, Tegtmeyer CJ. Peripheral angioplasty ballon technology. Cardiovasc Intervent Radiol 1993;16:135–143.

McNamara TO, Bomberger RA. Factors affecting initial and six month patency rates after intra-arterial thrombolysis with high dose urokinase. Am J Surg 1986;152:709–712.

McNamara TO, Fischer JR. Thrombolysis of peripheral and arterial graft occlusions: improved results using high-dose urokinase. AJR Am J Roentgenol 1985;144:769–775.

McShane MD, Proctor A, Spencer P, et al. Mesenteric angioplasty for chronic intestinal ischaemia. Eur J Vasc Surg 1992;6:333–336.

Moneta GL. Diagnosis of interinal ischemia. In: Rutherford RB, ed. Vascular Surgery, 5th edn. Philadelphia: WB Saunders; 2000.

Moneta GL, Yeager RA, et al. Duplex ultrasound criteria for diagnosis for splacnic artery stenosis or occlusion. J Vasc Surg 1991;14:511–516.

Moreira AM. Materiais. In: Carnevale FC, ed. Radiologia intervencionista e cirurgia endovascular. Rio de Janeiro: Revinter; 2006:33–55.

Nackman G, Walsh D, Fillinger M, Zwolak R, Bech F, Bettmann M, et al. Thrombolysis of occluded infrainguinal vein grafts: predictors of outcome. J Vasc Surg 1997;25:1023–1032.

Nelken N, Schneider PA. Advances in stent technology and drug-eluting stents. Surg Clin North Am 2004;84:1203–1236.

Norgren L, Hiatt WR, Dormandy JA, Nehler MR, Harris KA, Fowkes FGR. Inter-society consensus for the management of peripheral arterial disease (TASC II). Eur J Vasc Endovasc Surg 2007;33(suppl):S1–S75.

Okuda K, Ohtsuki T, Obata H, Tomimatsu M, Okazaki N, Hasegawa H, Nakajima Y, Ohnishi K. Natural history of hepatocellular carcinoma and prognosis in relation to treatment. Study of 850 patients. Cancer 1985;56:918–928.

Ouriel K. Current status of thrombolysis for peripheral arterial occlusive disease. Ann Vasc Surg 2002;16(6):797–804.

Ouriel K, Shortell CK, DeWeese JA, et al. A comparison of thrombolytic therapy with operative revascularization in the initial treatment of acute peripheral arterial ischemia. J Vasc Surg 1994;19:1021–1030.

Ouriel K, Veith FJ, Sasahara AA; Thrombolysis or Peripheral Arterial Surgery (TOPAS) Investigators. A comparison of recombinant urokinase with vascular surgery as initial treatment for acute arterial occlusion of the legs. N Engl J Med 1998;338:1105–1111.

Ouriel K, Kandarpa K, Schuerr DM, et al. Prourokinase versus urokinase for recanalization of peripheral occlusions, safety and efficacy: the PURPOSE trial. J Vasc Interv Radiol 1999;10:1083–1091.

Parikh S, Hyman D. Hepatocellular cancer: a guide for the internist. Am J Med 2007;120(3):194–202.

Park JH, Yoon DY, Han JK, Kim SH, Han MC. Retrieval of intravascular foreign bodies with the snare and catheter capture technique. J Vasc Interv Radiol 1992;3:581–582.

Peeters P, et al. Preliminary results after application of absorbable metal stents in patients with critical limb ischemia. J Endovasc Ther 2005;12:1–5.

Pell JP, Whyman MR, Fowkes FG, et al. Trends in vascular surgery since introduction of percutaneous transluminal angioplasty. Br J Surg 1994;81:832–835.

Prahlow JA, Obryant TJ, Barnard JJ. Cardiac perforation due to Wallstent embolization: a fatal complication of the transjugular intrahepatic portosystemic shunt procedure. Radiology 1997;205:170–172.

Razavi M, Chung H. Endovascular management of chronic mesenteric ischemia. Tech Vasc Interv Radiol 2004;7:155–159.

Results of a prospective randomized trial evaluating surgery versus thrombolysis for ischemia of the lower extremity. The STILE trial. Ann Surg 1994;220:251–266; discussion 266–268.

Richardson JD, Grover FL, Trinkle JK. Intravenous catheter emboli. Experience with twenty cases and collective review. Am J Surg 1974;128:722–727.

Rossi P, Salvatori FM, Fanelli F, et al. Polytetrafluoroethylene-covered nitinol stent-graft for transjugular intrahepatic portosystemic shunt creation: 3-year experience. Radiology 2004;231:820–830.

A Roussin, C Carter. Clinical guide – Thrombolytic therapy in peripheral arterial disease (December 2006).

Russo MW, Zacks SL, Sandler RS, Brown RS. Costeffectiveness analysis of transjugular intrahepatic portosystemic shunt (TIPS) versus endoscopic therapy for the prevention of recurrent esophageal variceal bleeding. Hepatology 2000;31: 358–563.

Saddekni S, Sniderman KW, Hilton S, et al. Percutaneous transluminal angioplasty of nonatherosclerotic lesions. AJR Am J Roentgenol 1982;135:975–982.

Sanchez RB, Roberts AC, Valji K, Lengle S, Bookstein JJ. Wallstent misplaced during transjugular placement of an intrahepatic portosystemic shunt: retrieval with a loop snare. AJR Am J Roentgenol 1992;159:129–130.

Savader SJ, Brodkin J, Osterman FA. In-situ formation of a loop snare for retrieval of a foreign body without a free end. Cardiovasc Intervent Radiol 1996;19:298–301.

Schaefer PJ, Schaefer FK, Muller-Huelsbeck S, Janke T. Chronic mesenteric ischemia. Stenting of mesenteric arteries. Abdom Imaging 2007;32:304–309.4.

Schellhammer F, Zahringer M, Lackner K. Nitinol microforceps for retrieval of intravascular objects: first in vitro experiences. Invest Radiol 2002;37:577–579.

Schreiber MJ, Pohl MA, Novick AC. The natural history of atherosclerotic and fibrous renal artery disease. Urol Clin North Am 1984;11:383–392.

Schwarten DE, Cutcliff WB. Arterial occlusive disease below the knee: treatment with percutaneous transluminal angioplasty performed with low-profile catheters and steerable guide wires. Radiology 1988;169:71–74.

Semba CP, Murphy TP, Bakal CW, et al. Thrombolytic therapy with use of alteplase (rt-PA) in peripheral arterial occlusive disease: review of the clinical literature. The Advisory Panel. J Vasc Interv Radiol 2000;11(2 pt 1):149–161.

Seong KC, Kim JK, Chung JW, Kim SH, Han JK, Kim HB, Park JH. Tubular foreign body or stent: safe retrieval or repositioning using the coaxialsnare tecnique. Korean J Radiol 2002;3: 30–37.

Sharafuddin MJ, Olson CH, Sun S, et al. Endovascular treatment of celiac and mesenteric arteries stenosis: applications and results. J Vasc Sur 2003;38:692–698.5.

Shortell CK, Queiroz R, Johansson M, et al. Safety and efficacy of limited-dose tissue plasminogen activator in acute vascular occlusion. J Vasc Surg 2001;34:854–859.

Siegel EL, Robertson EF. Percutaneous transfemoral retrieval of a free-floating titanium Greenfield filter with an Amplatz gooseneck snare. J Vasc Interv Radiol 1993;4:565–568.

Slonim SM, Dake MD, Razavi MK, et al. Management of misplaced or migrated endovascular stents. J Vasc Interv Radiol 1999;10:851–859.

Soder HK, et al. Prospective trial of infrapopliteal artery balloon angioplasty for critical limb ischemia: angiographic and clinical results. J Vasc Interv Radiol 2000;11:1021–1031.

Sos TA, Pickering TG, Sniderman K, et al. Percutaneous transluminal renal angioplasty in renovascular hypertension due to atheroma or fibromuscular dysplasia. N Engl J Med 1983;309:274–279.

Steinmetz E, Tatou E, Favier- Blavoux C, et al. Endovascular treatment as first choice in chronic mesenteric ischemia. Ann Vasc Surg 2002;16:693–699.

Swischuk JL, Fox PF, Young K, et al. Transcatheter intraarterial infusion of rt-PA for acute lower limb ischemia: results and complications. J Vasc Interv Radiol 2001;12:423–430.

Thanigaraj S, et al. Retrieval of an IV catheter fragment from the pulmonary artery 11 years after embolization. Chest 2000;117:1209–1211.

Tegtmeyer CJ, Selby JB, Hartwell GD, et al. Results and complications of angioplasty in fibromuscular disease. Circulation 1991;83(2 suppl):I155–I161.

The Cancer of the Liver Italian Program (CLIP) Investigators. A new prognostic system for hepatocellular carcinoma: a retrospective study of 435 patients. Hepatology 1998;28:751–755.

The Cancer of the Liver Italian Program (CLIP) Investigators. Prospective validation of the CLIP score: a new prognostic system for patients with cirrhosis and hepatocellular carcinoma. Hepatology 2000;31:840–845.

Thomas J, Sinclair-Smith B, Bloomfield D, et al. Nonsurgical retrieval of a broken segment of steel spring guide from the right atrium and inferior vena cava. Circulation 1964;30:106–108.

Uflaker R, Lima S, Melichar AC. Intravascular foreign bodies: percutaneous retrieval. Radiology 1986;160:731–735.

Viallet A, Marleau D, Huet M, et al. Hemodynamic evaluation of patients with intrahepatic portal hypertension. Relationship between bleeding varices and the portohepatic gradient. Gastroenterology 1975;69:1297–1300.

Weaver FA, Comerota AJ, Youngblood M, et al.; The STILE Investigators. Surgical revascularization versus thrombolysis for nonembolic lower extremity native artery occlusions: results of a prospective randomized trial. Surgery versus thrombolysis for ischemia of the lower extremity. J Vasc Surg 1996;24:513–521; discussion 521–523.

White C. Intermittent claudication. N Engl J Med 2007;356:1241–1250.

Wolf F, Thurnher S, Lammer J. Simon nitinol vena cava filters: effectiveness and complications. Rofo 2001;173:924–930.

Wolf F, Schernthaner RE, Dirisamer A, et al. Endovascular management of lost or misplaced intravascular objects: experiences of 12 years. Cardiovasc Intervent Radiol 2008;31:563–568.

Yazdi HR, Youness F, Laroia S, Shiliand S, Abada H, Sharafuddin M, Golzarian M. Mesenteric artery stenting for chronic mesenteric ischemia. Vasc Dis Manag 2007;4(6) (Digital Journal).

Yedlicka JF, Carlson JE, Hunter DW, et al. Nitinol gooseneck snare for removal of foreign bodies: experimental study and clinical evaluation. Radiology 1991;178:691–693.

Zanetti PH, Sherman FE. Experimental evaluation of a tissue adhesive as an agent for the treatment of aneurysm and arteriovenous anomalies. J Neurosurg 1972;36:72–79.

Zuckerman DA, Alderman MG, Idso MC, Pilgram TK, Sicard GA. Follow-up of infrainguinal graft thrombolysis. Analysis of predictors of clinical success. Arch Surg 2003;138:198–202.

Lower Extremity Arteries

4

Javier Peiró, Álvaro Iglesias, and Ramón Ribes

J.J. Muñoz and R. Ribes, *Learning Vascular and Interventional Radiology,* Learning Imaging,
DOI: 10.1007/978-3-540-87997-8_4, © Springer-Verlag Berlin Heidelberg 2010

Case 4.1

Severe Stenosis in the Left Common Iliac Artery

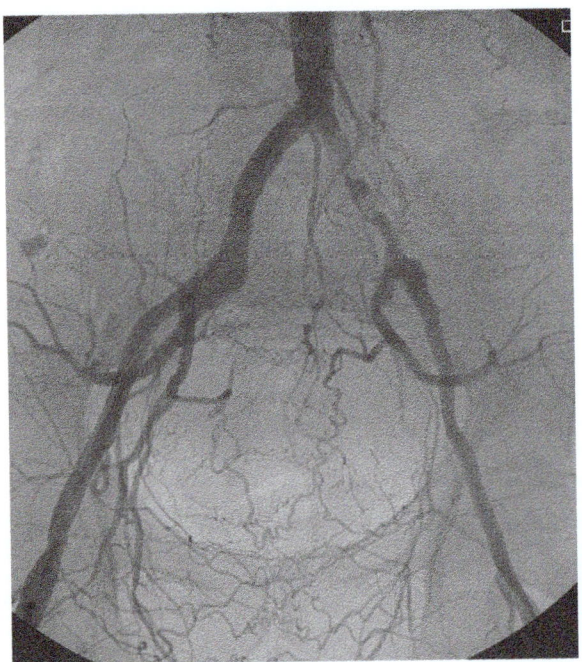

Fig. 4.1.1

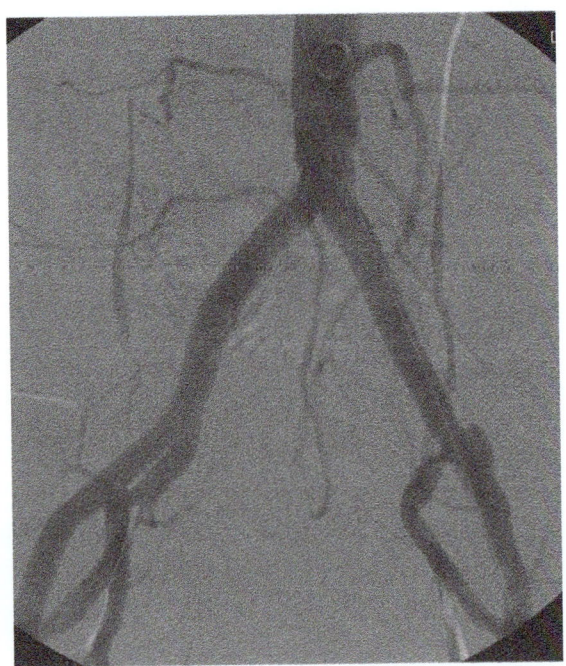

Fig. 4.1.2

Figure 4.1.1 Long stenosis of the left common iliac artery with a pronounced calcified component

Figure 4.1.2 Arteriogram after angioplasty and stent placement

A 55-year-old man with intermittent claudication (grade II B/Rutherford category 2) had severe stenoses in the right common iliac artery with no other involvement in the rest of the vascular bed of the lower limbs.

Comments

Iliac stenoses and obstructions are the most common vascular lesions in patients from 35 to 65 years of age, and stenosis is up to three times more common than obstruction.

Iliac stenosis or obstruction manifests as intermittent claudication, which can be both distal and proximal. Although proximal claudication can have a neurological or musculoskeletal origin, it is usually caused by iliac stenosis and obstruction. The femoral pulse is absent or a murmur and/or thrill is heard.

Iliac stenosis is usually well tolerated at first, thanks to collateral flow through branches of the lumbar, inferior mesenteric, or hypogastric arteries; however, the condition normally progresses continually, and without treatment, the recovery is torpid.

Another symptom that may be present is erectile dysfunction, which may or may not be associated to claudication.

Procedure

1. Perform a diagnostic study first. Approach through the right femoral artery using a 4F catheter.
2. Under fluoroscopic guidance, insert a 6F introducer sheath through the left femoral artery. Replace the catheter on the right side with a 6F introducer sheath.
3. Maneuver a 0.035 in. angled hydrophilic guidewire through the lesion. If necessary, use a hydrophilic vertebral catheter to help the guidewire through. Pass another hydrophilic guidewire through the right side.
4. Apply the "kissing technique," consisting of simultaneous bilateral dilation by inflating two PTA balloon catheters, one measuring 8×40 mm on the right side and another measuring 7×40 mm on the left.
5. Implant the 8 mm balloon-expandable stent (in case 3, a 9 mm balloon-expandable stent).
6. Check the outcome with a postprocedural arteriogram.

Equipment List

1. Prior diagnostic study: 4F femoral puncture.
2. Vascular recanalization:

- Left femoral puncture. 6F introducer sheath.
- Exchange the right 4F catheter for a 6F introducer sheath.
- Two 0.035 angled hydrophilic guidewires (180 and 260 cm long)
- "Kissing technique," bilateral PTA balloon catheters measuring 8×40 mm (right) and 7×40 mm (left).
- 8 mm balloon-expandable stent (37 mm case 1; 55 mm case 2)

Case 4.2
Bilateral Iliac Artery Lesions

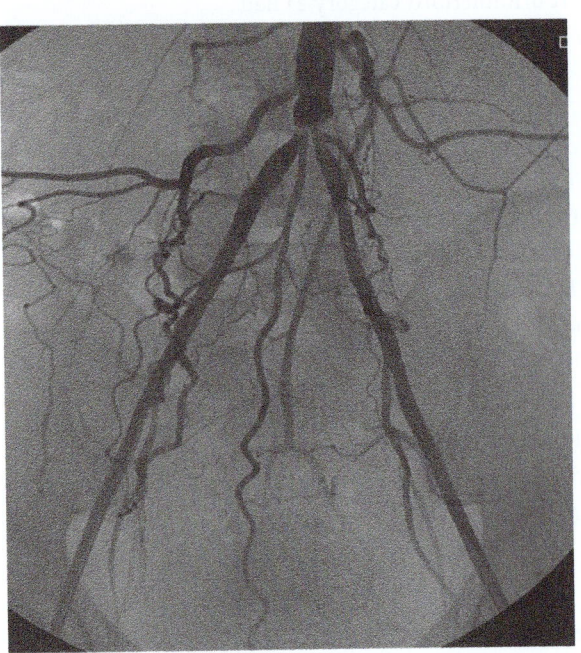

Fig. 4.2.1

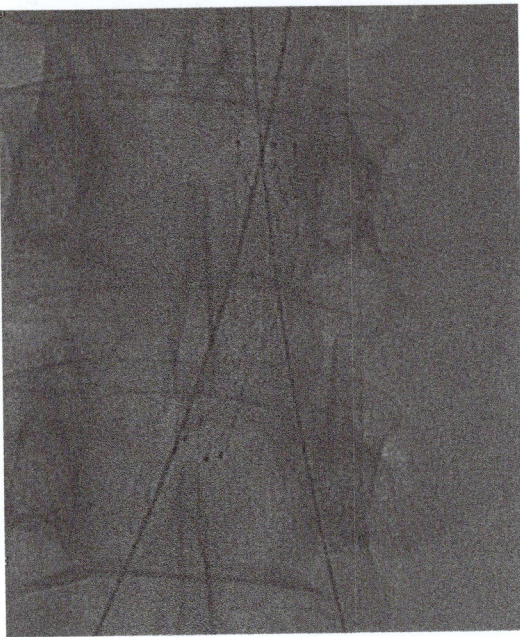

Fig. 4.2.2

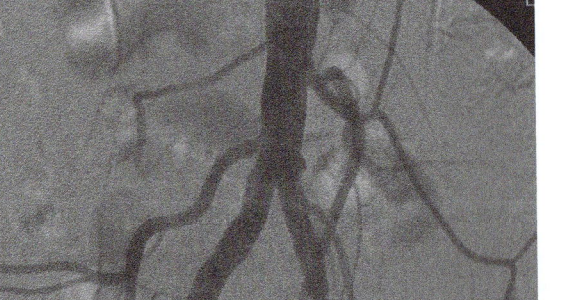

Fig. 4.2.3

Figure 4.2.1 Bilateral ostial stenoses of both common iliac arteries
Figure 4.2.2 Implanted right stent
Figure 4.2.3 Postprocedural arteriogram with two implanted stents

A 57-year-old man with intermittent bilateral claudication (grade II B/Rutherford category 2) of both lower limbs presented critical stenoses in the origins or both common iliac arteries with no other involvement in the rest of the vascular bed of the lower limbs.

Iliac stenoses and obstructions are the most common vascular lesions in patients from 35 to 65 years of age, and stenosis is up to three times more common than obstruction.

Iliac stenosis or obstruction manifests as intermittent claudication, which can be both distal and proximal. Although proximal claudication can have a neurological or musculo-skeletal origin, it is usually caused by iliac stenosis and obstruction. The femoral pulse is absent or a murmur and/or thrill is heard.

Iliac stenosis is usually well tolerated at first, thanks to collateral flow through branches of the lumbar, inferior mesenteric, or hypogastric arteries; however, the condition normally progresses continually, and without treatment, the recovery is torpid.

Another symptom that may be present is erectile dysfunction, which may or may not be associated to claudication.

1. Prior diagnostic study: 4F right femoral puncture.
2. Left femoral puncture under fluoroscopic guidance. Bilateral 6F introducer sheath.
3. Maneuver through the lesions using 180 and 260 cm angled 0.035 in. hydrophilic guide-wires. If necessary, use a 5F hydrophilic vertebral catheter to help in maneuvering.
4. Double-barrel bilateral stent.

- Implant two 8×40 mm self-expanding stents
- Dilation with two 8×40 mm PTA balloon catheters.

1. Prior diagnostic study: 4F right femoral puncture.
2. Vascular recanalization:

- 6F bilateral femoral introducer sheath
- Two 0.035 in. angled hydrophilic guidewires (180 and 260 cm)
- Two self-expanding stents (8×40 mm)
- Two 8×40 mm PTA balloon catheters.

Case 4.3
Recanalization of a Unilateral Obstruction of the Iliac Artery

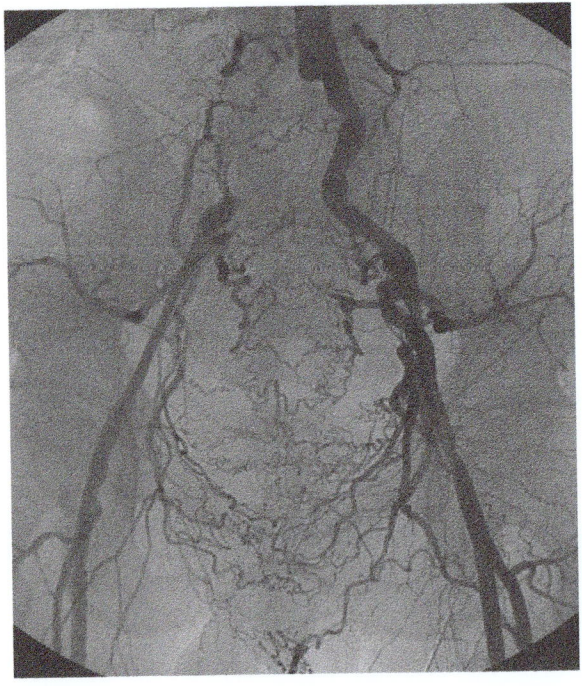

Fig. 4.3.1

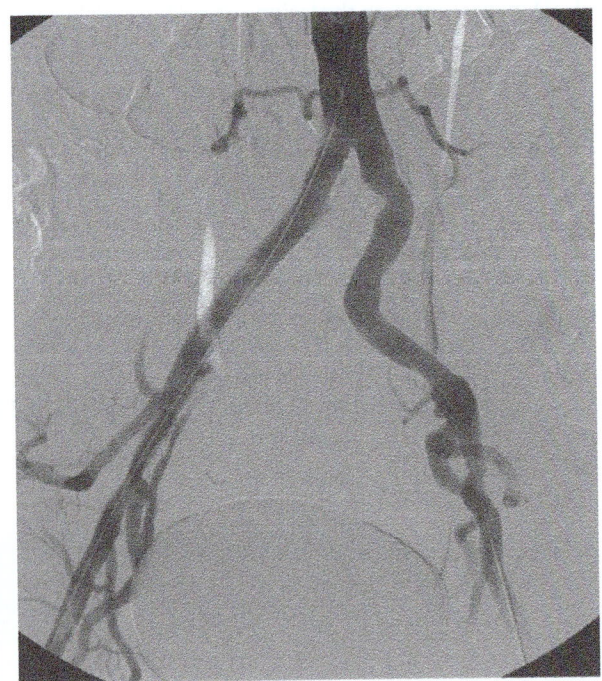

Fig. 4.3.2

Figure 4.3.1 Ostial obstruction of the right common iliac artery; near its bifurcation, blood flow is rechanneled through the hypogastric and lumbar arteries. There is minimal stenosis in the contralateral common iliac artery

Figure 4.3.2 Arteriogram obtained after recanalization

A 55-year-old man with intermittent severe claudication (Rutherford 3) presented unilateral iliac obstruction with no other involvement in the rest of the vascular bed of the lower limbs.

Iliac stenoses and obstructions are the most common vascular lesions in patients from 35 to 65 years of age, and stenosis is up to three times more common than obstruction.

Iliac stenosis or obstruction manifests as intermittent claudication, which can be both distal and proximal. Although proximal claudication can have a neurological or musculoskeletal origin, it is usually caused by iliac stenosis and obstruction. The femoral pulse is absent or a murmur and/or thrill is heard.

Iliac stenosis is usually well tolerated at first, thanks to collateral flow through branches of the lumbar, inferior mesenteric, or hypogastric arteries; however, the condition normally progresses continually, and without treatment, the recovery is torpid.

Another symptom that may be present is erectile dysfunction, which may or may not be associated to claudication.

1. Perform a diagnostic study first. Approach through the left femoral artery using a 4F catheter.
2. Under fluoroscopic guidance, puncture the right femoral artery and insert a 6F introducer sheath. Replace the catheter on the left side with a 6F introducer sheath.
3. Maneuver through the lesions using 180 and 260 cm angled 0.035 in. hydrophilic guidewires and a 5F hydrophilic vertebral catheter. Insert another hydrophilic guidewire with the same characteristics through the right side.
4. Apply the "kissing technique," consisting of simultaneous bilateral dilation by inflating two 8 × 40 mm PTA balloon catheters.
5. Implant the 8 × 55 mm balloon-expandable stents in the right side while simultaneously inflating the 8 × 40 mm PTA balloon catheter again on the left side.
6. Check the outcome with a postprocedural arteriogram.

1. Prior diagnostic study: 4F left femoral puncture.
2. Vascular recanalization:

- Right femoral puncture. 6F introducer sheath
- Exchange the catheter on the left for a 6F introducer sheath
- 5F hydrophilic vertebral catheter
- Two 0.035 angled hydrophilic guidewires (180 and 260 cm long)
- "Kissing technique": Two 8 × 40 mm PTA balloon catheters
- Balloon-expandable stent (8 × 55 mm)

Case 4.4
External Iliac Artery Lesions

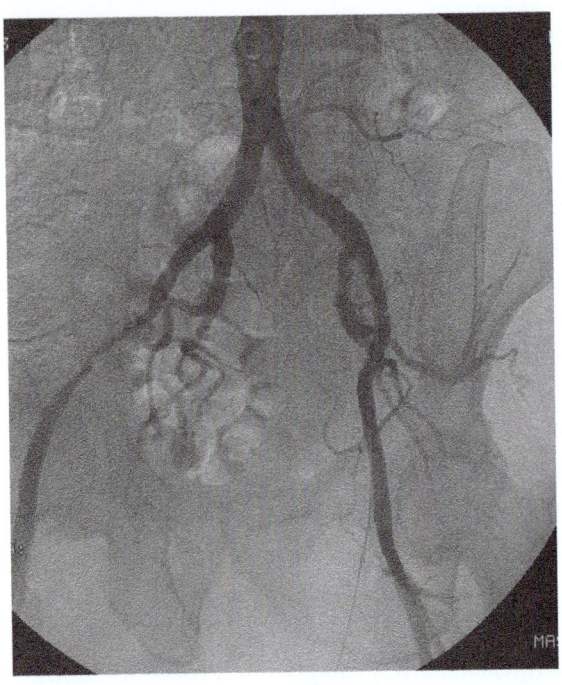

Fig. 4.4.1

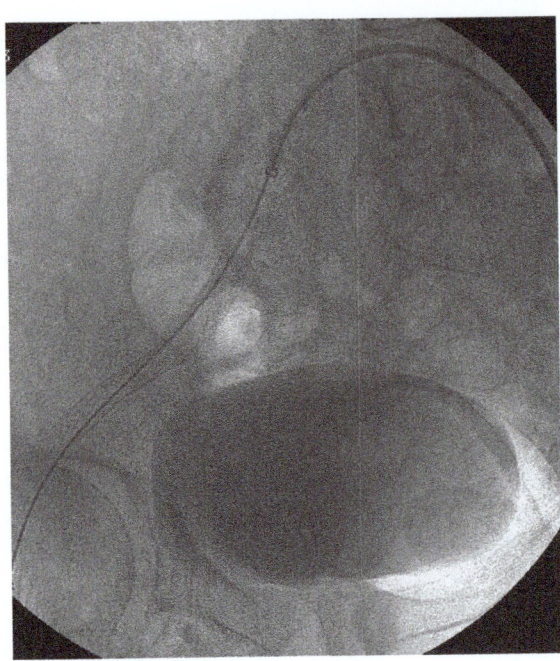

Fig. 4.4.2

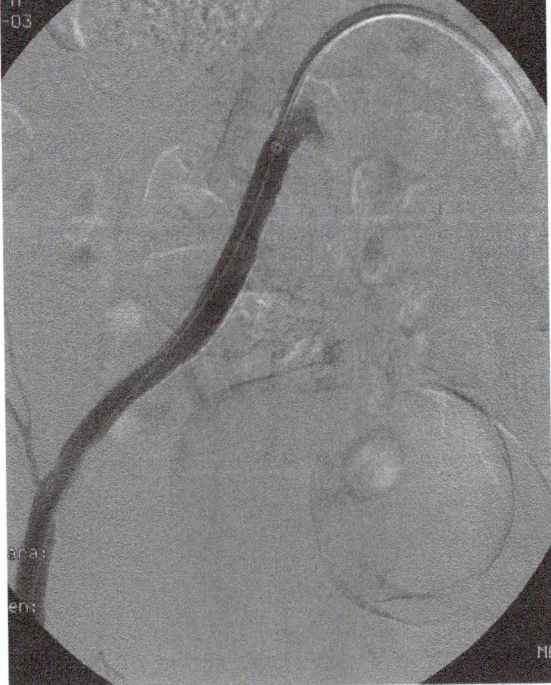

Fig. 4.4.3

Figure 4.4.1 Long stenosis at the level of the right external iliac artery

Figure 4.4.2 Passing a hydrophilic guidewire through the lesion, placing a curved hydrophilic introducer sheath, and implanting a self-expanding stent

Figure 4.4.3 Postprocedural arteriogram

A 59-year-old male patient presented with right lower limb claudication and pain limited to the right buttock and thigh; right femoral and distal pulses were absent.

Comments

The age at which external iliac artery lesions appear depends on the type of lesion: stenoses mainly affect patients older than 50 years of age, and obstructions normally appear in younger patients. In general, stenoses are more common than obstructions and are often associated with more distal lesions, especially at the level of the common femoral artery.

The disease manifests as intermittent claudication, which is often proximal, at the level of the buttock or thigh; together with an absent femoral pulse, murmur, and/or thrill, this presentation raises suspicion of external iliac artery lesions.

Collateral flow is established fundamentally through the branches of the hypogastric arteries and from connections with the circumflex artery. The patient's tolerance of external iliac artery lesions will depend on the degree of collateral circulation and the presence of associated lesions.

Procedure Steps

1. Access the femoral artery with a 4F catheter and perform a preprocedural diagnostic study.
2. Access the contralateral femoral artery with a 4F sidewinder catheter and insert a 260 cm long angled 0.035 in. hydrophilic guidewire through the lesions to the common femoral artery. Place a curved 6F hydrophilic introducer sheath.
3. Predilate the lesion with a PTA balloon catheter (6 mm in diameter and 40 mm long).
4. Implant the 7×40 mm self-expanding nitinol stents.
5. Postdilate the stent with a 7×40 mm PTA balloon catheter.
6. Confirm the outcome with a postprocedural arteriogram.

Equipment List

1. Prior diagnostic study: 4F femoral puncture.
2. Passing to the contralateral artery: 4F Sidewinder I hydrophilic catheter/4F Cobra II hydrophilic catheter

- 260 cm long 0.035 in. angled hydrophilic guidewire
- 6F curved hydrophilic introducer sheath

3. Vascular recanalization:

- Predilation with a 6×40 mm PTA balloon catheter
- 7×40 mm self-expanding nitinol stent
- Postdilation with a 7×40 mm PTA balloon catheter

Case 4.5
Stenosis in the Superficial Femoral Artery

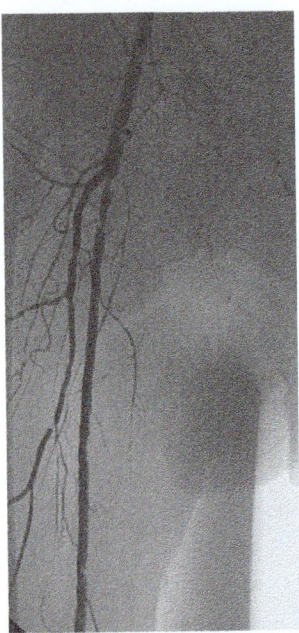

Fig. 4.5.1

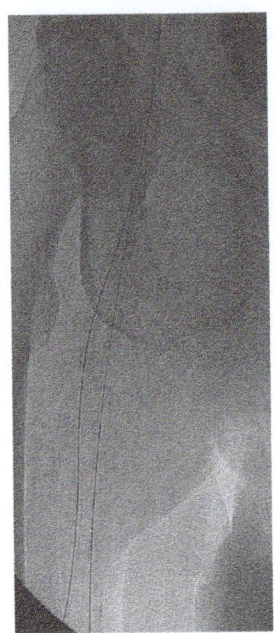

Fig. 4.5.2

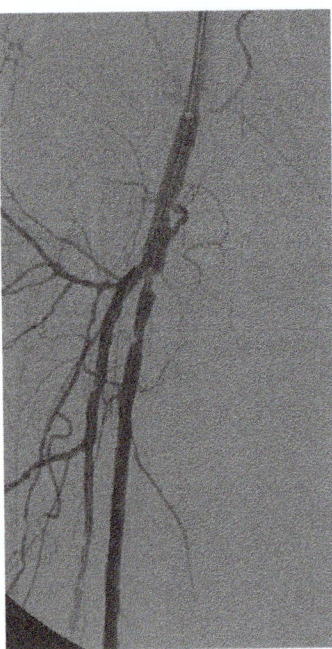

Fig. 4.5.3

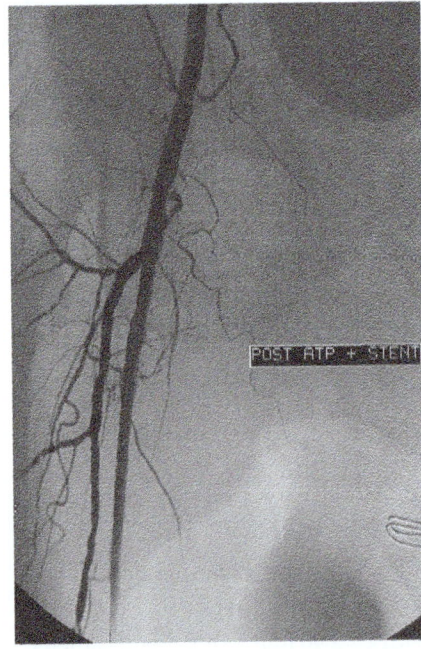

Fig. 4.5.4

Figure 4.5.1 The right superficial femoral artery has two stenoses at the ostial and proximal levels

Figure 4.5.2 Passing two guidewires, one through the superficial femoral artery and one through the deep femoral artery

Figure 4.5.3 Verification of the correct placement of both guidewires

Figure 4.5.4 Result obtained after angioplasty and stent implantation

Comments

Femoropopliteal artery lesions usually occur in patients older than 60 years of age and are three times more common than iliac artery lesions. They are usually located in Hunter's canal. Contrary to what occurs in iliac disease, femoropopliteal obstructions are three times more common than stenoses.

Femoropopliteal artery lesions present clinically as intermittent distal claudication at the level of the calves, and popliteal and distal pulses are absent. These lesions are usually well tolerated at first, thanks to collateral flow through branches of the deep femoral arteries, although the patient's evolution will depend on the appearance of associated lesions in other territories, basically at the level of the distal vascular bed.

Procedure Steps

1. Access the femoral artery with a 4F catheter and perform a preprocedural diagnostic study.
2. Access the contralateral femoral artery with a 4F sidewinder catheter and insert a 260 cm long angled 0.035 in. hydrophilic guidewire through the lesions to the common femoral artery. Place a curved 8F hydrophilic introducer sheath over the guidewire.
3. Approach the lesion with a 4F hydrophilic vertebral catheter using the angled guidewire.
4. Insert a 0.018 in. guidewire to the superficial femoral artery and a 0.014 in. guidewire to the deep femoral artery; verify that the guidewires have been correctly placed.
5. Insert a balloon-expandable stent over the guidewire in the superficial femoral artery and check that it is placed just at the origin of the superficial femoral artery before expanding it.
6. Implant the 6 × 28 mm stent.
7. Confirm the results of the procedure with a postprocedural arteriogram.

Equipment List

1. Prior diagnostic study: 4F femoral puncture.
2. Passing to the contralateral artery: 4F Sidewinder I hydrophilic catheter

- 260 cm long 0.035 in. angled hydrophilic guidewire
- 8F curved hydrophilic introducer sheath

3. Vascular recanalization:

- 4F hydrophilic vertebral catheter.
- 260 cm long 0.014 in. guidewire with a shapeable tip/260 cm long 0.018 in. guidewire with a shapeable tip.
- 6 × 28 mm balloon-expandable stent

Case 4.6

■

Deep Femoral Artery Arteriovenous Fistula and Pseudoaneurysm due to an Incised Wound

Figure 4.6.1 Branches of the deep femoral artery (*arrow*) are feeding a large hematoma (*open arrow*) in the left groin

Figure 4.6.2 Arterial phase DSA shows early opacification of the left common femoral vein, and external iliac veins (*arrows*)

Figure 4.6.3 Coronal MIP gadolinium-enhanced 3D MRA image clearly depicts the arteriovenous fistula and pseudoaneurysm (*arrow*). MRA allowed us to plan the percutaneous treatment noninvasively

Figure 4.6.4 DSA shows how the fistula was occluded and the hematoma was no longer present after the placement of coils in all the branches of the deep femoral artery.

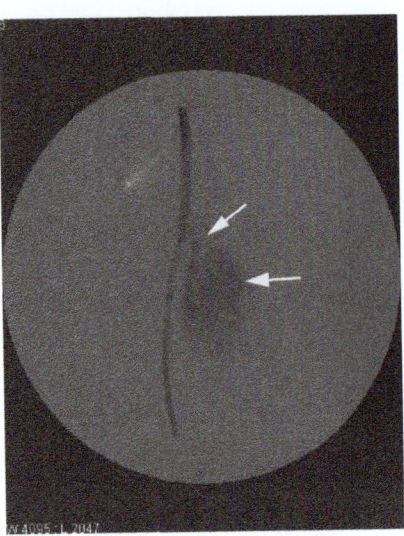

Fig. 4.6.1

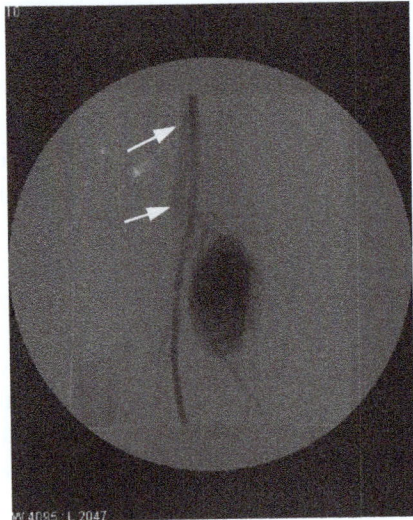

Fig. 4.6.2

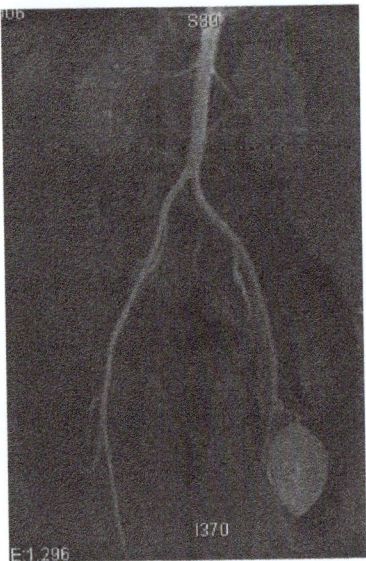

Fig. 4.6.3

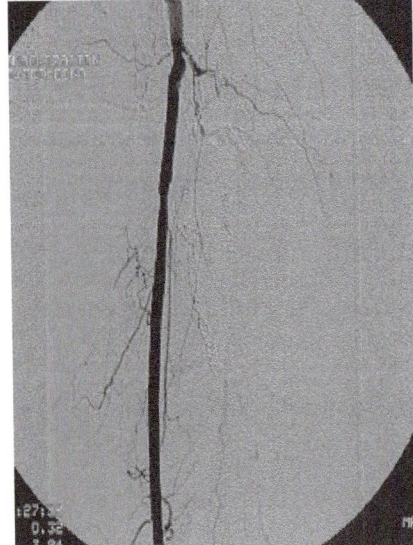

Fig. 4.6.4

We did not place a coil in the trunk of the deep femoral artery because there was a risk of coil migration to the run-off vessels due to its limited length.

A 44-year-old woman presented with pain and a symptomatic left-to-right shunt after a stab wound to her left groin. After a failed attempt to place a stent-graft in the proximal third of the left superficial artery, she underwent emergency surgery, and an end-to-end Dacron draft was placed in the superficial femoral artery. Despite the percutaneous and surgical approaches, both the arteriovenous fistula and hematoma remained unaltered. Direct percutaneous injection of thrombin after the placement of an occlusion balloon in the common femoral vein decreased the size of the pseudoaneurysm but did not occlude it completely. After the placement of coils in all branches of the left deep femoral artery, the arteriovenous communication was finally occluded.

Comments

Blood vessels are susceptible to a wide variety of traumatic injuries.

High-energy injuries such as rifle bullets disperse destructive energy to a vessel adjacent to but not within the area of greatest soft-tissue damage. Conversely, knife wounds create injury only to those tissues that interact directly with the blade.

Arteriovenous fistulas are almost always acquired point-to-point communications between an artery and a vein. Sometimes, as in our case, they are accompanied by hematomas and pseudoaneurysms that warrant either surgical or percutaneous treatment.

The most common etiology is traumatic; in the hospital setting, many arteriovenous fistulas and pseudoaneurysms are iatrogenic, occurring secondary to arterial catheterization or central line placement. Although small fistulas may remain asymptomatic or even close spontaneously, fistulas of all sizes can enlarge over time recruiting additional feeding vessels. Independent of the additional feeding vessels, the original communication usually remains point-to-point. Arteriovenous fistulas are pulsatile with a palpable thrill and an audible bruit. The presentation is usually similar to that of arteriovenous malformations: pain and symptomatic left-to-right shunt.

Procedure Steps

1. Access the femoral artery with a 4F catheter and perform a preprocedural diagnostic study.
2. Access the contralateral femoral artery with a 4F sidewinder catheter and insert a 260 cm long angled 0.035 in. hydrophilic guidewire through the lesions to the common femoral artery. Place a curved 8F hydrophilic introducer sheath over the guidewire.
3. Approach the lesion with a 4F hydrophilic vertebral catheter using the angled guidewire.
4. Implant coils (3 and 5 mm in diameter).
5. Confirm the results of the procedure with a postprocedural arteriogram.

Equipment List

1. 4F femoral artery puncture.
2. 4F Sidewinder I 4 hydrophilic catheter
3. 5F vertebral catheter
4. 260 cm long angled 0.035 hydrophilic guidewire
5. 8F curved hydrophilic introducer sheath
6. 3 and 5 mm coils

Case 4.7
Femoral Arteriovenous Fistula after Cardiac Catheterization

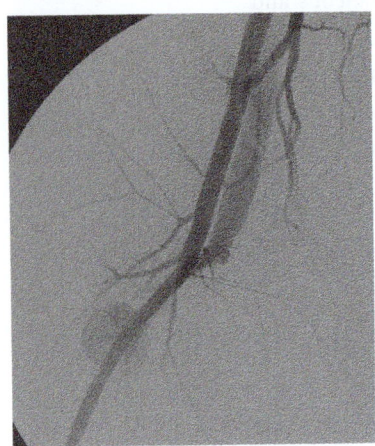

Fig. 4.7.1

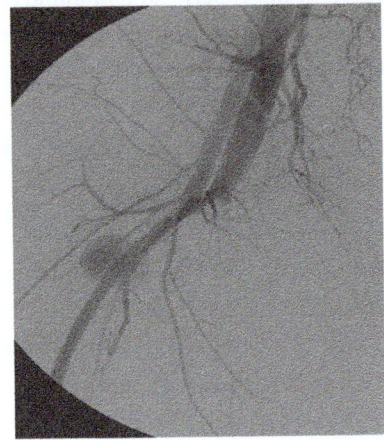

Fig. 4.7.2

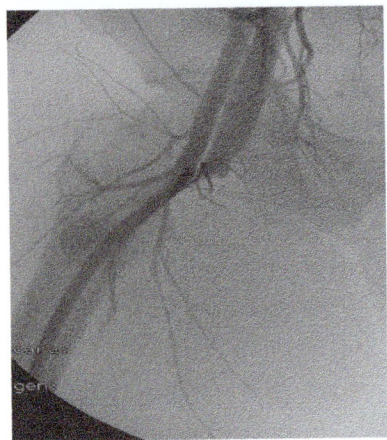

Fig. 4.7.3

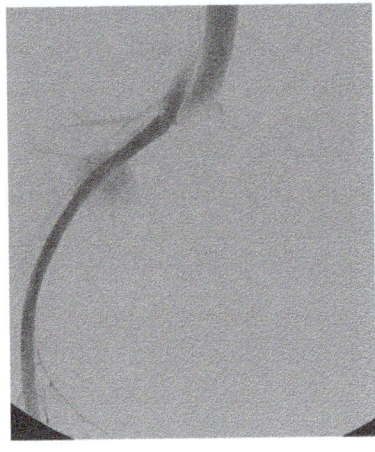

Fig. 4.7.4

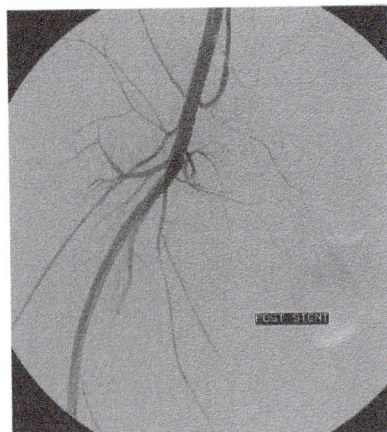

Fig. 4.7.5

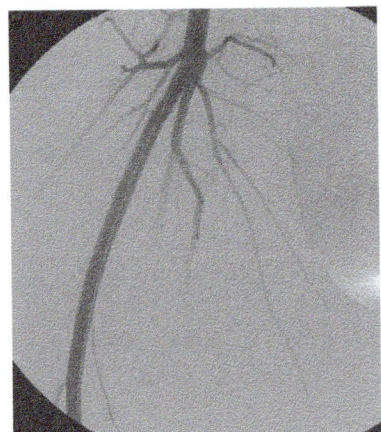

Fig. 4.7.6

Figure 4.7.1, 4.7.2, and 4.7.3 Selective arteriograms of the right iliofemoral axis acquired in different phases and projections show a pseudoaneurysmatic cavity and an arteriovenous fistula with early filling of the right femoral and iliac veins

Figure 4.7.4 Selective arteriogram of the right superficial femoral artery confirms the filling of both the pseudoaneurysmatic cavity and the arteriovenous fistula from the proximal portion of the artery

Figure 4.7.5 and 4.7.6 Postprocedural arteriogram after implantation of a coated stent at the level of the first segment of the superficial femoral artery

A 50-year-old male patient with a recent history of cardiac catheterization presented with abrupt onset pulsatile hematoma in the root of the right thigh.

An arteriovenous fistula is a direct communication between the arterial and venous systems without passing through the capillary bed. Arteriovenous fistulas can be congenital or acquired. Congenital arteriovenous fistulas result from a defect in embryological development and are usually multiple. Acquired arteriovenous fistulas are more common and are caused by penetrating injuries. Iatrogenic arteriovenous fistulas caused by invasive maneuvers are relatively common. Acquired arteriovenous fistulas can also arise spontaneously due to tumor or aneurysmatic growth that causes erosion of the vessel walls.

Arteriovenous communications cause peripheral and systemic effects in function of their size and location. Peripheral effects include ischemia due to the steal phenomenon, and systemic effects include heart failure due to overload, which is the final consequence in long-standing high-flow arteriovenous communications.

Procedure Steps

1. Access the left femoral artery with a 5F catheter and perform a preprocedural diagnostic study.
2. Access the contralateral femoral artery with a 5F sidewinder I or 5F cobra II hydrophilic catheter
3. Obtain various projections to visualize the point of entry into the pseudoaneurysmatic cavity and the arteriovenous fistula. Measure the diameter of the artery as accurately as possible to enable stent placement later.
4. Place a curved 8F hydrophilic introducer sheath over a 260 cm long stiff 0.035 in. hydrophilic guidewire.
5. Implant a 7×40 mm coated stent and dilate it with a 7×40 mm balloon catheter.
6. Confirm the results on a postprocedural arteriogram.

Equipment List

1. Prior diagnostic study: 5F femoral puncture.
2. Vascular intervention:

- 5F sidewinder I hydrophilic catheter
- 260 cm long angled stiff 0.035 in. hydrophilic guidewire
- 8F curved hydrophilic introducer sheath
- 5F hydrophilic vertebral catheter
- 7×50 mm coated stent
- 7×40 mm PTA balloon catheter

Figure 4.8.1 Three stenoses, two of which are preocclusive, in the middle and distal thirds of the right popliteal artery

Figure 4.8.2 Recanalization achieved through the implantation of a balloon-expandable stent in the most distal lesion and through a self-expanding stent in the two proximal lesions

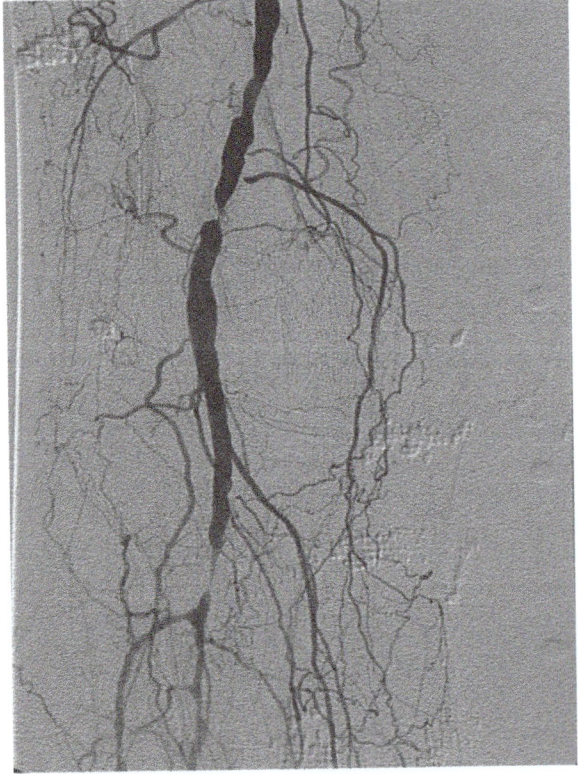

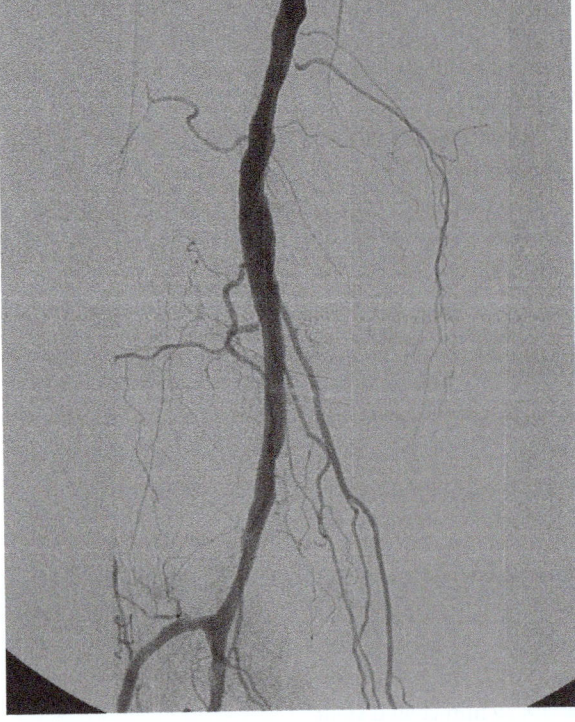

Fig. 4.8.1   **Fig. 4.8.2**

A 72-year-old man with a history of hypertension, smoking, and type II diabetes presented with ulcerous lesions in the fourth and fifth toes of his right foot.

The right femoral pulse was present, but the popliteal and distal pulses were absent (ankle-arm index = 0.4).

Femoropopliteal artery lesions usually occur in patients older than 60 years of age and are three times more common than iliac artery lesions. They are usually located in Hunter's canal. Contrary to what occurs in iliac disease, femoropopliteal obstructions are three times more common than stenoses.

Femoropopliteal artery lesions present clinically as intermittent distal claudication at the level of the calves, and popliteal and distal pulses are absent. These lesions are usually well tolerated at first, thanks to collateral flow through branches of the deep femoral arteries, although the patient's evolution will depend on the appearance of associated lesions in other territories, basically at the level of the distal vascular bed.

1. Access the right femoral artery with a 4F catheter and perform a preprocedural diagnostic study.
2. Access the contralateral femoral artery with a 4F sidewinder catheter. Pass a 260 cm long angled 0.035 in. hydrophilic guidewire until the common femoral artery and place a curved 5F hydrophilic introducer sheath over it.
3. Implant a 7 × 40 mm coated stent and dilate it with a 7 × 40 mm balloon catheter.
4. Approach the lesion with a 5F hydrophilic vertebral catheter using the angled guidewire.
5. Use a 300 cm long shapeable 0.014 in. guidewire to cross through the lesions and verify that they have been adequately reamed.
6. Predilate the proximal preocclusive lesion using the 4 mm diameter PTA balloon.
7. Implant the 5 × 40 mm self-expanding stent proximally.
8. Implant the 3 × 38 mm balloon-expandable stent distally.
9. Confirm the results on a postprocedural arteriogram.

1. Prior diagnostic study: 4F femoral puncture.
2. Passing to the other side: 4F Sidewinder I/4F Cobra II hydrophilic catheter

- 260 cm long angled 0.035 in. hydrophilic guidewire
- 5F curved hydrophilic introducer sheath

3. Vascular recanalization:

- 5F hydrophilic vertebral catheter
- 300 cm long shapeable tipped 0.014 in. guidewire
- 4 × 40 mm PTA balloon catheter
- 5 × 40 mm self-expanding nitinol stent
- 3 × 38 mm balloon-expandable stent

Case 4.9

Infrapopliteal Lesions: Proximal Obstruction of the Left Anterior Tibial and Peroneal Arteries

Figure 4.9.1 Proximal obstruction of the anterior tibial and peroneal arteries; the posterior tibial artery is patent, but multiple irregularities and stenoses are present throughout the artery

Figure 4.9.2 PTA balloon catheter in the posterior tibial artery

Figure 4.9.3 PTA balloon catheter in the anterior tibial artery

Figure 4.9.4 Arteriogram after dilation/stent placement

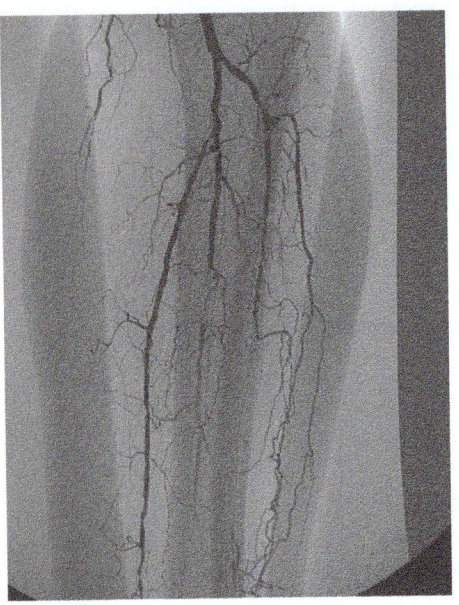

Fig. 4.9.1

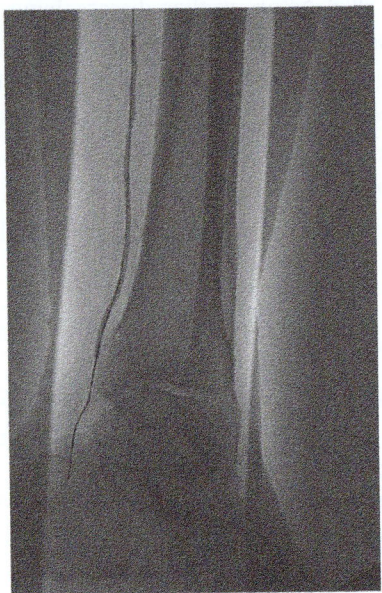

Fig. 4.9.2

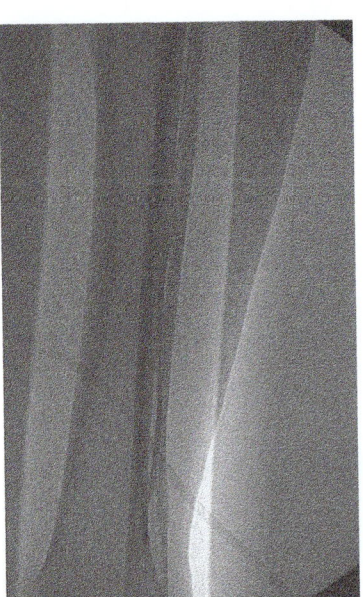

Fig. 4.9.3

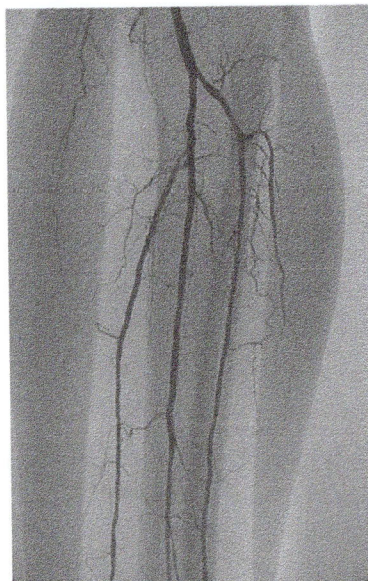

Fig. 4.9.4

A 62-year-old diabetic male patient presented with grade IV ischemia of his left leg and a necrotic lesion in the fourth toe of his left foot.

Femoral and popliteal pulses were present, but distal pulses were absent in both legs.

Infrapopliteal lesions usually occur in patients over 60 years old; the infrapopliteal vessels are a typical location for diabetic arterial lesions.

At first, no symptoms or signs of disease may be present, even in cases with an obstructed vessel (the peroneal artery is the one that usually remains patent), although the disease may present with distal claudication immediately followed by trophic disorders (trophic disorders may even be the initial manifestation) because it is difficult to develop good collateral flow at this level. Vascular examination confirms the absence of distal pulses.

Vascular disease manifests in diabetic patients in two ways: macroangiopathy, which affects large- and medium-caliber vessels, and microangiopathy, which affects capillaries and arterioles. Macroangiopathy is practically indistinguishable from arteriosclerosis and typically affects the distal vascular bed of the lower limbs. Nonetheless, there are both quantitative and qualitative differences between diabetic and nondiabetic patients. Among the qualitative differences, hyalinization of the intima and especially calcification of the tunica media are more common in diabetics. Among the quantitative differences, in diabetics, the prevalence is higher, the disease appears at a younger age, and several vascular territories may be simultaneously and more severely compromised.

Procedure Steps

1. Access the femoral artery with a 4F catheter and perform a preprocedural diagnostic study.
2. Access the contralateral femoral artery with a 4F sidewinder catheter. Pass a 260 cm long angled 0.035 in. hydrophilic guidewire until the common femoral artery and place a curved 5F hydrophilic introducer sheath over it.
3. Approach the trifurcation with a 5F hydrophilic vertebral catheter using an angled guidewire.
4. Insert a 300 cm long shapeable 0.014 in. guidewire to the posterior tibial artery and dilate the artery progressively from distal to proximal with a 2–2.5 mm × 210 mm conical PTA balloon catheter. Insert a 0.014 in. guidewire to the peroneal artery, dilate the artery with the conical balloon, and then implant a 4 × 80 mm self-expanding stent. Pass the 0.014 in. guidewire to the anterior tibial artery, recanalizing from distal to proximal again with the conical balloon and then implanting a 3 × 76 mm balloon-expandable stent.
5. Confirm the results on a postprocedural arteriogram.

Equipment List

1. Preprocedural diagnostic study: 4F right femoral puncture.
2. Paso a contralateral: 4F Sidewinder I/4F Cobra II hydrophilic catheter

- 260 cm long angled 0.035 stiff hydrophilic guidewire
- 5F curved hydrophilic introducer sheath

3. Vascular recanalization:

- 5F hydrophilic vertebral catheter
- 300 cm long 0.014 in. guidewire with a shapeable tip
- 2–2.5 × 210 mm conical PTA balloon catheter
- 4 × 80 mm self-expanding nitinol stent
- 3 × 76 mm balloon-expandable stent

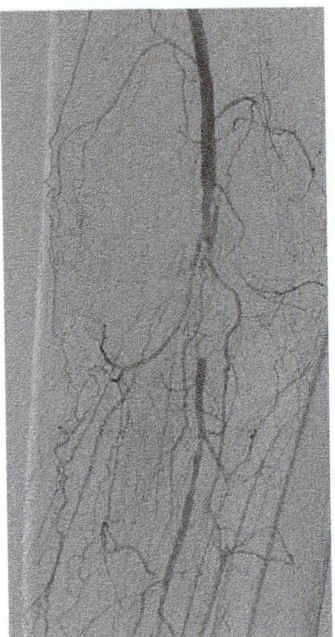

Case 4.10 ■ Infrapopliteal Lesions

Figure 4.10.1 3–4 cm obstruction in the distal third of the popliteal artery; the only patent infrapopliteal vessel is the peroneal artery

Figure 4.10.2 Arteriogram after popliteal recanalization by dilation and implantation of a self-expanding stent

Figure 4.10.3 Arteriogram after recanalization of the anterior tibial artery by dilation and implantation of a self-expanding stent

Fig. 4.10.1

A 71-year-old male patient with a history of hypertension and diabetes presented grade IV ischemia of the left lower limb and superficial necrotic lesions on the internal aspect of the hallux and heel. Distal pulses were absent in both limbs, and the ankle-arm index was 0.25 in both legs.

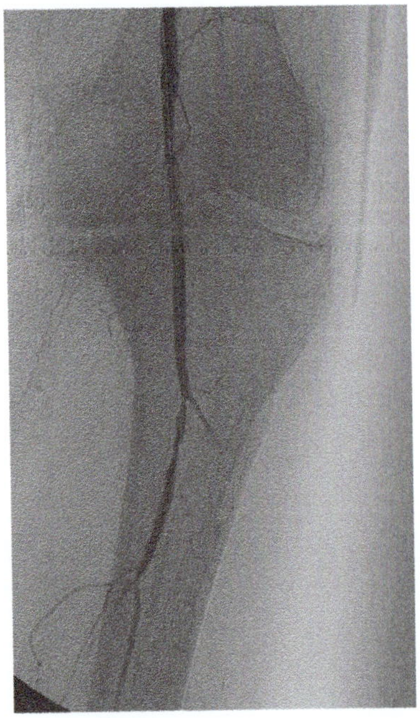

Fig. 4.10.2

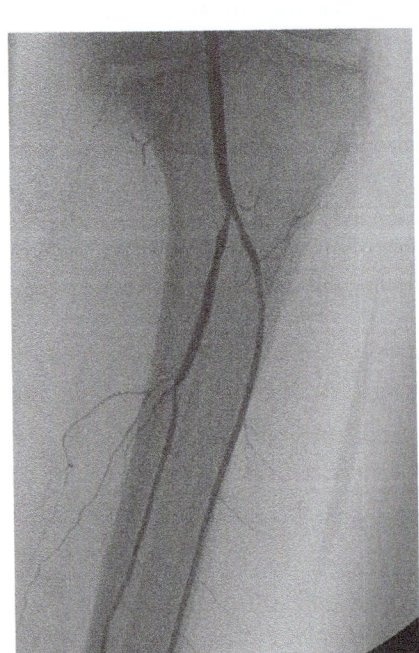

Fig. 4.10.3

Infrapopliteal lesions usually occur in patients over 60 years old; the infrapopliteal vessels are a typical location for diabetic arterial lesions.

At first, no symptoms or signs of disease may be present, even in cases with an obstructed vessel (the peroneal artery is the one that usually remains patent), although the disease may present with distal claudication immediately followed by trophic disorders (trophic disorders may even be the initial manifestation) because it is difficult to develop good collateral flow at this level. Vascular examination confirms the absence of distal pulses.

Vascular disease manifests in diabetic patients in two ways: macroangiopathy, which affects large- and medium-caliber vessels, and microangiopathy, which affects capillaries and arterioles. Macroangiopathy is practically indistinguishable from arteriosclerosis and typically affects the distal vascular bed of the lower limbs. Nonetheless, there are both quantitative and qualitative differences between diabetic and nondiabetic patients. Among the qualitative differences, hyalinization of the intima and especially calcification of the tunica media are more common in diabetics. Among the quantitative differences, in diabetics, the prevalence is higher, the disease appears at a younger age, and several vascular territories may be simultaneously and more severely compromised.

Comments

1. Access the femoral artery with a 4F catheter and perform a preprocedural diagnostic study.
2. Access the contralateral femoral artery with a 4F sidewinder catheter. Pass a 260 cm long angled 0.035 in. hydrophilic guidewire until the common femoral artery and place a curved 5F hydrophilic introducer sheath over it
3. Approach the popliteal lesion with a 5F hydrophilic vertebral catheter using an angled guidewire.
4. Run a 300 cm long 0.014 shapeable guidewire through the obstruction, dilate the vessel with a 4×40 mm PTA balloon catheter, and implant a 5×40 mm self-expanding stent. Check the results.
5. Insert a 0.014 guidewire to the anterior tibial artery and recanalize it from distal to proximal by expanding a 2×120 mm balloon and then implanting a 4×80 mm self-expanding stent.
6. Confirm the results on a postprocedural arteriogram.

Procedure Steps

1. Preprocedural diagnostic study: 4F right femoral puncture.
2. Passing to the other side: 4F Sidewinder I/4F Cobra II hydrophilic catheter

- 260 cm long angled 0.035 stiff hydrophilic guidewire
- 5F curved hydrophilic introducer sheath

3. Vascular recanalization:
   a. 5F hydrophilic vertebral catheter
   b. 300 cm long 0.014 in. guidewire with a shapeable tip

- Popliteal recanalization: 4×40 mm PTA balloon catheter
- 5×40 mm self-expanding nitinol stent
- Anterior tibial recanalization: 2×120 mm PTA balloon catheter
- 4×80 mm self-expanding nitinol stent

Equipment List

Further Reading

Becquemin J-P, et al. Systematic versus selective stent placement after superficial femoral artery balloon angioplasty: a multicenter prospective randomized study. J Vasc Surg 2003;37(3): 487–494.

Blum U, et al. Percutaneous recanalization of iliac artery occlusions: Results of a prospective study. Radiology 1993; 189:536–540.

Colapinto RF, et al. Transluminal angioplasty of complete iliac obstructions. AJR Am J Roentgenol 1986;146:859–862.

Conroy RM, et al. Angioplasty and stent placement in chronic occlusion of the superficial femoral artery: technique and results. J Vasc Interv Radiol 2000;11(8):1009–1020.

Dayananda L, et al. Infrapopliteal angioplasties for limb salvage in diabetic patients: does the clinical outcome justify its use? Indian J Radiol Imaging 2008;18(2):156–161.

Dotter CT, Judkins MP. Transluminal treatment of arterioesclerotic obstruction: description of a new technique and preliminary report of its application. Circulation 1964;30:654–670.

Ferreira M, et al. Superficial femoral artery recanalization with self-expanding nitinol stents: long-term follow-up results. Eur J Vasc Endovasc Surg 2007;34(6):702–708.

Gardiner GA Jr, et al. Quantification of elastic recoil after balloon angioplasty in the iliac arteries. J Vasc Interv Radiol 2001;12(12):1389–1393.

Gilles KA, et al. Infrapopliteal angioplasty for critical limb ischemia: relation of TransAtlantic InterSociety Consensus class to outcome in 176 limbs. J Vasc Surg 2008;48(1):128–136.

Gruntzig A, Hopff H. Percutane Rekanalisatin Chronischer Arterieller Verschlusse Mit Einem Neven Dilatations-Katheter. Dtsch Med Wochenschr 1974;99:2502.

Hood DB, Hodgson KJ. Percutaneous transluminal angioplasty and stenting for iliac artery occlusive disease. Surg Clin North Am 1999;79(3):575–596.

Jahnke T, et al. Endovascular placement of self-expanding nitinol coil stents for the treatment of femoropopliteal obstructive disease. J Vasc Interv Radiol 2002;13(3):257–266.

Kawano Y, et al. An unusual femoral arteriovenous fistula following cardiac catheterisation. Interv J Cardiol 2007;119(1):17–18.

Lampmann LE. Stenting in the femoral superficial artery: an overview. Eur J Radiol 1999;29:276–279.

Lemaire J-M, Dondelinger RF. Percutaneous coil embolization of iatrogenic femoral arteriovenous fistula or pseudo-aneurysm. Eur J Radiol 1994;18(2):96–100.

Long AL, et al. Percutaneous iliac artery stent: angiographic long-term follow-up. Radiology 1991;180:771–778.

Reyes R, et al. Treatment of chronic iliac artery occlusions with guide wire recanalization and primary stent placement. J Vasc Interv Radiol 1997;8(6):1049–1055.

Schillinger M, et al. Balloon angioplasty versus implantation of nitinol stents in the superficial femoral artery. N Engl J Med 2006;354:1879–1888.

Smith JC, et al. Angioplasty or stent placement in the proximal common iliac artery: is protection of the contralateral side necessary? J Vasc Interv Radiol 2001;12(12):1395–1398.

Sullivan TM, et al. Percutaneous transluminal angioplasty and primary stenting of the iliac arteries in 288 patients. J Vasc Surg 1997;25(5):829–839.

Tsetis D, Belli A-M. The role of infrapopliteal angioplasty. Br J Radiol 2004;77:1007–1015.

Waltman AC. Percutaneous transluminal angioplasty: iliac and deep femoral arteries. AJR Am J Roentgenol 1980;135(5): 921–925.

Yildirim S, Oguzkurt L. Endovascular treatment of traumatic femoral arteriovenous fistula. Eur J Radiol 2005;55(1):33–35.

Maribel Real and Marta Burrel

J.J. Muñoz and R. Ribes, *Learning Vascular and Interventional Radiology*, Learning Imaging,
DOI: 10.1007/978-3-540-87997-8_5, © Springer-Verlag Berlin Heidelberg 2010

Case 5.1

Hepatic Artery Aneurysm Treated with a Stent-Graft

Figure 5.1.1 Abdominal CT angiogram shows a partially thrombosed fusiform aneurysm (20 mm in diameter) in the first portion of the hepatic artery

Figure 5.1.2 Selective angiogram of the hepatic artery shows the hepatic artery branching directly from the aorta, an aneurysm of the common hepatic artery 5 mm from its origin, and a 12-mm patent lumen. The gastroduodenal artery and the hepatic artery itself and its bifurcating branches are all patent

Figure 5.1.3 Angiogram obtained prior to stent-graft release shows the introducer sheath at the level of the common hepatic artery, a semi-stiff guidewire at the level of the gastroduodenal artery, and the stent-graft at the level of the aneurysm

Figure 5.1.4 Selective angiogram of the hepatic artery immediately after the placement of the stent-graft shows exclusion of the aneurysm with good patency of the hepatic artery and its extra and intrahepatic branches

A 65-year-old man underwent CT angiography in the diagnostic workup for renal transplantation. A 22-mm diameter saccular aneurysm of the common hepatic artery

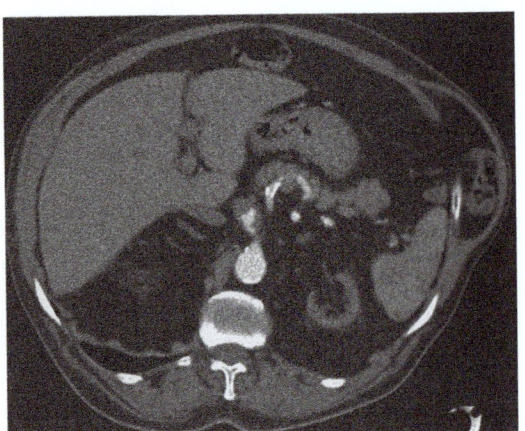

Fig. 5.1.1

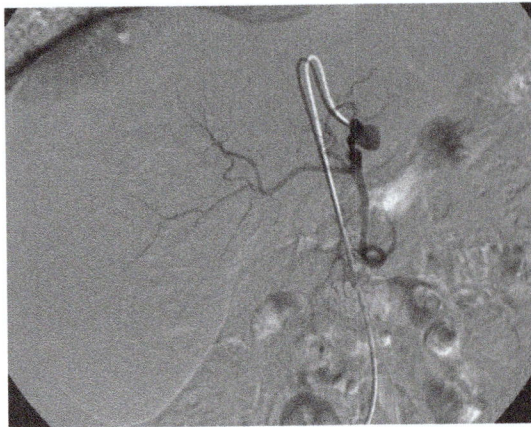

Fig. 5.1.2

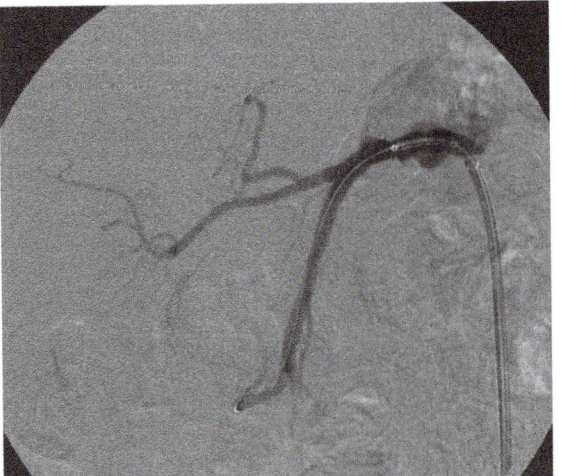

Fig. 5.1.3

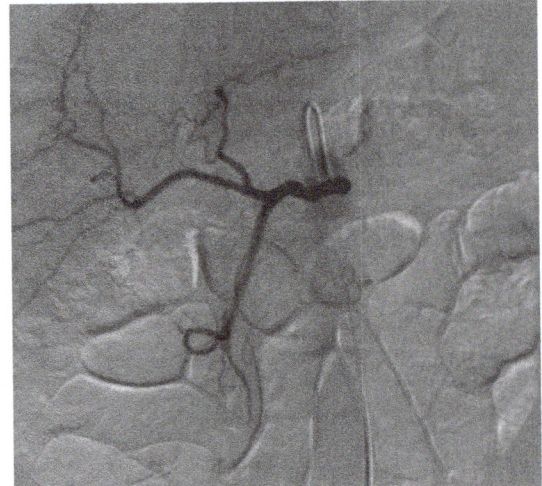

Fig. 5.1.4

was detected. The aneurysm was confirmed at angiography and treated by placing a coated stent.

Aneurysms of the visceral arteries can involve the celiac trunk, the superior mesenteric artery, and the inferior mesenteric artery as well as the branches of these three main trunks. The most common is the aneurysm of the splenic artery, which accounts for 60–80% of cases. Second in frequency is the aneurysm of the hepatic artery, which accounts for 20% of cases; most occur in men at the level of the hepatic artery and common hepatic artery. Intrahepatic aneurysms are usually of traumatic or iatrogenic origin. Extrahepatic aneurysms are usually degenerative or dysplastic and should be treated when their diameter is greater than 2 cm. Treatment options include surgical ligation and embolization. The risk of hepatic ischemia is relative due to flow from the portal vein. If the aneurysm affects the common hepatic artery, it can be treated by embolization of the aneurysmal sac if its neck is large enough, obstruction of the artery proximal and distal to the sac, or by exclusion with a coated stent. If the hepatic artery itself is affected, redirected flow to the intrahepatic arteries through the gastroduodenal artery should be taken into account. Intrahepatic lesions can generally be treated by embolization of the vessel, which will lead to segmental infarction without significant ischemic repercussions.

1. Puncture the right femoral artery and insert a 5F introducer sheath.
2. Perform selective angiography of the celiac trunk with a Simmons I catheter. In this case, we observed the hepatic artery arising directly from the aorta and an aneurysm of the common hepatic artery 5 mm from the ostium.
3. Catheterize the gastroduodenal artery with a hydrophilic guidewire and Cobra catheter. Use a semi-stiff FlexFinder guidewire to exchange materials.
4. Replace the 5F introducer sheath with a 45-cm-long 6F introducer sheath and place its tip at the level of the common hepatic artery distal to the aneurysm.
5. Insert the expandable coated stent. Once the stent is in place within the aneurysm, partially withdraw the introducer sheath until its tip is in the ostium of the hepatic artery.
6. Obtain an angiogram to confirm the correct placement of the stent before releasing it.
7. Release the stent and inflate the balloon using a manometer to control the pressure.
8. Check the position of the stent-graft and exclusion of the aneurysm by obtaining an angiogram through the introducer sheath.

1. 10-cm-long 5F introducer sheath.
2. 0.035 in. hydrophilic guidewire.
3. 5F Simmons I catheter.
4. 4F cobra II hydrophilic catheter.
5. 0.035 in. Nitrex semi-stiff guidewire (Ev3).
6. 45-cm-long 6F introducer sheath.
7. 6×22-mm Advanta® V12 coated stent (Atrium Europe B.V.).

Case 5.2

Hepatic Artery Graft Stenosis After Liver Transplantation Treated by Angioplasty

Figure 5.2.1 Angiogram of the celiac trunk shows greater than 90% stenosis of the hepatic artery at the level of the surgical anastomosis

Figure 5.2.2 Distal hepatic angiogram through the microcatheter after crossing the arterial stenosis

Figure 5.2.3 Angioplasty balloon inflated at the level of the arterial stenosis

Figure 5.2.4 Angiogram obtained after angioplasty confirms that the caliber of the vessel has been restored

A 41-year-old woman who received a liver transplant for autoimmune hepatitis presented worsening liver function with hypertransaminasemia and cholestasis 2 weeks after transplantation. Doppler US showed signs of anastomotic stenosis

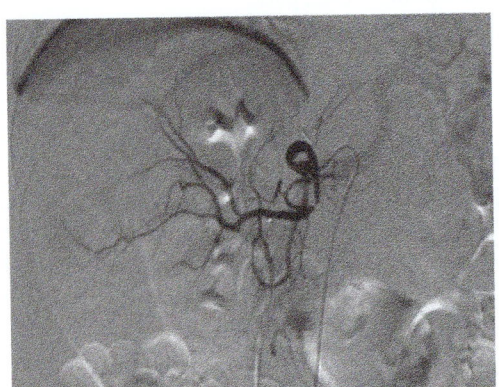

Fig. 5.2.1

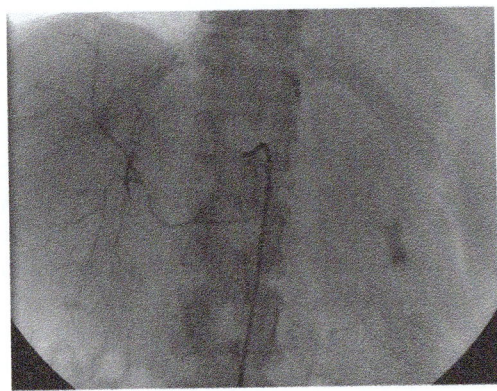

Fig. 5.2.2

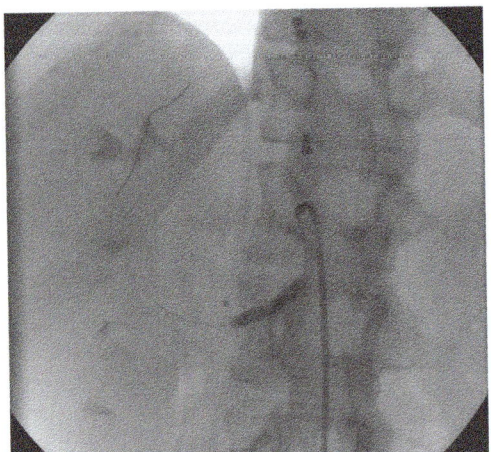

Fig. 5.2.3

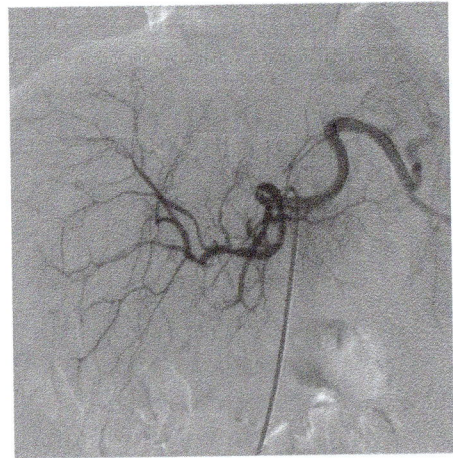

Fig. 5.2.4

in the hepatic artery. One month after transplantation she underwent angiography and angioplasty of the arterial stenosis.

Comments

Major arterial complications in liver transplantation include thrombosis, stenosis, anastomotic pseudoaneurysm, and splenic artery steal syndrome. Stenosis of the hepatic artery is the second most common complication, and it usually affects the surgical anastomosis. When the stenosis is mild and allows arterial blood flow, this condition sometimes causes no symptoms and does not require treatment. However, severe stenoses significantly decrease the flow through the hepatic artery and result in damage to the bile tract. They can also lead to thrombosis. Therefore, severe stenoses should be diagnosed and treated early. In cases with suspicion of arterial stenosis at US, arteriography is indicated to confirm the diagnosis and enable endovascular treatment (angioplasty or stenting) in the same session. Due to the fragility of the sutures, endovascular treatment is relatively contraindicated in patients transplanted less than 21 days before. Simple dilation initially resolves the stenosis in a high percentage of cases, although mid- and long-term patency is not guaranteed. The latest generation of stents promises improved outcomes; however, no prospective studies have compared their implantation with surgical reconstruction. .

Procedure Steps

1. Puncture the right femoral artery and insert a 5F introducer sheath.
2. Perform selective angiography of the celiac trunk with a Simmons I catheter. In this case, 90% anastomotic stenosis of the hepatic artery was confirmed.
3. Place the guiding catheter at the level of the celiac trunk.
4. Selectively catheterize the hepatic artery and go through the anastomotic stenosis with a microcatheter and hydrophilic micro-guidewire.
5. With the tip of the microcatheter in the left hepatic artery, exchange the hydrophilic micro-guidewire for a 0.014-in. guidewire through the catheter.
6. Introduce the balloon catheter using the 0.014 in. guidewire and place the balloon at the level of the stenosis.
7. Confirm the correct placement of the balloon by angiography through the guiding catheter.
8. Perform angioplasty, inflating the balloon with the manometer at its nominal pressure.
9. Obtain an angiogram to confirm that the caliber of the vessel has been restored.

Equipment List

1. 10-cm-long 5F introducer sheath.
2. 0.035 in. hydrophilic guidewire.
3. 5F Simmons I catheter.
4. 10-cm-long 6F introducer sheath.
5. 55-cm-long 6F guiding catheter.
6. Progreat microcatheter (BOSTON SCIENTIFIC) with a 0.021-in. hydrophilic guidewire.
7. 0.014 in. micro-guidewire
8. 4×20-mm Viatrac 14 plus balloon catheter (ABBOT)

Case 5.3
Splenic Trauma Treated by Embolization

Figure 5.3.1 Abdominal CT angiogram shows a significant area of splenic contusion/laceration with free perisplenic fluid compatible with hemoperitoneum

Figure 5.3.2 Selective angiogram of the celiac trunk shows foci of extravasation of contrast material in the lower and middle portions of the spleen

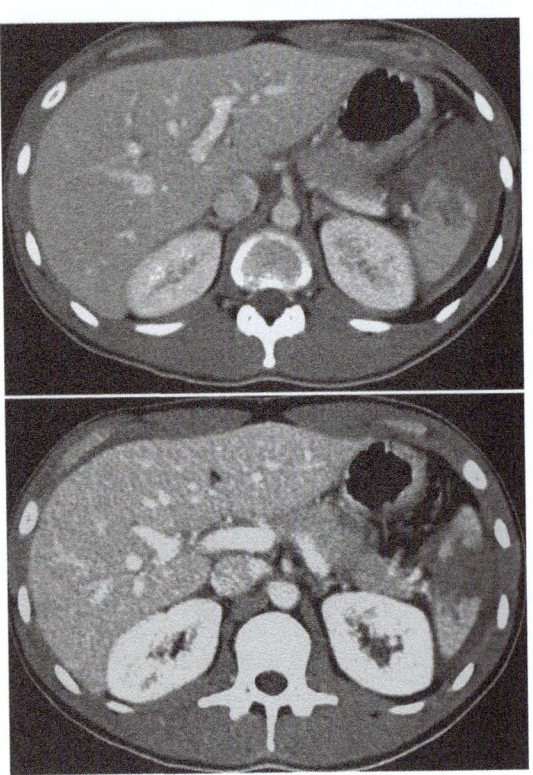

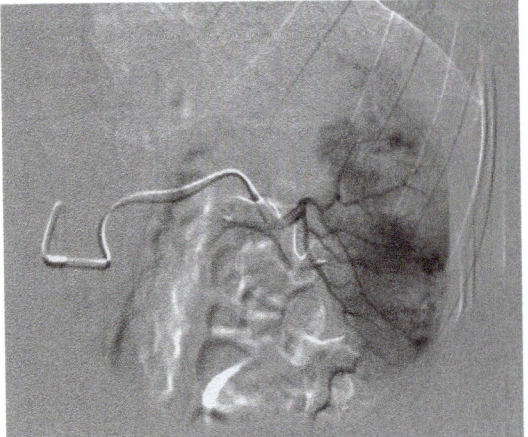

Fig. 5.3.1

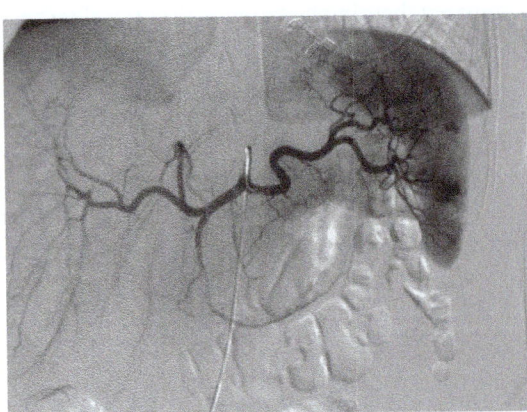

Fig. 5.3.2

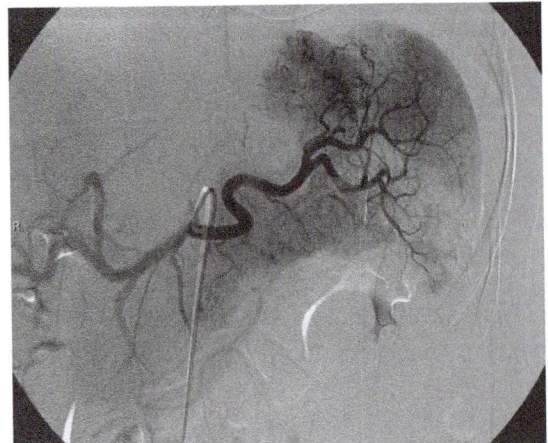

Fig. 5.3.3

Fig. 5.3.4

Figure 5.3.3 Superselective catheterization of the bleeding arterial vessels obtained with a microcatheter

Figure 5.3.4 Angiogram of the celiac trunk after embolization shows the occlusion of the bleeding arteries and the patency of the remaining splenic arteries

After a traffic accident, a 22-year-old man presented at the emergency department with right hypochondrial pain and guarding. Abdominal CT showed contained splenic laceration and hematoma with slight hemoperitoneum. Given the patient's hemodynamic stability, we decided to embolize the splenic artery.

Comments

Due to the high risk of infection after splenectomy, the management of splenic trauma is becoming more conservative.

In patients with hemorrhagic splenic lesions and high risk of hypovolemic shock, embolization enables partial preservation of the spleen. Abdominal CT enables determination of the type of lesion and indication of the type of treatment. Lesions that can be treated with embolization include pseudoaneurysm, arteriovenous fistula, disruption of an arterial branch, and extravasation of contrast material. Active intraparenchymal bleeding can manifest with "parenchymal staining," and embolization is also indicated in these cases.

Embolization should be performed as distal as possible at the level of the intrasplenic branches. In general, proximal embolization will not be effective, as it is equivalent to ligature of the splenic artery and results in retrograde supply to the parenchyma through branches of the gastric artery. Some groups perform hemostatic proximal embolization using Spongostan particles and coils to reduce the overall blood supply to the spleen in cases of splenic laceration without associated arterial lesions. In cases of splenic trauma, arterial embolization achieves hemostasis without the need for later surgery in 87–95% of cases.

Procedure Steps

1. Puncture the right femoral artery and insert a 5F introducer sheath.
2. Use a 5F Simmons I catheter to selectively study the celiac trunk. In this case, several intrasplenic foci of contrast material extravasation were confirmed in the middle and lower thirds of the spleen.
3. Use a 2.7F microcatheter to perform superselective catheterization.
4. Use 500–700 micra PVA microspheres to embolize the distal intrasplenic branches that give rise to the hemorrhagic foci.
5. Check the results by angiography. In this case, no signs of active bleeding were present, and we observed areas of infarction in the middle and lower portions of the spleen (approximately 30% of the parenchyma).

Equipment List

1. 10-cm-long 5F introducer sheath
2. 0.035 in. hydrophilic guidewire
3. 5F Simmons I catheter
4. 2.7F Progreat microcatheter with a 0.021-in. hydrophilic guidewire (BOSTON SCIENTIFIC)
5. BeadBlock 500–700 micra PVA embolization particles

Case 5.4

Surgical Marking for Acute Digestive Hemorrhage Due to an Ileal Ulcer

Figure 5.4.1 Angiogram of the superior mesenteric artery shows active bleeding in the ileal zone evidenced by extravasation of contrast material

Figure 5.4.2 Late-phase angiogram of the superior mesenteric artery confirms extravasation of contrast material from an ileal branch

Figure 5.4.3 Selective angiogram obtained with a microcatheter shows the bleeding ileal artery

Figure 5.4.4 Surgical marking by staining the bleeding ileal zone with methylene blue through the microcatheter

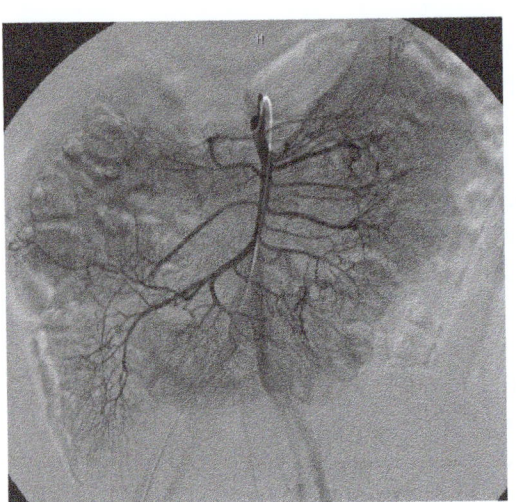

Fig. 5.4.1

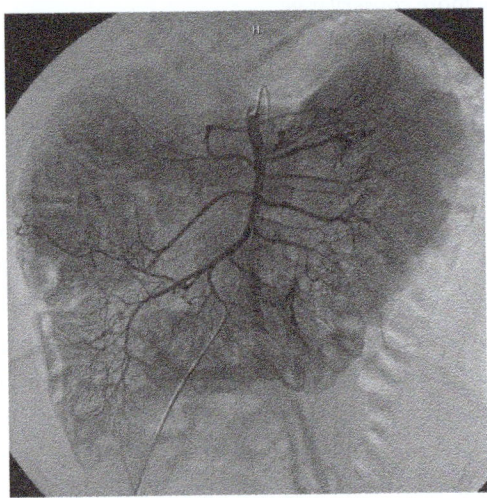

Fig. 5.4.2

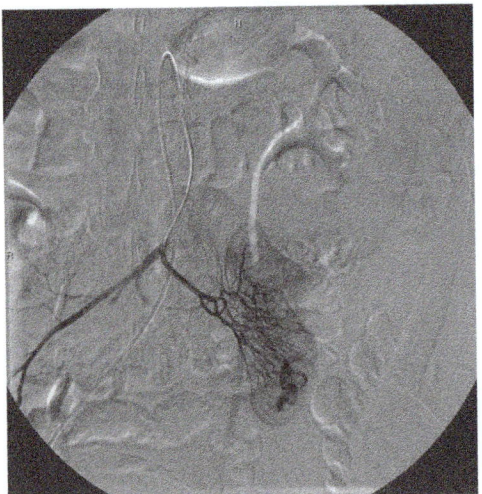

Fig. 5.4.3

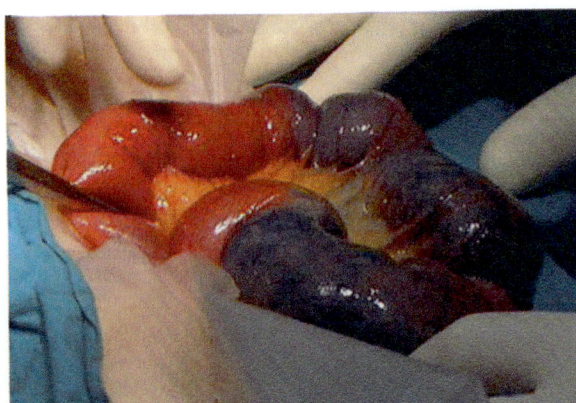

Fig. 5.4.4

A 45-year-old HIV-positive man was admitted for fever of unknown origin. While hospitalized, he presented intestinal bleeding, and his hematocrit dropped eight points. Endoscopic examination was negative, so he underwent urgent angiography.

Comments

Small bowel bleeding accounts for 5% of all acute digestive hemorrhage. Endoscopic capsules and multidetector CT are two minimally invasive techniques that enable the entire small bowel to be studied. In cases of acute bleeding, it is necessary to find the bleeding points quickly. Both CT and angiography can locate the bleeding point in acute digestive hemorrhage. Angiography has the advantage of combining diagnosis with treatment by arterial embolization or surgical marking with methylene blue. Bleeding lesions in the small bowel like ulcers or vascular malformations that do not cause a mass effect are difficult to locate during surgery, especially when there is a large amount of blood in the intestinal lumen. In these patients, although CT and angiography locate the hemorrhage at the level of the jejunum or ileum, minimal surgical resection without leaving the bleeding lesion is difficult. Surgical marking by selectively catheterizing the bleeding vessel and injecting methylene blue through a microcatheter facilitates the location of the area to be resected during the surgical intervention.

Procedure Steps

1. Puncture the right femoral artery.
2. Obtain an angiogram of the superior mesenteric artery. In this case, extravasation of contrast material from an ileal artery was evident.
3. Use a microcatheter to selectively catheterize the ileal branches and identify the bleeding arterial branch.
4. Once the bleeding artery is identified, place the tip of the catheter as close to the extravasation of contrast material as possible.
5. Fix the microcatheter in place and move the patient to the operating room for the surgical intervention.
6. Once the intestine has been surgically exposed, inject 2 cc of methylene blue through the microcatheter; this will immediately stain the bleeding area of the intestine.
7. Resect the 20 cm of the ileum stained with methylene blue.
8. Remit the specimen for histologic study; in this case, histologic study revealed intestinal toxoplasmosis with ulceration of the mucosa.

Equipment List

1. 10-cm-long 5F introducer sheath
2. 0.035 in. hydrophilic guidewire
3. 5F Simmons I catheter
4. 4F Cobra II hydrophilic catheter
5. 2.7F Progreat microcatheter with an 0.021-in. hydrophilic guidewire (BOSTON SCIENTIFIC)
6. Methylene blue (2 cc)

Case 5.5

■

Lower Digestive Tract Bleeding. Treatment of Rectorrhagia by Embolization

Figure 5.5.1 *Left* Angiogram of the abdominal aorta and iliac sector shows severe aortoiliac atheromatosis, more than 70% stenosis of the left common iliac artery, and proximal obstruction of the left hypogastric artery. *Right* Selective angiography of the inferior mesenteric artery shows normal vascularization of the descending colon

Figure 5.5.2 Angiogram of the inferior mesenteric artery centered on the rectum shows an arteriovenous fistula at the level of the terminal portion of the left superior rectal branches

Figure 5.5.3 Superselective angiogram of the superior rectal arteries obtained with a microcatheter shows extravasation of contrast material due to active rectal bleeding

Figure 5.5.4 Selective angiogram of the inferior mesenteric artery obtained after embolization shows metallic coils occluding the bleeding vessels at the level of the left superior rectal artery

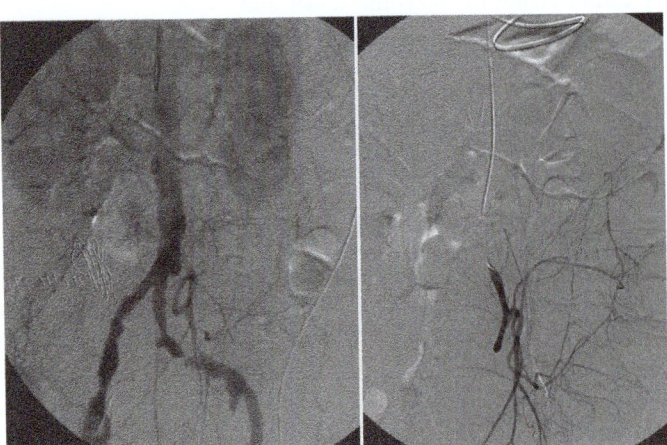

Fig. 5.5.1

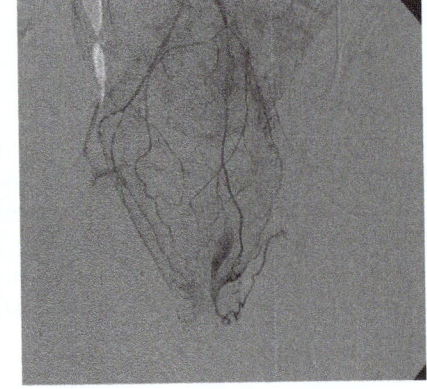

Fig. 5.5.2

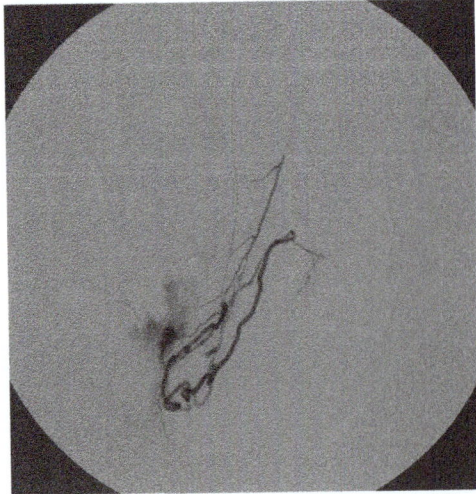

Fig. 5.5.3

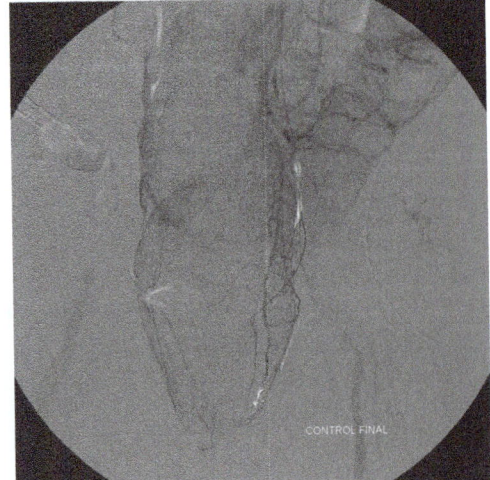

Fig. 5.5.4

A 68-year-old man with a history of hypertension and ischemic stroke was admitted for signs of lower digestive tract bleeding. Findings at upper gastrointestinal endoscopy were normal. Colonoscopy revealed internal hemorrhoids and diverticula. While hospitalized, he had an episode of rectal bleeding with hemodynamic instability, so urgent angiography was performed.

Lower digestive tract bleeding is defined as hemorrhage below the angle of Treitz. Colorectal bleeding is the most common, and the most common causes of colorectal bleeding are diverticular disease and angiodysplasias. Anorectal hemorrhage accounts for 7–11% of all lower digestive tract bleeding.

Rectal blood supply depends on the superior rectal arteries, which branch from the inferior mesenteric artery, and on the medial and inferior rectal arteries, which branch from the anterior bifurcation of the hypogastric artery.

Consequently, it is important to note that the inferior mesenteric artery and the hypogastric arteries must be included in the study of rectal lesions.

The surgical treatment of a rectal lesion can be invalidating and sometimes requires abdominoperineal resection. Distal embolization of the afferent arteries can be very useful and involves little or no risk of intestinal wall ischemia.

Embolization of lower digestive tract bleeding generally achieves optimal initial outcomes, with 95% hemostasis on average. The main problem is early rebleeding, which affects 21% of patients, whereas major ischemic complications occur in only 2% of cases.

The recommended material for embolization is microcoils placed as near as possible to the hemorrhage and PVA particles in cases in which it is foreseen that coils will not be effective.

Procedure Steps

1. Puncture the right humeral artery and insert a long 5F introducer sheath.
2. Obtain an angiogram of the abdominal aorta and iliac sector using a 5F pigtail catheter. In this case, severe atheromatosis of the aorta and both iliac sectors, stenosis greater than 70% of the left common iliac artery, and proximal obstruction of the left hypogastric artery were seen.
3. Perform a selective study of the inferior mesenteric artery. In this case, an arteriovenous fistula was seen at the level of the terminal portion of the left superior rectal branches.
4. Perform a superselective study with a microcatheter. In this case, we saw contrast extravasation due to active bleeding.
5. Use 500–700 micra particles and two microcoils to achieve distal embolization.
6. Check the outcome by angiography – in this case, the angiogram confirmed correct occlusion of the embolized vessels.

Equipment List

1. 45-cm-long 5F introducer sheath.
2. 0.035 in. hydrophilic guidewire.
3. 5F Simmons I catheter.
4. 2.5F Excelsior microcatheter.
5. 0.014 in. Syncro micro-guidewire.
6. 500–700 micra PVA particles.
7. Two Vortx microcoils (3 × 28 mm) Boston scientifc.

Case 5.6

■

Embolization to Treat Hematuria Due to Pelvic Trauma Treated

Figure 5.6.1 Angiogram of the aortoiliac sector shows extravasation of contrast material from an area supplied by the left hypogastric artery

Figure 5.6.2 Selective angiogram of the left hypogastric artery shows active bleeding with extravasation of contrast material from an area supplied by the vesicoprostatic artery

Figure 5.6.3 Superselective angiography of the vesicoprostatic artery obtained with a microcatheter allows direct visualization of the extravasation of contrast material

Figure 5.6.4 *Left* Superselective angiogram of the vesicoprostatic artery after embolization shows two metallic coils occluding the bleeding vessel. *Right* Angiogram of the hypogastric artery obtained after embolization shows that the bleeding artery has been occluded while the remaining branches of the left hypogastric artery remain patent

After a traffic accident, a 22-year-old man was admitted to the emergency department with an extensive fracture of the pelvis involving the obturator foramina. He was hemodynamically

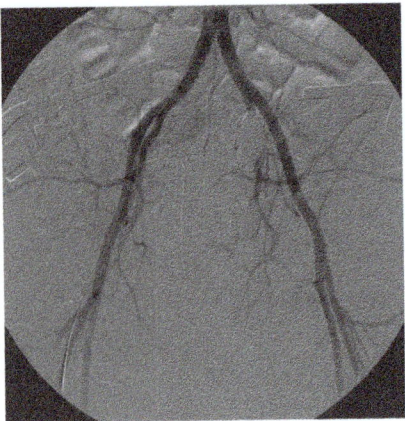

Fig. 5.6.1

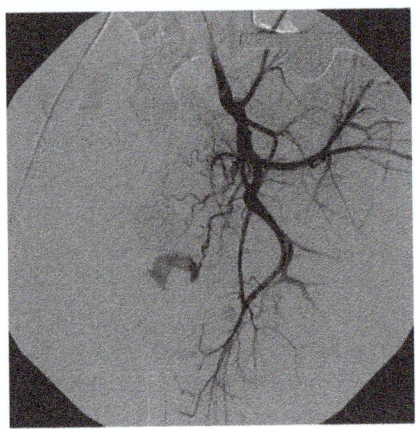

Fig. 5.6.2

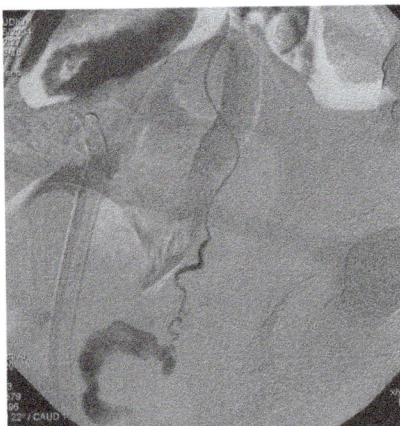

Fig. 5.6.3

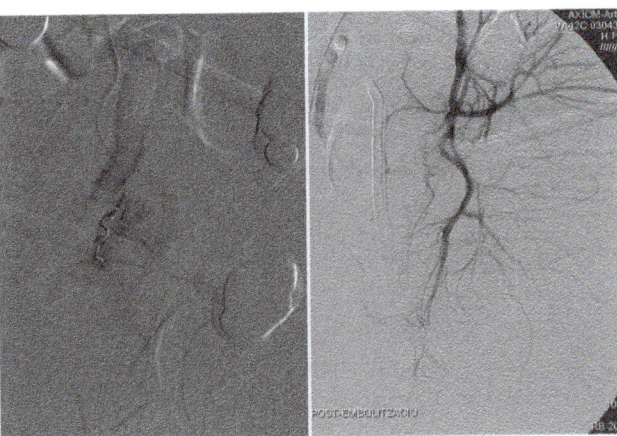

Fig. 5.6.4

stable, and CT found no active bleeding. The patient presented hematuria, and urethroscopy showed arterial bleeding in the prostatic urethra. Urethroscopy was unable to bring about hemostasis, so we performed angiography with embolization of the vesicoprostatic arteries.

Comments

Bleeding is the most life-threatening complication of pelvic fractures and is associated to a high rate of mortality. Blood loss occurs after lesions to the hypogastric arteries or their branches. In posterior pelvic fractures, the gluteal arteries and the lateral sacral arteries are the most commonly affected branches, whereas in anterior fractures, the pudendal and obturator arteries are the most commonly affected.

Embolization is the treatment of choice in patients with arterial bleeding secondary to pelvic fracture. Embolization is indicated when contrast extravasation is seen at CT. Multidetector CT is currently the most useful technique for the rapid diagnosis of pelvic trauma and for planning endovascular treatment. Multidetector CT provides information about the location of active bleeding and which vessels are involved; it can orient embolization and thus avoid repeated examinations of different pelvic vessels. In cases of intermittent bleeding, CT can show the hematoma without detecting active bleeding; these patients require watchful waiting and, if the patient's condition deteriorates, embolization (whether after repeated CT examination or not). Embolization should be as selective as possible. The most frequently employed embolizing agents in trauma cases are Spongostan® and metallic coils. Embolization successfully controls arterial bleeding in 85–95% of cases. The rate of complications from embolization is less than 10%, and most of these occur in cases with bilateral hypogastric embolizations. Reported complications include ischemia, infarction, infection, and impotence.

Procedure Steps

1. Puncture the right femoral artery.
2. Perform angiography of the aortoiliac sector. In this case, active bleeding in the territory of the left hypogastric artery was seen.
3. Perform selective angiography of the left hypogastric artery. In this case, contrast extravasation was seen in the area supplied by the vesicoprostatic artery.
4. After the appropriate projection to locate the ostium of the bleeding artery, use a microcatheter to perform selective catheterization and angiographic study of the vesicoprostatic artery to confirm contrast extravasation.
5. Embolize the bleeding vessel with two VortX metallic coils (3 × 28 mm) and Spongostan particles.
6. Confirm the outcome with angiography. In this case, angiography showed correct occlusion of the bleeding vessel.

Equipment List

1. 10-cm-long 5F introducer sheath
2. 0.035 in. hydrophilic guidewire
3. 5F straight catheter with side holes
4. 5F Simmons I
5. 4F Cobra II hydrophilic catheter
6. 2.7F Progreat microcatheter with 0.021 in. micro-guidewire (BOSTON SCIENTIFIC)
7. Two VortX microcoils (3 × 28 mm) (Boston Scientific)
8. Spongostan particles

Case 5.7
■
Obstetric Bleeding Treated with Embolization

Figure 5.7.1 Selective angiogram of the right hypogastric artery shows contrast extravasation in the area supplied by the right cervicovaginal arteries

Figure 5.7.2 Selective angiogram of the cervicovaginal arteries shows extravasation of contrast material at the vaginal level

Figure 5.7.3 Selective angiogram obtained after embolization shows occlusion of the bleeding vessels

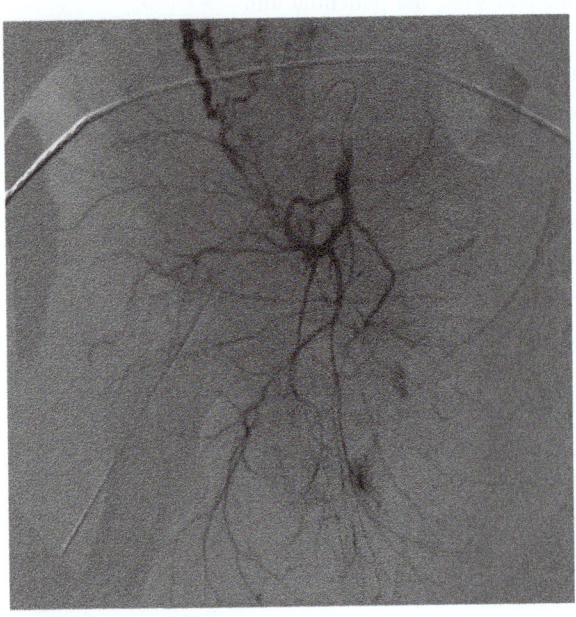

Fig. 5.7.1

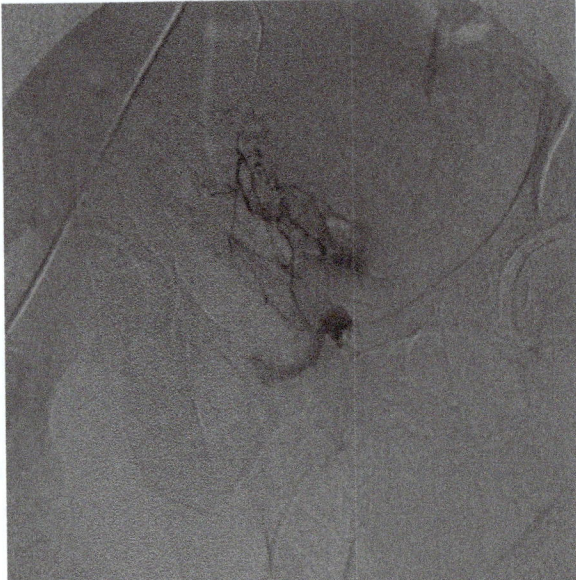

Fig. 5.7.2

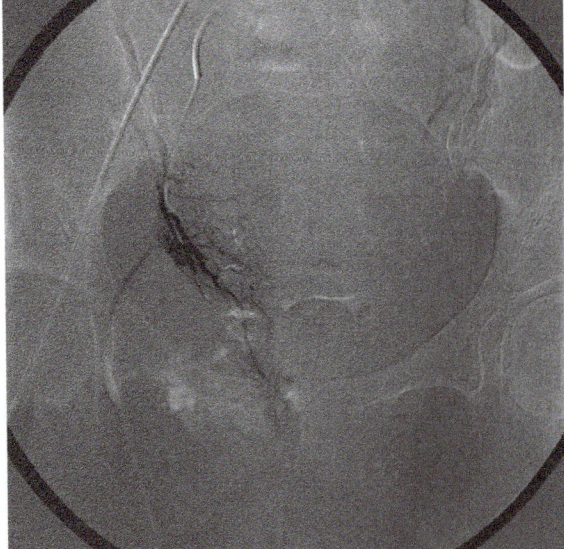

Fig. 5.7.3

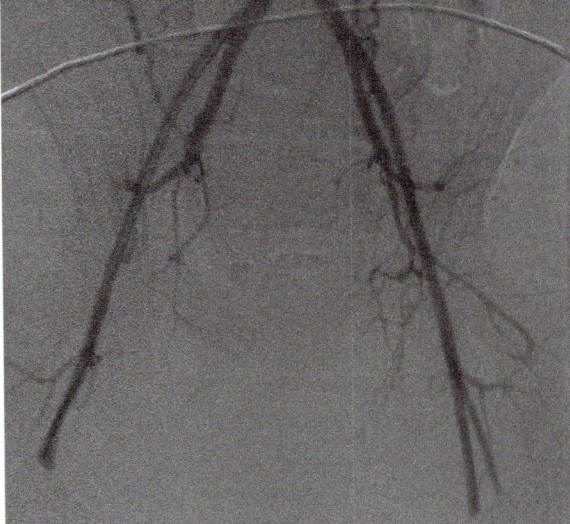

Fig. 5.7.4

Figure 5.7.4 Angiogram of the entire iliac sector shows hypertrophy of the uterine arteries in the abdominal cavity that supply the uterus and the occlusion of the bleeding vessels

After a normal delivery, a 31-year-old woman presented vaginal hematoma and bleeding at the level of the episiorrhaphy in the immediate postpartum period. She was hemodynamically stable, with hemoglobin 7.5, hematocrit 20%, and transfusion requirement of seven RBC units. We performed angiography and embolization of the cervicovaginal arteries.

Postpartum bleeding is the first cause of maternal death worldwide. Uterine atony is the most frequent cause of postpartum bleeding, accounting for 75% of cases. Other causes include tears, lacerations, and hematomas in the birth canal, the presence of placental remains, uterine inversion, and alterations in placental insertion. Arterial embolization is indicated for the treatment of postpartum bleeding when conservative obstetric measures fail. The uterus and vagina are supplied by the uterine, vaginal, and pudendal arteries, which are all branches of the anterior bifurcation of the hypogastric artery. There are anastomoses between the uterine arteries and the ovarian arteries on both sides, as well as between the uterine and vaginal arteries. Angiographic study in cases of postpartum bleeding should include the hypogastric and ovarian arteries as well as the vaginal, vulvar, and perineal circulations. Spongostan is the most frequently used material for embolization in postpartum bleeding. In cases with super-selective catheterization or pseudoaneurysms, PVA particles or metallic coils can be used. Arterial embolization achieves hemostasis in 89–100% of cases, and the rate of complications is very low in groups with experience. Other indications for arterial embolization include bleeding after gynecological surgery or abortion and secondary or late postpartum bleeding.

Comments

1. Puncture the right femoral artery.
2. Perform angiography of the aortoiliac sector; in this case, active bleeding was seen in the area supplied by the right hypogastric artery.
3. Perform selective angiography of the right hypogastric artery; in this case, active bleeding was seen in the area supplied by the right cervicovaginal artery.
4. Use a microcatheter for superselective catheterization of the bleeding arteries.
5. Use Spongostan particles to selectively embolize the bleeding arteries.
6. Confirm the outcome with angiographic study of the treated hypogastric artery and of the aortoiliac sector; in this case, the correct occlusion of the bleeding vessel and absence of collateral vessels were confirmed.

Procedure Steps

1. 5F introducer sheath
2. 180-cm-long 0.035 in. hydrophilic guidewire
3. 65-cm-long 5F straight catheter with side holes
4. 5F Simmons I
5. 80-cm-long 4F Cobra II hydrophilic catheter
6. 2.7F microcatheter
7. 0.021 in. micro-guidewire
8. Spongostan particles – manually cut and mixed with iodinated contrast material

Equipment List

Case 5.8

■

Embolization to Treat Hemoperitoneum Due to Ruptured Hepatocellular Carcinoma

Figure 5.8.1 Abdominal CT shows a 75-mm subcapsular nodule suggestive of hepatocellular carcinoma at the tip of the left liver lobe, hyperdense fluid compatible with hemoperitoneum, and signs of cirrhosis

Figure 5.8.2 Selective angiogram of the common hepatic artery shows a hypervascular nodular lesion in the lateral segments of the left liver lobe. There are no signs of active bleeding

Figure 5.8.3 Selective angiogram of the left hepatic artery shows a hypervascular tumor in the left liver lobe supplied by the arteries in segments two and three

Figure 5.8.4 Hepatic angiogram after embolization shows occlusion of the arteries that feed the tumor and patency of the rest of the intrahepatic circulation and of the gastroduodenal artery

A 77-year-old man with a history of acute hepatitis C at age 40 was admitted for abdominal pain radiating to the shoulders and hypotension with a tendency toward hemodynamic

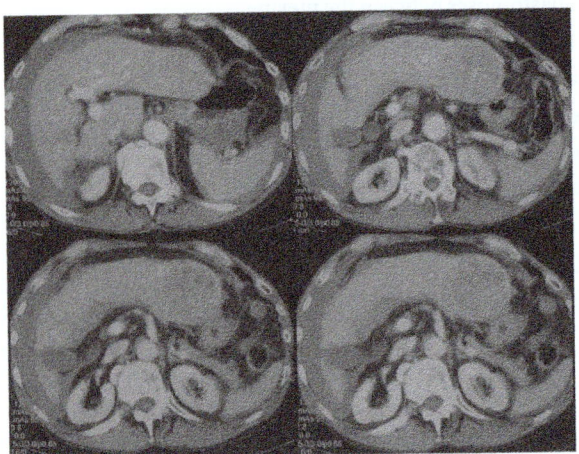

Fig. 5.8.1

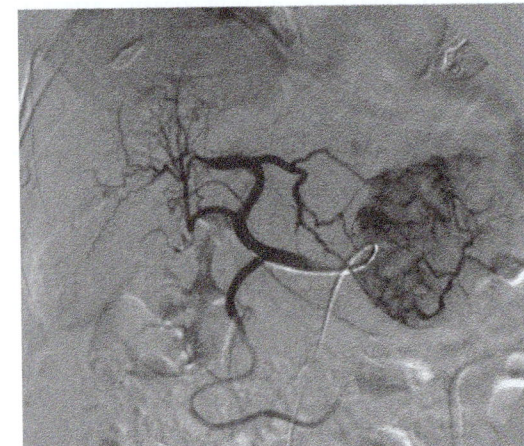

Fig. 5.8.2

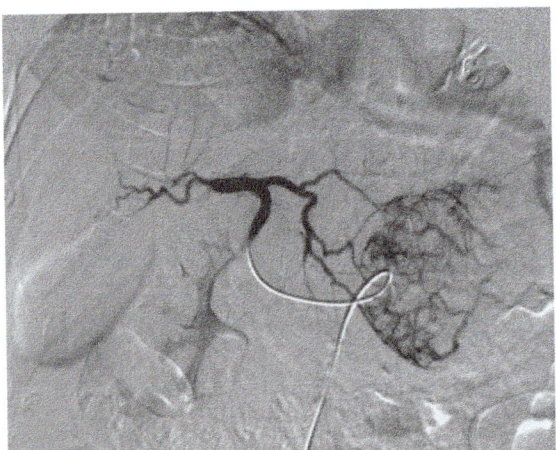

Fig. 5.8.3

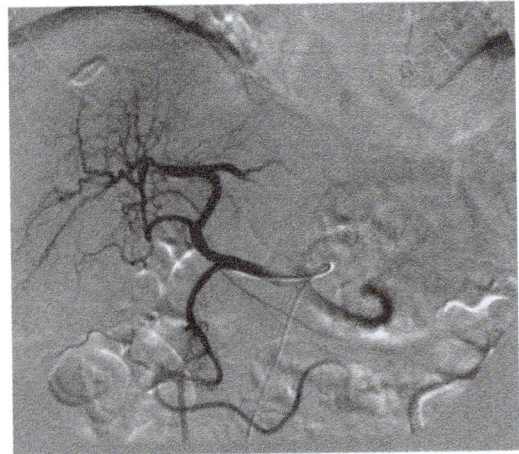

Fig. 5.8.4

instability. Blood tests showed leukocytosis, 23% hematocrit, and preserved liver function classified as Child-Pugh A. CT showed signs compatible with ruptured hepatocellular carcinoma (HCC) and secondary hemoperitoneum. We performed angiography and embolization.

Comments

The incidence of spontaneous rupture of HCC is 2%. The causes of HCC rupture are related with the tumor's rapid growth, with tumor necrosis, and with increased pressure within the tumor secondary to the vascular invasion of the hepatic veins.

The diagnosis of ruptured HCC can be difficult, especially in patients with no history of cirrhosis, and 20–30% of cases are diagnosed during exploratory laparotomy.

US and CT are useful for diagnosing hemoperitoneum and liver tumors and for assessing portal patency.

Conservative treatment results in 85% mortality, and surgical treatment in the acute phase results in 65% mortality.

In cases in which hemodynamic shock can be controlled, selective arterial embolization is a fast and safe way to achieve hemostasis.

The angiographic technique makes it possible to locate the point of active bleeding, assess portal patency, and embolize the bleeding vessel in the same intervention. The best material for embolization in this scenario is Spongostan, although metal coils and PVA particles have also been successfully employed.

Although embolization successfully stops the bleeding in most cases of ruptured HCC, the procedure is contradicted in cases of thrombosis of the main trunk of the portal vein because the risk of liver failure leads to 26–36% mortality 7 days after arterial embolization.

Two recently published studies reported better outcomes and concluded that arterial embolization is efficacious for achieving hemostasis in the acute phase. These studies report higher success rates compared to open surgery and lower 30-day mortality (0–37 vs. 28–75%). Both studies also concluded that outcomes are better in cases in which scheduled resection is performed after embolization that in those in which the HCC is resected in the acute phase.

Procedure Steps

1. Puncture the right femoral artery and insert a 5F introducer sheath.
2. Perform selective angiography of the celiac trunk and superior mesenteric artery with a 5F Simmons I catheter.
3. Use a hydrophilic guidewire and a cobra II catheter to selectively catheterize the common hepatic artery and the left hepatic artery.
4. Use a 2.7F coaxial microcatheter to perform superselective catheterization of the arteries that feed the tumor from the left hepatic artery.
5. Embolize the arteries that feed the tumor with 300–500 micra PVA microspheres.
6. Perform angiography to check that the tumor has been completely devascularized.

Equipment List

1. 10-cm-long 5F introducer sheath
2. 0.035 in. hydrophilic guidewire
3. 5F Simmons I catheter
4. 4F Cobra II hydrophilic catheter
5. 2.7F Progreat microcatheter with 0.021 in. micro-guidewire (BOSTON SCIENTIFIC)
6. Two VortX microcoils (3 × 28 mm) (Boston Scientific)
7. PVA particles (300–500 micras)

Case 5.9

■

Embolization to Treat Renal Hematoma Due to Angiomyolipoma

Figure 5.9.1 Abdominal CT shows a fatty tumor in the lower pole of the *right* kidney; it has exophytic growth (9 × 19 × 8 cm) and is compatible with angiomyolipoma. There is a hematoma inside the angiomyolipoma, foci of active bleeding, and perirenal hematoma with thickening of the right pararenal fascia

Figure 5.9.2 Selective renal angiogram shows a hypervascular tumor in the lower pole of the right kidney and a pseudoaneurysm within the lesions without signs of active bleeding

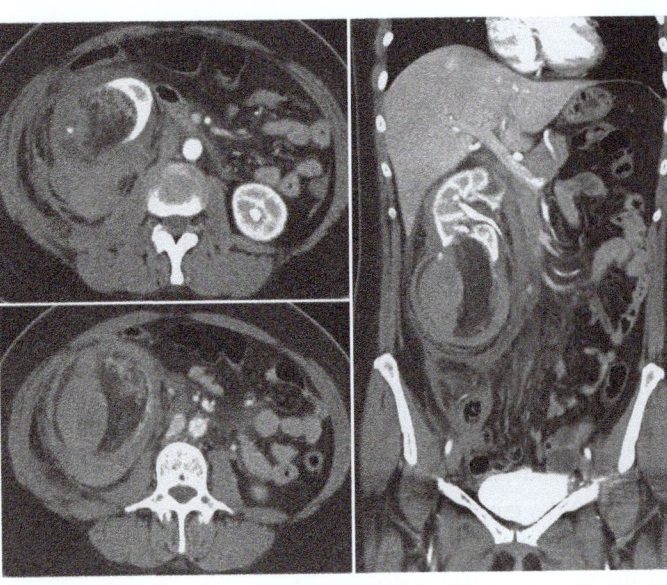

Fig. 5.9.1

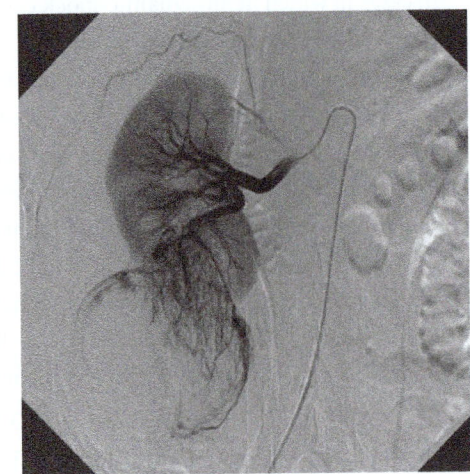

Fig. 5.9.2

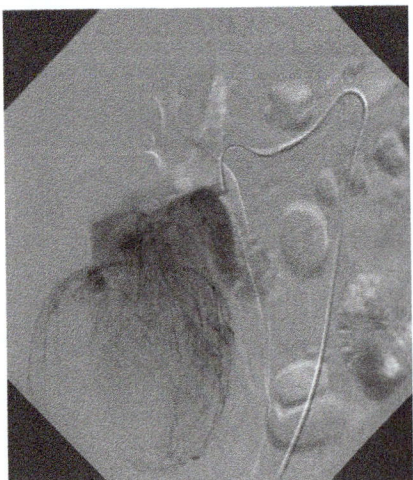

Fig. 5.9.3

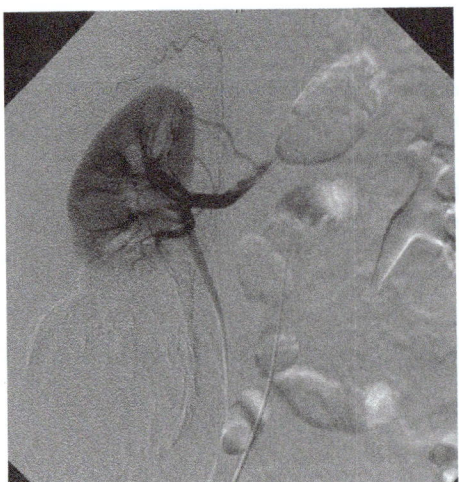

Fig. 5.9.4

Figure 5.9.3 Selective angiogram of the inferior segmental arteries confirms the vascularization of the tumor and the pseudoaneurysmatic lesion

Figure 5.9.4 Selective renal angiogram obtained after embolization shows the total devascularization of the tumor and patency of the rest of the renal vessels

A 58-year-old woman presented at the emergency department with low back pain of abrupt onset, sweating, vomiting, and nausea. At physical examination, she was hemodynamically stable with pale skin and mucosa and had right abdominal pain on palpation. Her hematocrit was 26%. CT at admission showed a heterogeneous tumor in the lower pole of the right kidney compatible with an angiomyolipoma and signs of hemorrhage within the lesion. We performed angiography and embolization.

Comments

A renal angiomyolipoma is a benign hamartomatous tumor that contains various proportions of fat, smooth muscle, and anomalous vessels. It usually arises from the renal cortex and has an exophytic growth pattern. The main complication associated with renal angiomyolipoma is bleeding, which can be life threatening. The main risk factors for bleeding are size, the presence of aneurysms greater than 5 mm in diameter, an angiogenic component, association with tuberous sclerosis, and pregnancy.

Embolization is clearly established as the treatment of choice in emergency cases. For elective treatment, tumors larger than 4 cm should be treated because their risk of hemorrhage is 50–60%. Recent publications recommend embolization before surgical resection, as the results overlap and the rates of organ preservation are higher with embolism. However, there is a greater risk of recurrence in patients with tuberous sclerosis, and these patients require long-term follow-up.

Procedure Steps

1. Puncture the right femoral artery and insert a 5F introducer sheath.
2. Use a 5F Simmons I catheter to perform selective angiography of the right renal artery. In this case, the tumor on the lower pole was confirmed. It had moderate vascularization, with hypertrophy of the segmental artery that fed the lesion and an aneurysmatic dilation measuring 1 cm. There were no signs of active bleeding.
3. Use a 2.7F Progreat coaxial microcatheter to selectively catheterize the arteries that supply the tumor.
4. Embolize the arteries that feed the tumor using 300–500 micra PVA microspheres, four controlled-release IDC microcoils (4×40 mm), and two VortX microcoils (3×38 mm).
5. Perform selective renal angiography after embolization to confirm complete devascularization of the tumor.

Equipment List

1. 10-cm-long 5F introducer sheath.
2. 0.035 in. hydrophilic guidewire.
3. 5F Simmons I.
4. 2.7F Progreat microcatheter with 0.021 in. micro-guidewire (BOSTON SCIENTIFIC).
5. PVA particles (300–500 micras).
6. Four IDC microcoils (4×40 mm) and two VortX microcoils (3×28 mm).

Case 5.10
Renal Artery Stenosis Treated with Stenting

Figure 5.10.1 Aortorenal angiogram shows stenosis >80% of the proximal third left renal artery

Figure 5.10.2 Aortorenal angiogram prior to releasing the renal stent shows the correct placement of the 0.014 in. guidewire through the stenosis in the left renal artery

Figure 5.10.3 Digitally subtracted and native image during the release of the renal stent

Figure 5.10.4 Angiogram obtained after releasing the stent in the renal artery shows the complete restoration of the caliber of the left renal artery

A 63-year-old man with a history of hypertension, type II diabetes, dyslipemia, hyperuricemia, and renal lithiasis and an 18-month history of renal failure with creatinine stable at 2 mg/dL presented with deteriorating renal function (creatinine 3.9 mg/dL). Doppler US

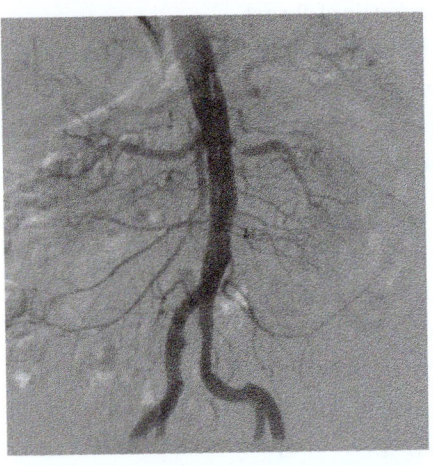

Fig. 5.10.1

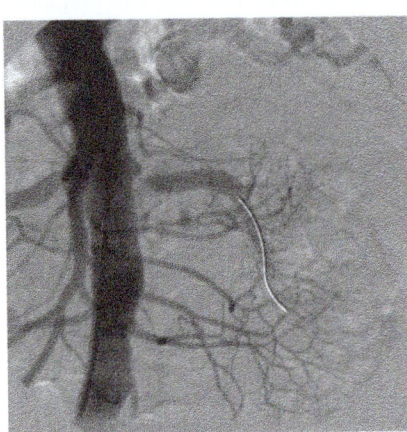

Fig. 5.10.2

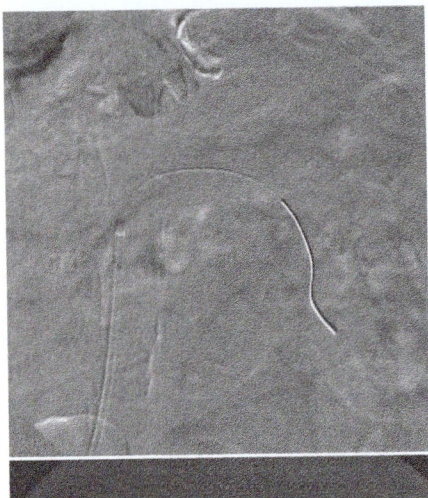

Fig. 5.10.3

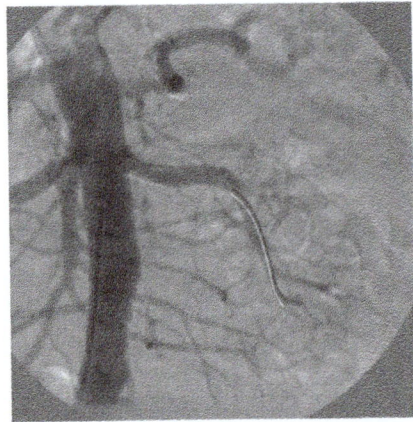

Fig. 5.10.4

showed renal asymmetry (right kidney 10.6 cm, left kidney 8.4 cm) and findings suggestive of significant stenosis of the proximal third of the left renal artery (right renal artery velocity 170 cm/s; left renal artery velocity 287 cm/s), so angiography was performed to see if stenting was necessary.

Percutaneous renal revascularization is indicated in cases in which renal artery stenosis is clearly suspected as the cause of the symptoms. Symptoms include fast-developing malignant hypertension in a single kidney or that responds poorly to medical treatment, as well as renal failure and congestive heart failure in certain cases. In general, asymptomatic renal artery stenosis should not be treated. The diagnosis is anatomic and functional. MR angiography, CT angiography, and arteriography are the morphological examinations. The functional tests are Doppler US, creatinine clearing, renins, and measuring the intra-arterial pressure gradient.

In renal stenosis of arteriosclerotic origin, the treatment of choice is stent placement. Several random controlled trials have shown the significant superiority of stenting over simple angioplasty, both in terms of the initial technical success (98 vs. 77%, respectively) and of the percentage of restenosis (14–17 vs. 26–48%, respectively).

In fibromuscular dysplasia, the treatment of choice is simple angioplasty. Factors influencing good outcome include age below 50 years, absence of associated coronary or carotid disease, and hypertension of less than 2 years' evolution. Stenting should be reserved for cases refractory to simple angioplasty or with complications secondary to simple angioplasty, such as arterial dissection. In fibromuscular dysplasia, angioplasty achieves clinical improvement or cure in 74–79% of cases.

Procedure Steps

1. Puncture the right femoral artery and insert a 5F introducer sheath.
2. Insert an Accu-Vu multiperforated angiographic catheter and obtain an aortogram. In this case, stenosis >80% of the proximal left renal artery was confirmed.
3. Insert a 45-cm-long 6F introducer sheath.
4. Pass a hook catheter and hydrophilic guidewire through the stenosis.
5. Replace the hydrophilic guidewire with a 0.014-in. guidewire.
6. Place a 6 × 18-mm Herculink balloon-expandable stent at the level of the stenosis and inflate the balloon using a manometer at its nominal pressure.
7. Check the results by angiography performed through a straight 4F multiperforated catheter to confirm the restoration of the caliber of the vessel and the absence of residual stenosis.

Equipment List

1. 10-cm-long 5F introducer sheath.
2. 0.035 in. hydrophilic guidewire.
3. 5F Accu-Vu angiographic catheter.
4. 45-cm-long 6F introducer sheath.
5. 4F hook catheter
6. 0.014 in. micro-guidewire.
7. Herculink balloon-expandable stent (6 × 18 mm) (ABBOT).
8. Straight 4F multiperforated catheter.

Further Reading

Abbas MA, Fowl RJ, Stone WM, Panneton JM, Oldenburg WA, Bower TC et al. Hepatic artery aneurysm: factors that predict complications. J Vasc Surg 2003;38(1):41-45.

Anderson SW, Soto JA, Lucey BC, Burke PA, Hirsch EF, Rhea JT. Blunt trauma: Feasibility and clinical utiliy of pelvic CT angiography performed with 64-detector row CT. Radiology 2008:246:410-419.

Banovac F, Lin R, Shah D, White A, Pelage JP, Spies J. Angiographic and interventional options in obstetric and gynecologic emergencies. Obstet Gynecol Clin North Am 2007;34(3): 599-616.

Ben-Menachem Y, Coldwell DM, Young JWR, Burgess AR. Hemorrhage associated with pelvic fractures: causes, diagnosis, and emergent management. AJR 1991;157:1005-1014.

Berczi V, Gopalan D, Cleveland TJ. Embolization of a hemorrhoid following 18 hours of life-threatening bleeding. Cardiovasc Intervent Radiol 2008;31(1):183-185.

Buczkowski AK, Kim PT, Ho SG et al. Multidisciplinary management of ruptured hepatocellular carcinoma. J Gastrointest Surg 2006;10:379-386.

Christopher White J. Catheter-based therapy for atherosclerotic renal artery stenosis. Circulation 2006;113:1464-1473.

David Trost MD. Renovascular disease: the role of IR in diagnosis, treatment and managenent. *2005 SIR 30th Annual Scientific Meeting.*

Defreyne L, Verstraeten V, De Potter C, Pattyn P, DeVos M, Kunnen M. Jejunal arteriovenous malformation, diagnosed by angiography and treated by embolization and catheter-guided surgery: case report and review of literature. Abdom Imaging 1998;23:127-131.

Demetriades D, Hadjizacharia P, Constantinou C, Brown C, Inaba K, Rhee P et al. Selective nonoperative management of penetrating abdominal solid organ injuries. Ann Surg 2006;244(4):620-628.

Dobson CC, Nicholson AA. Treatment of rectal hemorrhage by coil embolization. Cardiovasc Intervent Radiol 1999;22(2): 143-146.

Eriksson LG, Mulic-Lutvica A, Jangland L, Nyman R. Massive postpartum hemorrhage treated with transcatheter arterial embolization: technical aspects and long-term effects on fertility and menstrual cycle. Acta Radiol 2007;48(6):635-642.

Gady JS, Reynolds H, Blum A. Selective arterial embolization for control of lower gastrointestinal bleeding: recommendations for a clinical management pathway. Curr Surg 2003;60:344-347.

Jain A, Costa G, Marsh W, Fontes P, Devera M, Mazariegos G et al. Thrombotic and nonthrombotic hepatic artery complications in adults and children following primary liver transplantation with long-term follow-up in 1000 consecutive patients. Transpl Int 2006;19(1):27-37.

Kondo H, Yamada T, Kanematsu M, Kako N, Goshima S, Yamamoto N. Embolization for massive urethral hemorrhage. Abdom Imaging 2007;32:262-263.

Kothary N, Soulen MC, Clark TW, Wein AJ, Shlansky-Goldberg RD, Crino PB et al. Renal angiomyolipoma: long-term results after arterial embolization. J Vasc Interv Radiol 2005;16(1): 45-50.

Kramer SC, Gorich J, Rilinger N, Siech M, Aschoff AJ, Vogel J et al. Embolization for gastrointestinal hemorrhages. Eur. Radiol. 2000;10(5):802-5.

Lai EC, Lau WY. Spontaneous rupture of hepatocellular carcinoma: a systematic review. Arch Surg 2006;141:191-198.

Laing CJ, Tobias T, Rosenblum DI, Banker WL, Tseng L, Tamarkin SW. Acute gastrointestinal bleeding: emerging role of multi-detector CT angiography and review of current imaging techniques. Radiographics 2007;27:1055-1070.

Marmery H, Shanmuganathan K, Alexander MT, Mirvis SE. Optimization of selection for nonoperative management of blunt splenic injury: comparison of MDCT grading systems. AJR Am J Roentgenol 2007;189(6):1421-1427.

Muray S, Martin M, Amoedo ML, Garcia C, Jornet AR, Vera M, Oliveras Am, Gomez X, Craver L, Real MI, Garcia L, Botey A, Montanya X, Fernandez E. Rapid decline in renal function reflects reversibility and predicts the outcome after angioplasty in renal artery stenosis. Am J Kidney Dis 2002;39(1):60-66.

Neuma HB, Zarzaur BL, Meyer AA, Cairns BA, Rich PB. Superselective catheterization and embolization as first-line therapy for lower gastrointestinal bleeding. Am Surg 2005; 71:539-544.

Nosher JL, Chung J, Brevetti LS, Graham AM, Siegel RL. Visceral and renal artery aneurysms: a pictorial essay on endovascular therapy. Radiographics 2006;26(6):1687-704.

Okazaki M, Higashihara H, Koganemaru F et al. Intraperitoneal hemorrhage from hepatocellular carcinoma: emergency chemoembolization or embolization. Radiology 1991;180: 647-651.

Orons PD, Sheng R, Zajko AB. Hepatic artery stenosis in liver transplant recipients: prevalence and cholangiographic appearance of associated biliary complications. AJR Am J Roentgenol 1995;165(5):1145-1149.

Ramon J, Rimon U, Garniek A, Golan G, Bensaid P, Kitrey ND et al. Renal Angiomyolipoma: long-term results following selective arterial embolization. Eur Urol 2009;55(5):1155-1161.

Rodríguez Jornet A, Ibeas J, Ribera L, Real J, Perendreu J, Falcó J, Vallespín J, Allegué N, Giménez Gaibar A, García M. Nefropatía isquémica: ¿revascularización o tratamiento médico conservador? Nefrologia 2005;25(3):258-268.

Saad WE, Davies MG, Sahler L, Lee DE, Patel NC, Kitanosono T et al. Hepatic artery stenosis in liver transplant recipients: primary treatment with percutaneous transluminal angioplasty. J Vasc Interv Radiol 2005;16(6):795-805.

Ueno T, Jones G, Martin A, Ikegami T, Sanchez EQ, Chinnakotla S et al. Clinical outcomes from hepatic artery stenting in liver transplantation. Liver Transpl 2006;12(3):422-427.

Weldon DT, Burke SJ, Sun S, Mimura H, Golzarian J. Interventional management of lower gastrointestinal bleeding. Eur Radiol 2008;18(5):857-867.

Wu SC, Chow KC, Lee KH, Tung CC, Yang AD, Lo CJ. Early selective angioembolization improves success of nonoperative management of blunt splenic injury. Am Surg 2007;73(9): 897-902.

Zuckerman DA, Gaz RD. Catheter-guided intraoperative localization of a jejunal angiodysplasia using the Tracker-18 coaxial catheter system: case report. Cardiovasc Intervent Radiol 1991;14:358-359.

Upper Extremity, Central Thoracic and Abdominal Veins

José M. Abadal, and José Urbano

J.J. Muñoz and R. Ribes, *Learning Vascular and Interventional Radiology*, Learning Imaging,
DOI: 10.1007/978-3-540-87997-8_6, © Springer-Verlag Berlin Heidelberg 2010

Case 6.1

■

Venous Angioplasty of a Hemodialysis Fistula

Figure 6.1.1 Brachiocephalic arteriovenous fistula seen at fistulography and ultrasonography shows the stenotic segment of the cephalic vein. Note the collateral circulation and the length and diameter of the stenosis

Figure 6.1.2 Doppler US shows increased peak systolic flow (up to 212 cm/s) at the point of maximum stenosis

Figure 6.1.3 US-guided percutaneous angioplasty at the level of the anastomosis. Note the notch in the middle third of the balloon due to the stenosis

Figure 6.1.4 Doppler US after angioplasty shows adequate flow in the color mode and reduction of flow velocity to 92 cm/s

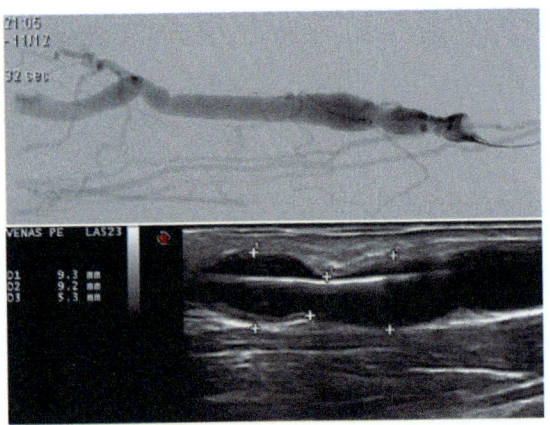

Fig. 6.1.1

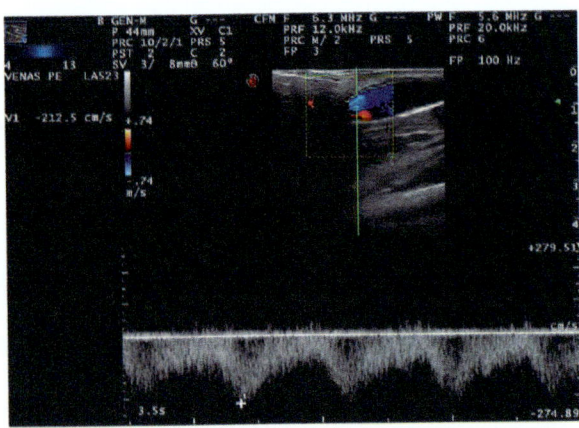

Fig. 6.1.2

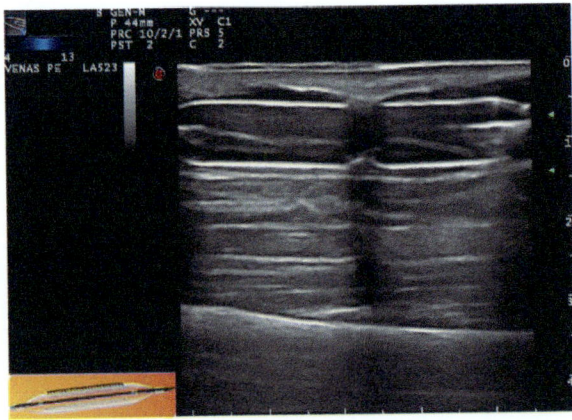

Fig. 6.1.3

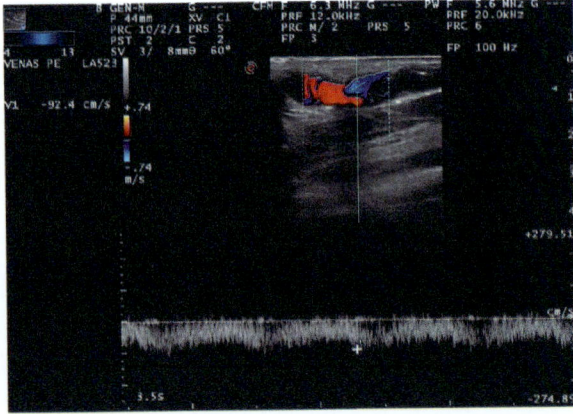

Fig. 6.1.4

A 48-year-old male patient with an autologous brachiocephalic hemodialysis fistula was referred for fistulography to evaluate poor function, including flow rate below 150 mL/min, prolonged dialysis time (>5 h), and difficulties in puncture.

Fistulography and Doppler US detected significant cephalic vein stenosis.

Comments

Autologous arteriovenous fistulas have proven the longest-lasting solution for dialysis with the lowest rate of complications; thus, they should be the first approach in patients with favorable anatomic conditions. Radiocephalic fistulas at the level of the wrist have the best patency; when these fail, a second option is to go up one venous segment to the elbow.

Changes in venous pressures during dialysis should raise suspicion of stenosis in the fistula. Stenosis usually occurs in the venous segments (85%) near the anastomoses.

Fistulography and Doppler US make it possible to detect and quantify the stenosis, as well as to plan treatment to avoid progression from stenosis to thrombosis of the access.

When it is anatomically and technically feasible, balloon angioplasty is indicated. This minimally invasive technique makes it possible to restore the stenosed vascular lumen. Midpressure-range (12–14 atm) balloons or high-pressure (up to 24 atm) balloons with dimensions about 10% greater than the diameter of the vein are normally used. In cases with refractory stenosis, balloons with atherotomes and, less frequently, stents can be used. Restenosis is not uncommon after angioplasty, so the fistula requires continual monitoring and possible reintervention to ensure long-term patency.

Complications are rare; these include venous rupture/extravasation, dissection, spasm, and thrombosis. Most complications can be resolved with endovascular techniques.

Procedure Steps

1. After infiltrating anesthetic into the skin, puncture the fistula. Be sure to leave enough space between the tip of the introducer sheath and the stenosis. Consider whether to use a retrograde venous approach, antegrade venous approach, or arterial approach on the basis of the location of the stenosis.
2. Under fluoroscopic guidance, pass a hydrophilic guidewire through the stenosis.
3. Insert an introducer sheath to enable endovascular material to be passed through.
4. Once the anastomosis is located, administer 4,000–5,000 U heparin prior to angioplasty. Then center the balloon within the stenosis and inflate it until the nominal pressure is reached, taking care not to reach the rupture pressure. The balloon can be repeatedly inflated for 30–60 s each time until the stenosis is resolved.
5. After checking the results, withdraw the introducer sheath, taking into account that the patient has been heparinized.

Equipment List

1. Needle for venous puncture.
2. 0.035 in. Terumo hydrophilic guidewire
3. 5–7F vascular introducer sheath
4. Angioplasty balloon (5–8 mm in diameter). Manometer to inflate the balloon.
5. Heparin (4,000–5,000 U). Iodinated contrast material

Case 6.2

■

Permanent Femoral Catheter for Hemodialysis

Figure 6.2.1 Hemodialysis patient with a malfunctioning catheter and edema of the upper limbs and neck. Phlebogram of the right arm shows the hemodialysis catheter with its tip in the superior vena cava. The flow of contrast material is detained at the level of the subclavian vein. Note the extensive cervical collateral circulation. These findings demonstrate catheter-related thrombosis in the superior vena cava

Figure 6.2.2 Because the patient needed dialysis, a permanent femoral catheter was implanted. Treatment planning. Note the Dacron sleeve of the catheter

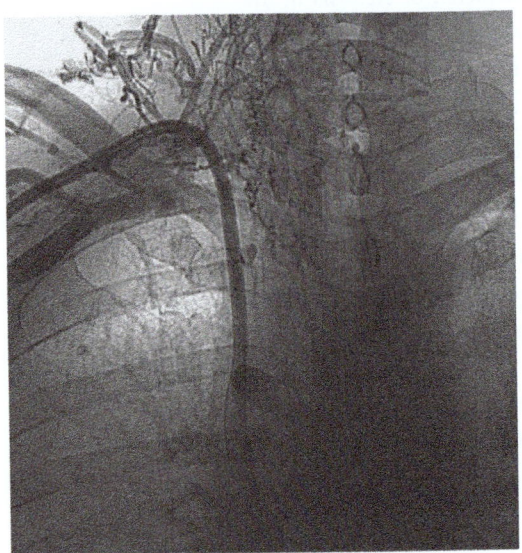

Fig. 6.2.1

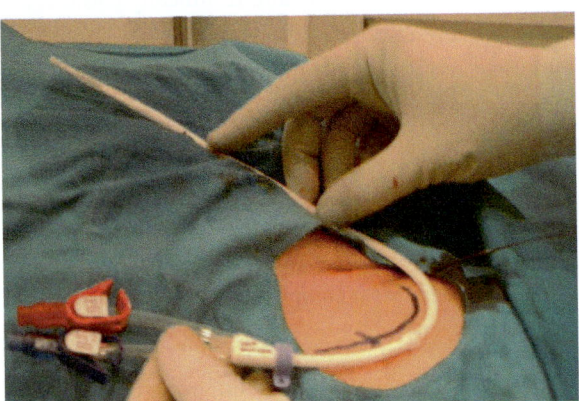

Fig. 6.2.2

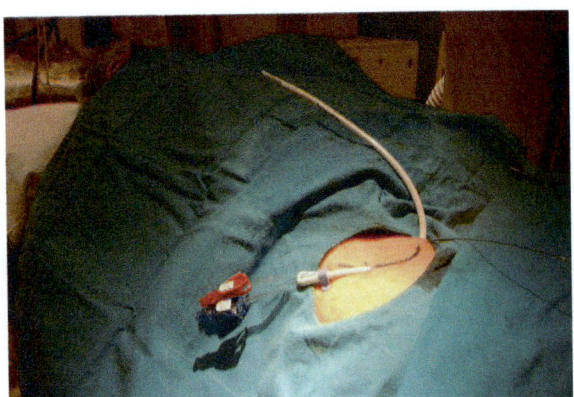

Fig. 6.2.3

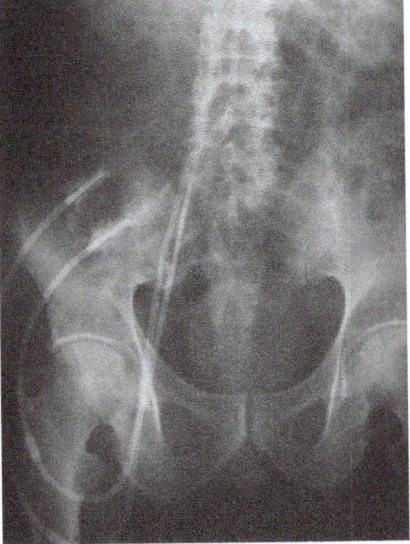

Fig. 6.2.4

Figure 6.2.3 Lateral ascending subcutaneous tunneling of the catheter to ensure patient comfort and prevent catheter migration

Figure 6.2.4 Abdominal X-ray shows the catheter with its distal tips in the inferior vena cava

A 50-year-old man undergoing dialysis through a permanent jugular catheter presented edema of the neck and right upper arm. Dialysis through the catheter was difficult, with long dialysis times and low flow. Phlebography showed thrombosis of the superior vena cava. We implanted a permanent femoral catheter and withdrew the jugular catheter.

The implantation of a permanent femoral catheter is a technically and clinically valid option in certain hemodialysis patients.

It is indicated in the following cases:

1. Dialysis in a patient with thrombosis in the superior vena cava.
2. To avoid jugular-subclavian thrombosis associated to any catheter placed through the jugular, and to serve as a bridge for hemodialysis while the arteriovenous fistula matures.

The average patency of femoral catheters is lower than in jugular catheters, so this option should be considered only for midterm dialysis. Due to the possible risk of lower limb thrombosis, prophylaxis with low molecular-weight heparin is recommended. Other possible complications such as infection or catheter migration are less likely when the ascending tunneling technique is used.

1. Catheterize the common femoral vein and leave a guidewire in the inferior vena cava.
2. Place a catheter on top of the patient and calculate its position using fluoroscopy. Draw the path of the subcutaneous tunnel on the patient's skin.
3. After infiltrating anesthesia, create the tunnel with a curved tunneler.
4. Dilate and place a peel-away sheath in the femoral vein.
5. Introduce a catheter through the peel-away sheath. Check the position of the distal tip in the infrarenal inferior vena cava and of the Dacron sleeve. Close the inguinal incision with silk sutures.

1. Hemodialysis Catheter Kit (includes puncture needle, guidewire, tunneler, and hemodialysis catheter).
2. Note 1: For ascending curved tunneling, manually bend the straight tunneler included in the kit.
3. Note 2: The length of the catheter must be adjusted to fit the patient. The distal tip must remain in the inferior vena cava. As a rule of thumb, the distance between the Dacron sleeve and the tip of the catheter should be greater than 30 cm.

Case 6.3
■

Percutaneous Extraction of an Intrapulmonary Foreign Body

Figure 6.3.1 Posteroanterior chest X-ray shows a foreign body projected over the left pulmonary hilum

Figure 6.3.2 Catheter trapped by the snare. Tip of the introducer sheath in the right ventricle and safety guidewire in the left pulmonary artery keeping the introducer sheath correctly oriented

Figure 6.3.3 The foreign body extracted. Detail of the snare (*upper right corner*)

Figure 6.3.4 Posteroanterior chest X-ray after the procedure

When a 47-year-old woman with a history of colon cancer treated with surgery and chemotherapy, asymptomatic and in complete remission, had the subcutaneous reservoir removed 1 year later, only the reservoir and a small segment of the catheter

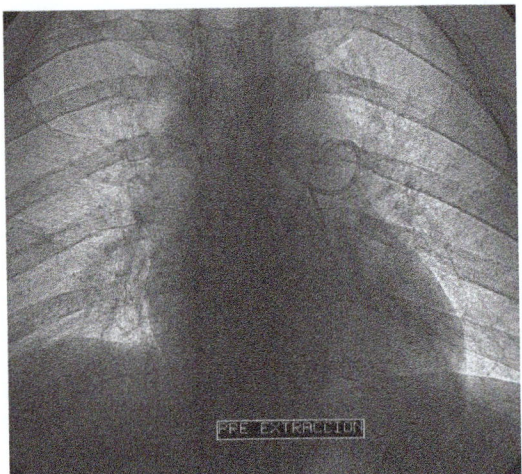

Fig. 6.3.1

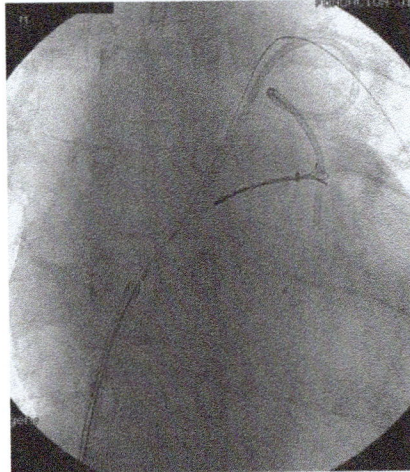

Fig. 6.3.2

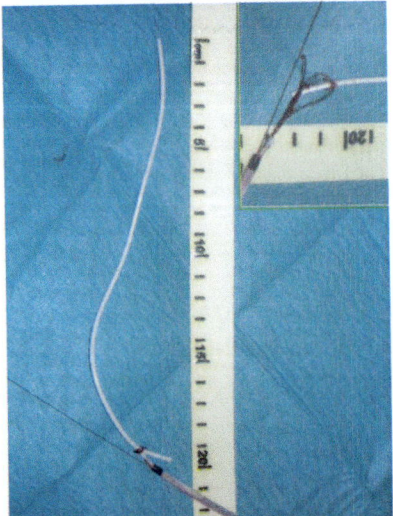

Fig. 6.3.3

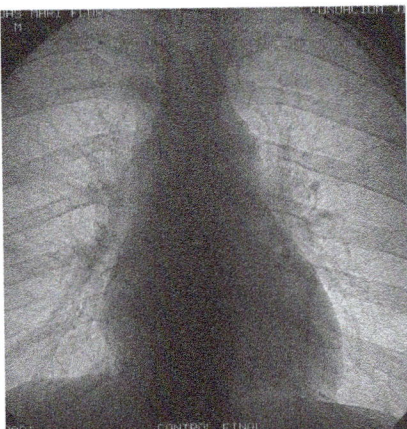

Fig. 6.3.4

were recovered. Chest X-ray showed that a fragment of the catheter had migrated to the pulmonary circulation, and the patient was referred to a tertiary hospital to have it removed.

The presence of an intravascular foreign body always carries the risk of infection, endocarditis, cardiac or vascular perforation, septic embolisms, hemorrhage, thrombosis, or cardiac arrhythmias. Percutaneous extraction is effective in approximately 90% of cases and has largely replaced surgical extraction.

The migration or fragmentation of catheters, central lines, guidewires, coils, stents, or vena cava filters is the most common. Pins, projectiles, or sharp objects in general can also occasionally be found lodged within blood vessels.

Tunneled central lines can break and migrate due to inappropriate manipulation during placement or withdrawal or to the "pinch-off" syndrome, which occurs when the catheter is trapped and compressed between the clavicle and the first rib while it is being introduced through the subclavian vein.

Endovascular retrieval may require forceps, baskets, and balloons, but snares are the most frequently employed instruments because they are efficacious and easy to manage. Originally, a single nitinol snare fits on the tip of the retrieval catheter; nowadays, three snares simultaneously unfold in three different directions. Turning and advancing the catheter will easily trap the foreign body. It is a good idea to place a thick introducer sheath to receive the recovered foreign body and occasionally also to coaxially introduce an auxiliary guidewire. Although this procedure is generally safe, it can be complicated by perforation or lesion of the vessel, arrhythmias, distal migration, and lodging of the foreign vessel making it impossible to extract.

1. Catheterize the pulmonary artery with a hydrophilic guidewire and 4F pigtail catheter.
2. Determine the exact location of the foreign body using pulmonary angiography in various projections.
3. Replace the hydrophilic guidewire with a stiff guidewire to advance a long 8F introducer sheath through the main left pulmonary artery.
4. Exchange it for a finer guidewire that makes it possible to introduce a snare coaxially.
5. Withdraw the tip of the introducer sheath until it is situated in the cone of the pulmonary artery; the guidewire will ensure that it remains in the correct orientation. From this position, pass the snare over the foreign body that does not fit in the introducer sheath until it becomes trapped.
6. Without releasing the tension over the snare, remove the introducer sheath and the snare simultaneously and extract the foreign body through the groin.

1. 55 cm long 8F introducer sheath
2. 180 cm long J-shaped hydrophilic guidewire
3. 4F pigtail catheter
4. 180 cm long J-shaped 0.035 in. Amplatz guidewire
5. 190 cm long 0.018 in. steel guidewire
6. 3D nitinol gooseneck snare

Case 6.4
■
Embolization of a Renal Arteriovenous Malformation

Figure 6.4.1 Intravenous contrast-enhanced CT in the arterial phase shows a 3 cm hypervascular nodular image in the right renal sinus. Catheterization confirmed the image corresponding to an arteriovenous malformation (AVM) and ruled out other diagnostic possibilities

Figure 6.4.2 Selective catheterization of the interlobar branch reveals an aneurysmatic component that continues with hypertrophic varicose drainage. Contrast material passes rapidly through the renal vein

Figure 6.4.3 Selective embolization of the AVM with bucrylate. With the aim of slowing flow to the vein, we performed embolization with an angioplasty balloon to occlude the renal vein

Figure 6.4.4 Follow-up image shows the exclusion of the AVM. The upper third of the kidney is slightly hypovascularized after embolization. The rest of the kidney shows normal vascularization. Note: there was a very slight iatrogenic dissection of the right renal artery

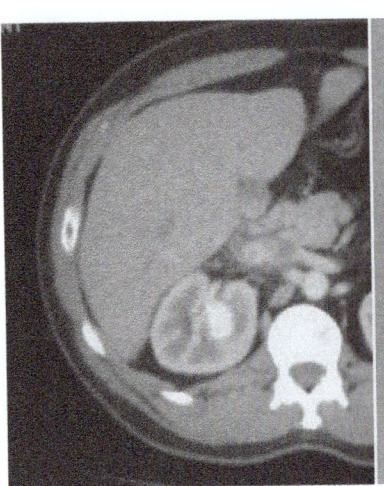
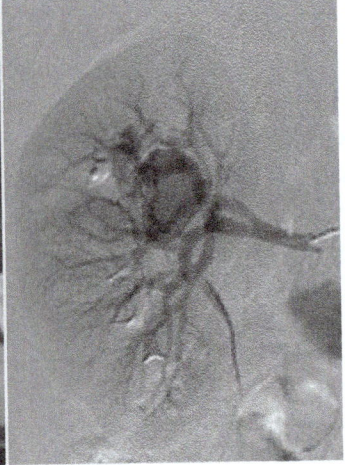

Fig. 6.4.1

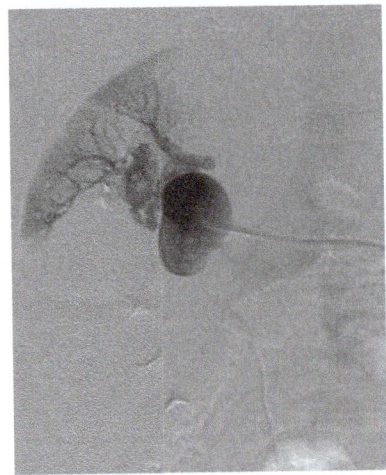

Fig. 6.4.2

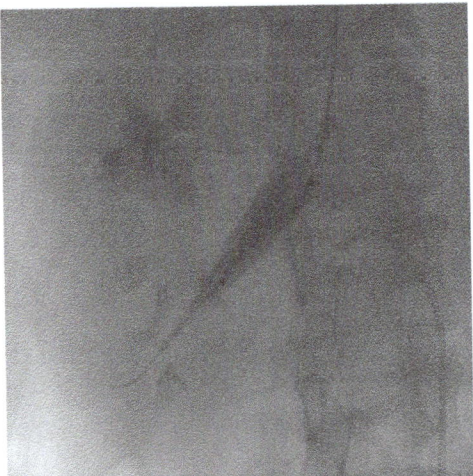

Fig. 6.4.3

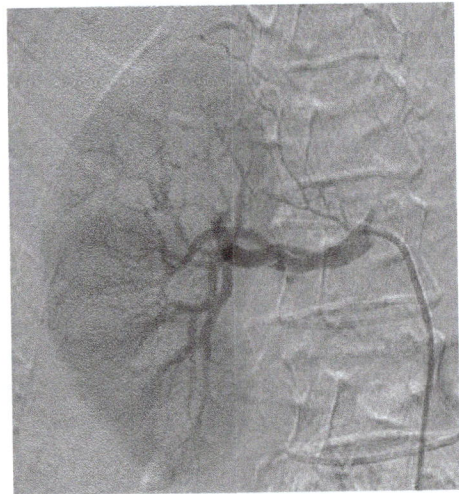

Fig. 6.4.4

A 55-year-old man presented moderate hypochondrial pain and microhematuria. The only relevant history was his mother's death after renal biopsy for hemorrhage.

Ultrasonography identified a lesion with a cystic appearance, but Doppler imaging showed intense vascular enhancement with an erratic high-flow curve with loss of the cyclic systolic–diastolic pattern. CT and catheterization confirmed a renal arteriovenous malformation (AVM). Embolization with bucrylate yielded good angiographic results and allowed the vascularization of the kidney to be conserved.

Comments

Renal AVMs are uncommon and tend to be one of three types: Congenital, acquired, or idiopathic. Acquired AVMs are the most common, accounting for 70% of all renal AVMs; they usually develop after trauma, surgery, biopsy, tumors, or inflammatory processes. Congenital AVMs have the classical presentation (cirsoid type, with hematuria) or the aneurysmatic presentation (abdominal murmur, hypertension, and high-flow heart failure). Idiopathic AVMs are the rarest, accounting for only 3% of all renal AVMs.

At ultrasonography, care should be taken not to confuse AVMs with other processes (hydronephrosis, parapelvic cysts...), especially if percutaneous or surgical intervention is contemplated.

Embolization with sclerosing agents succeeds in 68–100% of cases. This requires the complete occlusion of the arteriovenous fistula; otherwise, recanalization is not uncommon. High-flow AVMs are difficult to resolve because multiple veins and arteries are involved, the risk of occluding arteries with functional responsibilities is present, and the sclerosing agents have a very short contact with the endothelium. Despite the high success rate of embolization of arteriovenous fistulas (40% cured, 28% in partial remission), complications have been reported in 52% of cases. Complications reported include renal failure, tissular necrosis, venous thrombosis, pulmonary embolism, tachycardia, fever, and recanalization.

When embolization fails, persistent hematuria-hemorrhage calls for surgery.

Procedure Steps

1. Perform arterial catheterization with selective canalization of the arterial branch that supplies the AVM. Study the flow velocity and venous return to choose the sclerosing agent and to calculate the velocity of infusion.
2. Perform catheterization through the femoral or jugular vein with the aim of reducing the velocity of venous return with balloon catheters.
3. Infuse the sclerosing agent under continuous fluoroscopic/roadmap guidance until the AVM is completely occluded. Be careful to minimize the occlusion of vessels not included in the AVM.

Equipment List

1. Needle, guidewires, introducer sheaths, catheters.
2. Embolizing agents: Bucrylate, Onyx, alcohol...
3. Angioplasty balloons to occlude vascular flow.

Figure 6.5.1 (**a**) Ascending phlebogram obtained 20 years before the current episode shows a normal left iliac vein. (**b**) Current phlebogram shows chronic obstruction of the left common iliac vein with extensive collateral circulation through the lumbar and pelvic plexuses. (**c**) Extensive postphlebitic changes and left femoral vein insufficiency

Figure 6.5.2 Left calf with edema and hyperpigmentation

Figure 6.5.3 (**a**) Releasing the nitinol stent. (**b**) Partial recanalization with incomplete expansion of the stent. (**c**) Remodeling and intrastent PTA with a 14 mm balloon

Figure 6.5.4 Confirmatory phlebogram shows that the obstruction has been resolved and the collateral circulation has disappeared

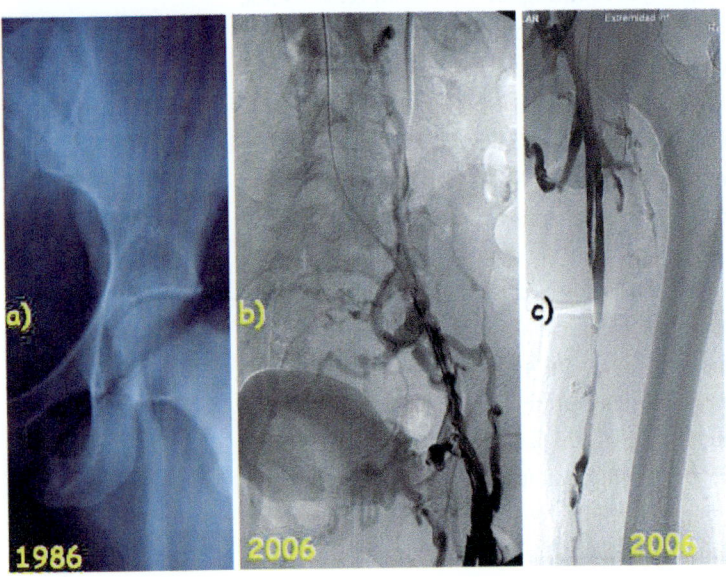
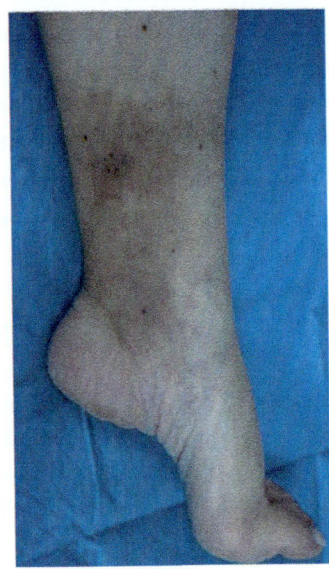

Fig. 6.5.1

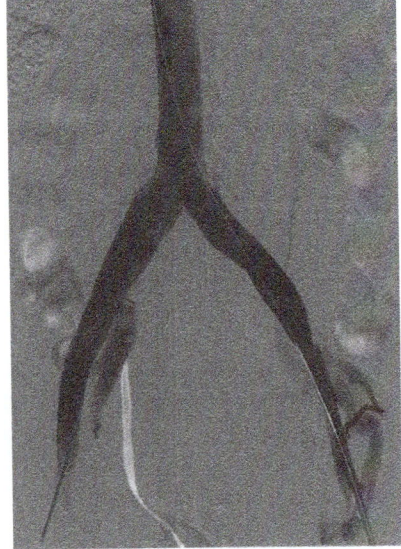

Fig. 6.5.2

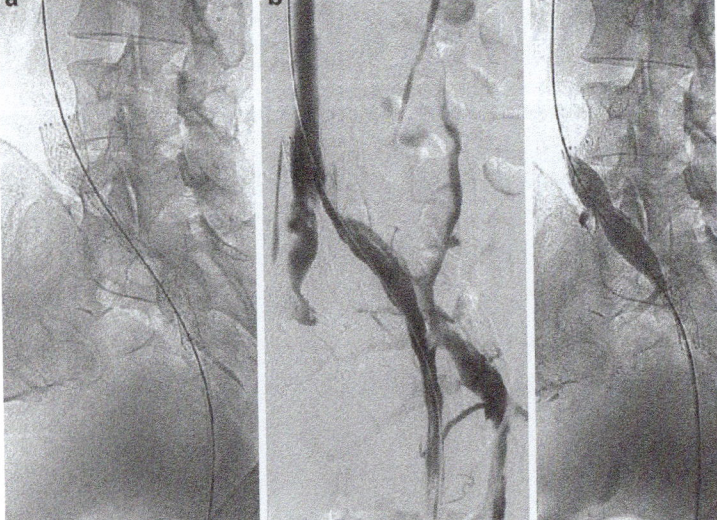

Fig. 6.5.3

Fig. 6.5.4

A 58-year-old woman with three prior episodes of deep vein thrombosis , the first 20 years earlier in relation to a torn calf muscle, and a history of pulmonary thromboembolism was referred after her postthrombotic syndrome continued to progress despite treatment with compression stockings. A varicose ulcer resolved, but chronic lower limb pain persisted. She also had cutaneous atrophy, sclerosis, and hyperpigmentation in the medial aspect of her left calf.

Comments

Recent MRI studies show that up to 66% of the population has asymptomatic compression of the left common iliac vein caused by the crossing of the right common iliac artery. This can partly explain why the incidence of deep vein thrombosis is greater in the left leg than in the right. When this compression is symptomatic, it is known as May–Thurner syndrome. This condition is most prevalent in middle-aged women. It presents as progressive lower limb edema with episodes of pain and can become chronic. These patients will normally have several episodes of deep vein thrombosis in their left legs in the course of their lives. Chronic edema with scleroderma, cutaneous atrophy, hyperpigmentation, and venous ulcers are the final manifestations of a clinical picture in which the postthrombotic syndrome is more severe due to the component of venous insufficiency added to the obstructive component.

A complete cure is improbable, and treatment aims to alleviate symptoms and delay the progression of venous insufficiency. Thus, it is important to reestablish adequate direct venous drainage. Recanalization by stenting is currently the best treatment option, as the results of surgery in this territory are poor. Self-expanding flexible nitinol stents that adapt to the lesion are best; self-expanding steel stents and balloon-expandable stents have worse results. It is also important to choose a large-caliber (14–16 mm) stent to increase the size of the vein and achieve long-lasting patency. The stent should surpass the lesion on both ends by at least 1.5 cm. Placement of the distal end of the stent into the inferior vena cava does not usually have consequences.

Procedure Steps

1. Obtain a phlebogram of the left femoroiliac sector (in this case, through a catheter introduced through the right jugular vein 6 weeks before the intervention). Locate the obstruction and determine its extension. Study the collateral supply. In this case, we also demonstrated that a hydrophilic guidewire could cross the obstructed segment.
2. Puncture the right common femoral vein and insert a 7F introducer sheath.
3. Administer 5,000 IU heparin.
4. Pass a hydrophilic guidewire and a straight 4F catheter through the obstruction.
5. Replace the hydrophilic guidewire with a 180 cm long 0.035 in. Amplatz guidewire with a J-shaped tip.
6. Insert a 6 cm long 14 mm nitinol stent.
7. Dilate and adapt the stent with a 14 mm × 4 cm catheter-balloon at a pressure of 12 atm.
8. Prescribe clopidogrel for 3 months.

Equipment List

1. 23 cm long 7F introducer sheath
2. 180 cm long 0.035 in. hydrophilic guidewire with a J-shaped tip
3. 65 cm long straight 4F catheter
4. 180 cm long stiff 0.035 in. guidewire with a J-shaped tip
5. Large-caliber self-expanding nitinol stent (Smart-Control®, Cordis)
6. Noncompliant angioplasty balloon (14 mm × 4 cm)

Case 6.6

◼

Paget–Schroetter Disease Resolved with Fibrinolysis

Figure 6.6.1 Phlebogram of the left arm shows a filling defect in the axillary vein and complete occlusion of the subclavian vein. The collateral circulation is minimal. Acute deep vein thrombosis was confirmed

Figure 6.6.2 Normal findings at thoracocervical CT rule out underlying disease

Figure 6.6.3 Straight multiperforated catheter inserted through the antecubital vein crosses the fresh thrombus (*arrow*). Phlebography showed that the left subclavian vein and trunk of the innominate vein were permeable and normal. We perfused fibrinolytic drugs through the catheter

Figure 6.6.4 Follow-up phlebogram 36 h later shows complete clinical and radiologic resolution

A 28-year-old woman with no relevant history presented at the emergency department with edema, pain, and paresthesias in her left arm of 24 h' evolution. Doppler US diagnosed acute thrombosis of the axillosubclavian vein. The patient was a

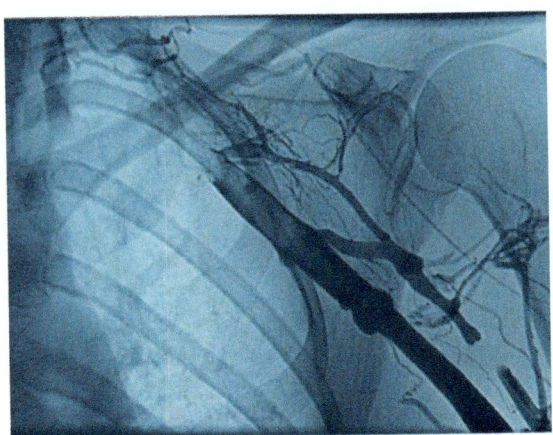

Fig. 6.6.1

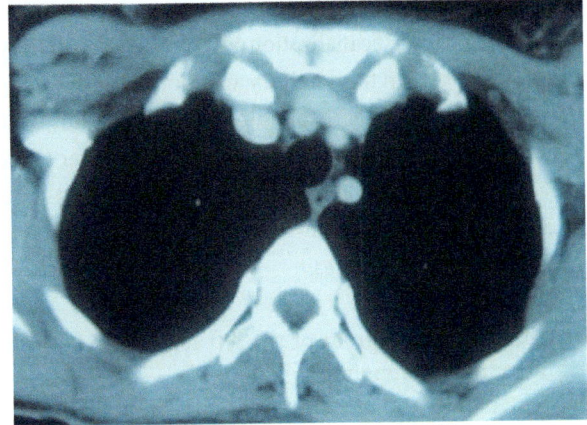

Fig. 6.6.2

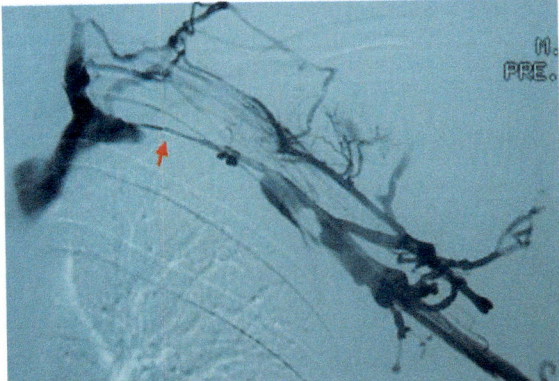

Fig. 6.6.3

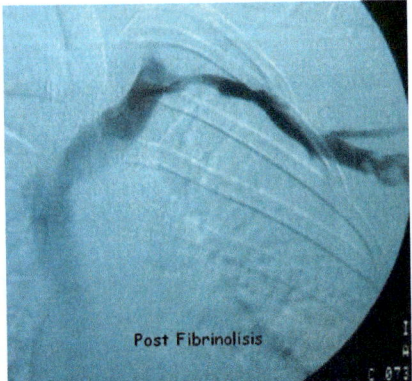

Fig. 6.6.4

nonsmoker and did not use birth control pills, and later studies ruled out thrombophilia. She worked restocking shelves in a shopping center. Effort-induced thrombosis was diagnosed, and direct fibrinolytic treatment was initiated.

Effort-induced thrombosis or Paget–Schroetter disease is acute thrombosis of the upper limb that occurs in healthy young people with no other triggering factor except recent, often strenuous, intense physical exercise. Pain, edema, weakness, and limited mobility are the symptoms. The physiopathological basis is endothelial damage secondary to mechanical trauma, caused by repeated compression of the subclavian vein between the first rib and the clavicle during repeated hyperabduction maneuvers of the upper limb. Classical treatment with anticoagulation and rest leads to chronic edema in 70% of cases. Nowadays, more aggressive treatment is recommended to establish early recanalization and prevent the postphlebitic syndrome. Fibrinolysis is efficacious provided that the thrombus has been present for less than 2 weeks. Adding mechanical thrombolysis by fragmentation or aspiration to pharmacological fibrinolysis is recommended to achieve better and faster results. Breaking up and aspirating the thrombus help increase the surface area of the thrombus in contact with the fibrinolytic drug. If treatment is delayed, there is a high risk of chronic thrombosis of the subclavian vein, in which case only general measures aimed at alleviating pain and edema can be applied.

Once the clinical symptoms have resolved, surgical resection of the anterior portion of the first rib to decompress the vein should be considered. There is no consensus regarding when this should be done, but it seems that decompression within a month of the episode yields better long-term results. In principle, recanalization by stenting is not very efficacious for late chronic obstruction, as nearly 100% become reobstructed.

Procedure Steps

1. Puncture the antecubital vein, confirm the diagnosis by phlebography, and determine the extent of the thrombosis. Obtain a phlebogram of the central vessels.
2. Insert a short 4F introducer sheath and pass a hydrophilic guidewire and straight catheter through the thrombus.
3. Administer heparin for anticoagulation using a pump through a peripheral line: the target should be to maintain the INR between 2 and 2.5.
4. Place the tip of the catheter inside the thrombus and anchor it firmly to the skin and to the introducer sheath to avoid displacement.
5. Inject a bolus of 200,000 IU of urokinase and perfuse urokinase through the catheter at a rate of 50,000–100,000 IU/h.
6. Check the results by phlebography every 12 h.

Equipment List

1. 5.5 cm short 4F introducer sheath in the left antecubital vein
2. 150 cm long J-shaped 0.035 in. hydrophilic guidewire
3. Straight 4F multiperforated catheter
4. Anticoagulation using a pump to infuse heparin through a peripheral line in the contralateral arm
5. Urokinase

Case 6.7

■

Treatment of Superior Vena Cava Syndrome with Metallic Stents

Figure 6.7.1 Bilateral phlebogram shows thrombosis of the right subclavian vein, brachiocephalic trunk, innominate vein, and superior vena cava, with extensive collateral circulation. A guidewire and catheter are passed through the left basilic vein into the superior vena cava and inferior vena cava

Figure 6.7.2 Implanting stents (Wallstents®) along the thrombosed segment

Figure 6.7.3 Balloon dilation until angiography shows the lumen open to at least 10 mm in diameter

Figure 6.7.4 Follow-up angiography of the vena cava shows the absence of proximal reflux and preferential flow through the vena cava rather than through the collateral vascular bed

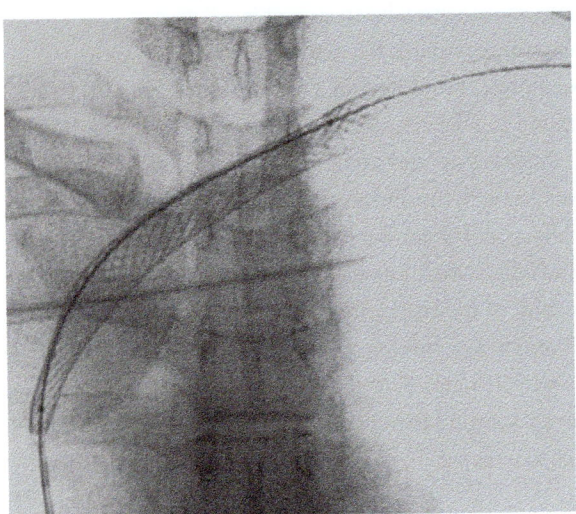

Fig. 6.7.1

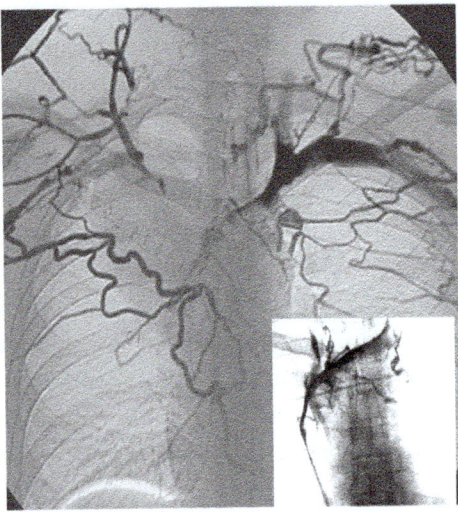

Fig. 6.7.2

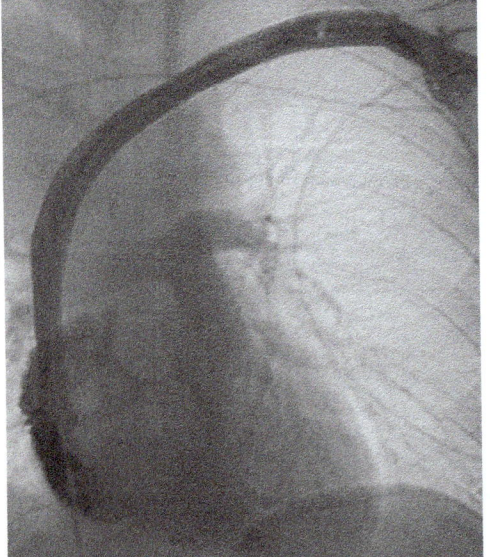

Fig. 6.7.3

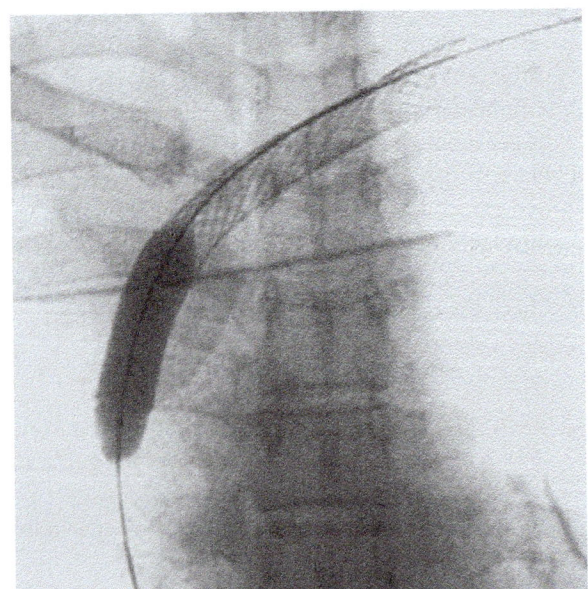

Fig. 6.7.4

A 58-year-old woman with a mediastinal leiomyosarcoma presented with recent onset edema and venous congestion in the upper half of the body. After confirming thrombosis/obstruction of the superior vena cava, we implanted stents in the obstructed venous segment. Clinical symptoms resolved within 2 days.

The superior vena cava syndrome is usually caused by a tumor compressing the vessel, and lung tumors are the most common cause of the syndrome. Although benign causes are less common, the increased use of permanent or semipermanent catheters and pacemakers has made them more common.

The traditional management includes medical therapy based on changing positions, diuretics, anticoagulants, corticoids, radiotherapy, and chemotherapy.

Another alternative is surgery to reconstruct the vein with a bridge between the right jugular or left innominate vein and the right atrium, which requires thoracotomy.

Metallic stents have been implanted as an effective palliative treatment in these cases, bringing about rapid improvement in symptoms due to obstruction.

The reported morbidity and mortality range from 0 to 23% and 0 to 6.7%, respectively. Complications include stent migration, pulmonary edema due to increased venous return, pulmonary embolism, acute thrombosis of the stent, and hemorrhage, among others. Technical success in different series with follow-up between 2.9 and 17 months ranges from 95 to 100%, clinical success from 90 to 100% (with clinical resolution in 2–6 days), primary patency from 77 to 92%, and secondary patency from 85 to 100%.

In cases of reobstruction, the same endovascular techniques can be used to treat the patient again.

Comments

1. Obtain a phlebogram of the superior vena cava to confirm stenosis/obstruction.
2. Approach the stenosis with shapeable angiographic catheters and hydrophilic guidewires through the basilic or jugular vein.
3. Implant a stent in the area of the obstruction/stenosis.
4. Expand the stent, with an angioplasty balloon if necessary.

Procedure Steps

1. Needle for puncture, introducer sheath, catheters, guidewires for navigation (Terumo®) and support (Amplatz®).
2. Self-expanding stents with diameters between 10 and 18 mm (Wallstent®). Sometimes multiple stents are necessary.
3. Angioplasty balloons (10–18 mm in diameter).

Equipment List

Case 6.8

Percutaneous Thrombectomy of a Hemodialysis Access

Figure 6.8.1 Brachioaxillary graft in the thrombosed left arm. Proximal puncture and scant injection of contrast material. There is no flow; filling defects occupy the access lumen

Figure 6.8.2 Mechanical thrombectomy using an Arrow-Trerotola device (*arrow*). The insert shows the final outcome, still without flow

Figure 6.8.3 Angioplasty over the underlying stenosis in the venous anastomosis

Figure 6.8.4 Final confirmation phlebogram shows the absence of both thrombosis and residual stenosis. A pulse and thrill were palpated at physical examination

A 72-year-old woman with terminal renal failure undergoing hemodialysis with a 6 mm Goretex vascular access placed 18 months earlier presented with a few weeks' history of increased venous pressure during dialysis and absent pulse in the vascular access of 24 h' evolution. The access was rescued using percutaneous mechanical thrombectomy, and the pulse and thrill were restored. This procedure was performed on an outpatient basis and enabled the patient to undergo her habitual dialysis session.

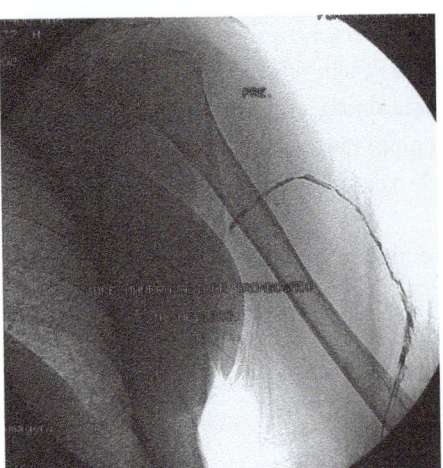

Fig. 6.8.1

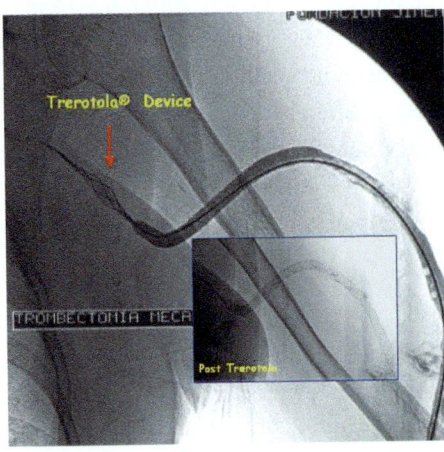

Fig. 6.8.2

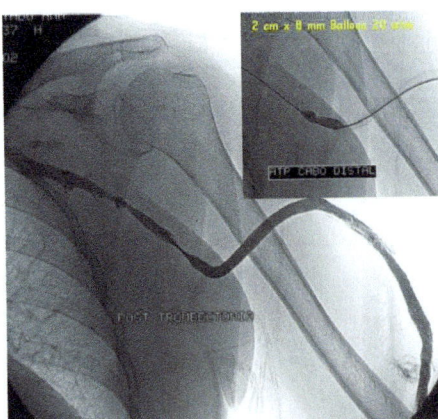

Fig. 6.8.3

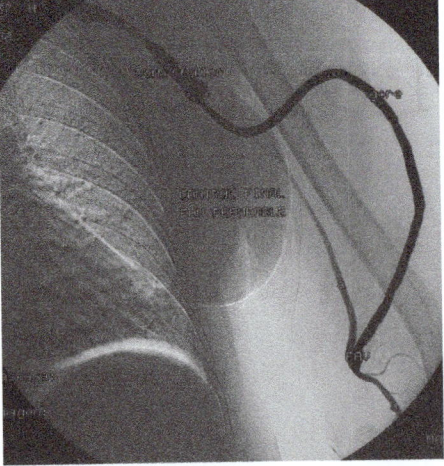

Fig. 6.8.4

Interventional radiologists must perform periodic angioplasties to maintain and prolong the patency of vascular accesses. When acute thrombosis occurs, interventional procedures also have an important role in treatment. One of the main advantages over surgical thrombectomy is that the access can be used immediately after percutaneous treatment. Diverse techniques are all more or less valid; we will choose the one that is most available and which we have the most experience in. In most cases, there is very severe underlying stenosis causing the thrombosis, and it is essential to locate it and treat it with angioplasty. Thrombectomy can be performed using fibrinolytic drugs or thrombectomy devices with hydrodynamic aspiration systems or mechanical fragmentation systems. Another effective approach involves inserting a thick introducer sheath and manually aspirating the thrombus through it. Several of these techniques are often combined.

When acute thrombosis affects a synthetic fistula, the Arrow-Trerotola device is efficacious. It works by fragmenting, macerating, and dislodging the thrombus from the wall of the graft, converting it into microparticles measuring $300\,\mu$ or less that are pushed toward the systemic circulation without causing any damage. The venous anastomosis should be dilated either before or after treatment with the Arrow-Trerotola, because severe stenosis is nearly always the cause of the dysfunction and thrombosis of the access. Lastly, the thrombus "plug" that remains in the arterial end must be removed; this is achieved by retrogradely advancing a deflated balloon up to the humeral artery and inflating it at a low pressure, then withdrawing it to allow the blood to flow.

1. Puncture the arterial end of the thrombosed fistula.
2. While compressing the arterial anastomosis, carefully inject contrast material through the thrombus to define its extension.
3. Advance the Arrow-Trerotola system. Once finished, wash out the anastomosis carefully, pushing the microfragments into the circulatory flow.
4. Perform PTA of the stenosis in the venous anastomosis with a 7–8 mm balloon.
5. Through the femoral vein, catheterize the axillary vein first and then continue through the Goretex until the humeral artery is reached retrogradely. Inflate a 6 mm balloon at low pressure and pull it through the entire access.

1. Percutaneous thrombectomy is an outpatient procedure performed under local anesthesia. Anticoagulation and fibrinolytics are only necessary if the thrombus extends into the axillosubclavian axis.
2. 5.5 cm long 6F introducer sheath for brachial access.
3. 180 cm long hydrophilic guidewire with a J-shaped tip.
4. Angioplasty balloons (7 and 8 mm) with a 50 cm instrument for dilating the venous anastomosis. 7 mm cutting balloon (optional).
5. 65 cm Arrow-Trerotola PTD® without a guidewire
6. 90 cm long 6F introducer sheath to access from the femoral vein.
7. 125 cm multipurpose catheter and 260 cm straight-tipped Amplatz guidewire with a 3 cm "flopppy" tip.
8. 6 mm × 2 cm balloon and 135 cm instrument for the final retrograde thrombectomy.

Case 6.9
Inferior Vena Cava Thrombolysis

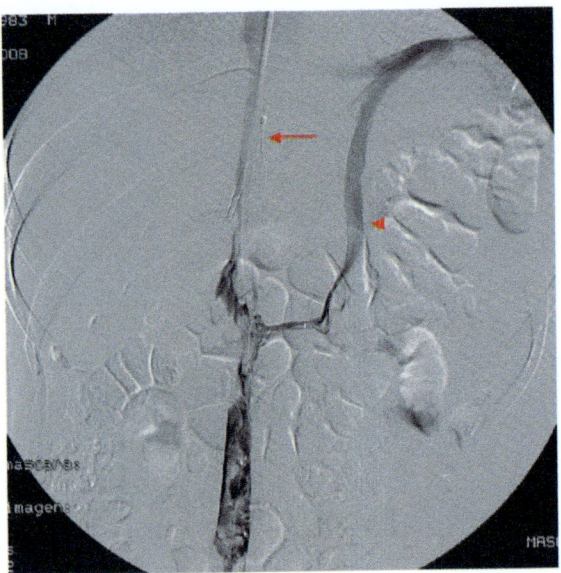

Fig. 6.9.1

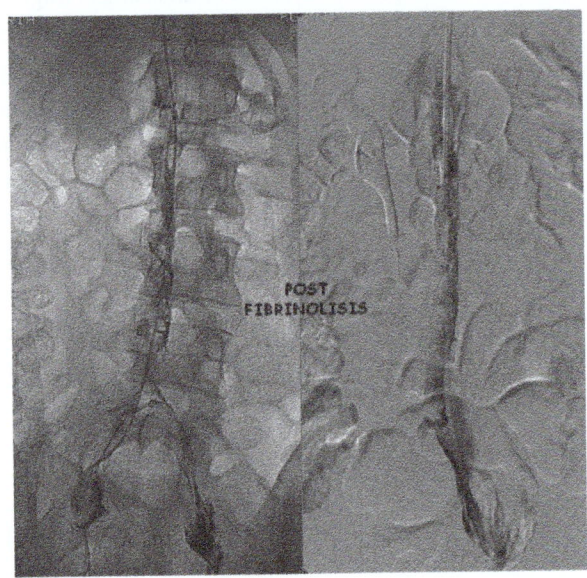

Fig. 6.9.2

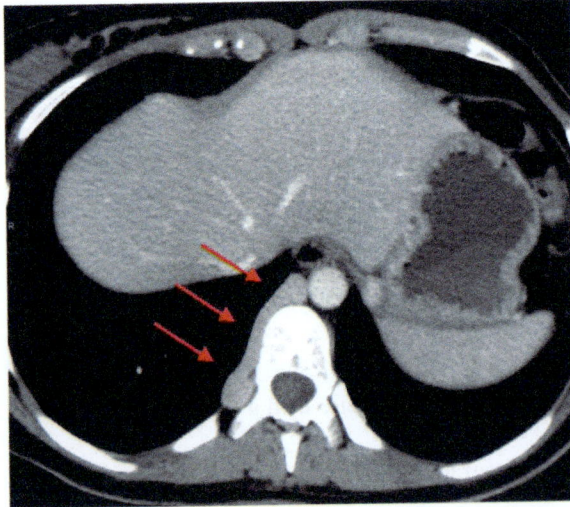

Fig. 6.9.3

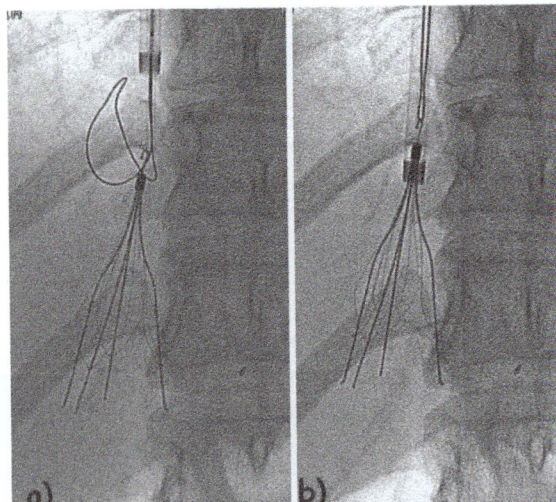

Fig. 6.9.4

Figure 6.9.1 Angiogram of the vena cava obtained using a jugular approach shows extensive filling defects in the inferior vena cava and the origin of the left renal vein. The left renal vein drains through a thick retroperitoneal collateral vessel (*arrow head*). A filter has been placed in the suprarenal vena cava (*arrow*). The right renal vein (not shown) was patent

Figure 6.9.2 Phlebogram obtained 36 h after fibrinolytic treatment shows little change

Figure 6.9.3 Intravenous contrast-enhanced CT shows dense retroperitoneal collateral circulation (*arrows*)

Figure 6.9.4 Removal of the filter from the vena cava: (**a**) Capture with a snare, (**b**) while maintaining smooth traction of the snare, the introducer sheath is advanced, folding the filter and dislodging it from the inferior vena cava

A previously healthy 25-year-old woman with a 3-week history of low back pain treated with NSAIDs presented after 2 days' clinical worsening including extensive edema in both lower limbs accompanied by pain, paresthesias, claudication, and coldness. At physical examination, the femoral pulses were palpated, but the pedal pulses were absent. Diagnosed with phlegmasia cerulea dolens, she was administered anticoagulation and fibrinolytic treatment resulting in little radiologic improvement but appreciable clinical improvement.

Comments

Symptomatic extensive proximal thrombosis of the iliocaval venous sector leads to significant long-term morbidity, so early recanalization is recommended. Young, active patients with occlusive thrombosis and phlegmasia cerulea are the most widely accepted indications for early recanalization.

In addition to conventional fibrinolytic treatment, mechanical fragmentation or thromboaspiration will improve the efficacy of treatment, although these procedures will also increase the risk of pulmonary thromboembolism. For this reason, several authors recommend the temporary placement of a vena cava filter prior to treatment. Several mixed models have been commercialized. These mixed models are similar to conventional filters that can be left in place permanently; however, the mixed models can be removed percutaneously before their struts become integrated into the walls of the inferior vena cava. It is also important to consider the age of the thrombus; treatment of thrombi older than 14–21 days is rarely successful. This partially explains the treatment failure in the present case, in which the presence of a well-developed collateral circulation shows that this was a new acute episode involving an old thrombus. In most cases, some residual thrombus remains; however, treatment should aim to bring about clinical improvement by reestablishing flow through the obstructed vessel rather than to achieve optimal angiographic results.

In selected cases, placing a large-caliber self-expanding stent is justifiable.

Procedure Steps

1. Administer anticoagulation using a heparin pump through a peripheral vein with a target PTT of 60–90 s.
2. Admit the patient to the ICU during fibrinolysis.
3. Puncture the right internal jugular vein, insert a 4F introducer sheath and a pigtail catheter over a hydrophilic guidewire, and smoothly advance retrogradely through the iliocaval thrombus.
4. Obtain an angiogram of the iliocaval sector to locate the thrombus and determine its extension by manually injecting contrast material.
5. Taking into account the extension of the thrombus, place a removable vena cava filter in the suprarenal vena cava for prophylaxis.
6. Insert a straight multiperforated catheter into the thrombus and inject a bolus of 200,000 IU of urokinase.
7. Perfuse urokinase 150,000 IU/h during the first 10 h and then 70,000 IU/h during the next 26 h.
8. Remove the vena cava filter 7 days later.

Equipment List

1. 4F introducer sheath
2. 4F pigtail catheter
3. 180 cm long J-shaped 0.035 in. hydrophilic guidewire
4. Günter-Tulip® (CooK) removable vena cava filter over an 8.5F jugular system
5. Straight multiperforated catheter
6. Urokinase
7. Filter extraction system with a 60 cm long 11F introducer sheath and a snare

Case 6.10

■

Endovascular Treatment of a Varicocele

Figure 6.10.1 Steps involved in spermatic phlebography: Canalization of the left renal vein (**a**) and seeking the ostium of the spermatic vein (**b**), navigation through and injection of contrast material into the spermatic vein (**c**), and visualization of the course of the internal spermatic vein and its collateral vessels up to the testis (**d**)

Figure 6.10.2 Releasing coils into the vein

Figure 6.10.3 Contrast-enhanced follow-up showing the occlusion/thrombosis of the vein

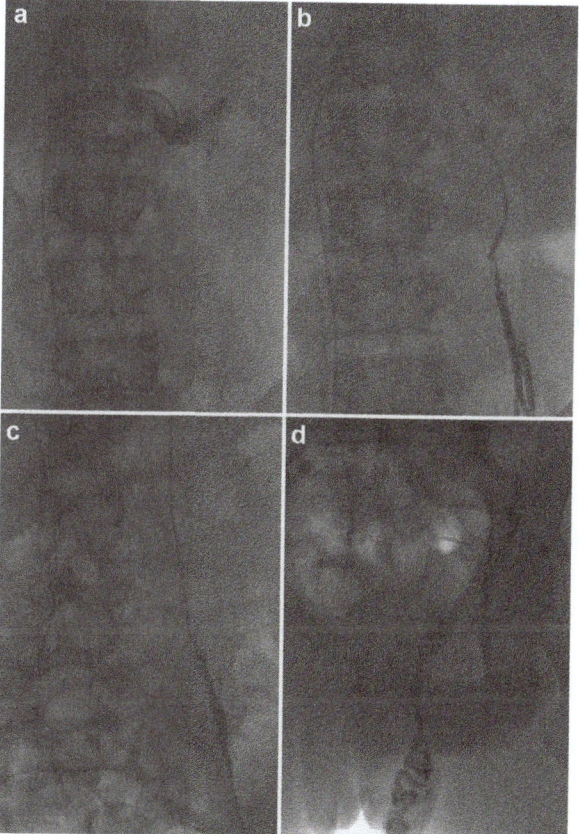

Fig. 6.10.1

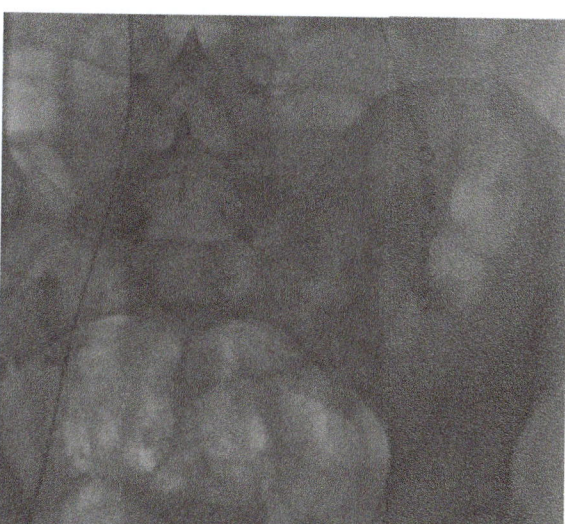

Fig. 6.10.2

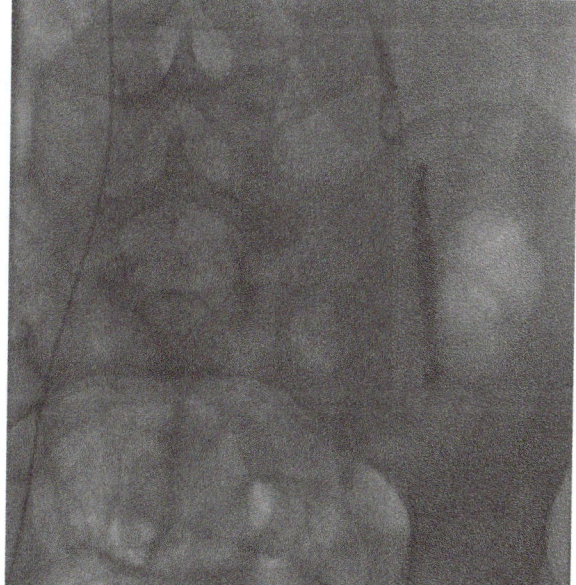

Fig. 6.10.3

A 25-year-old man consulting for infertility presented with intermittent testicular pain. At physical examination, a cord was palpated in the scrotal sac, and it was accentuated on standing and during the Valsalva maneuver. Doppler US showed venous dilation and reversal of flow during the Valsalva maneuver.

Comments

A varicocele is an abnormal dilation of the pampiniform plexus that can extend from the spermatic vein to the level of the renal vein. In most cases, there is an incompetence of the venous valvular system. Varicoceles are usually primary though they may occur secondary to compression at different venous levels. Their incidence ranges between 8 and 23% in young men. The left side is affected in 70–100%.

The most common indications for the correction of varicoceles are

- Infertility lasting at least 2 years, with oligoasthenospermia and no other apparent cause of infertility (the etiology and indication of the treatment are controversial)
- Pain and/or testicular mass
- Testicular atrophy in boys or adolescents
- Recurrence of the varicocele after surgery.

Treatment options include surgery and embolization. One advantage of embolization is that it is minimally invasive, and phlebography is usually used to plan treatment in any case.

The most common technical problems and complications of embolization are difficulties in the canalization of the testicular vein and its tributaries, perforation of the wall of the vein, and migration of embolizing material. The estimated mean dose of radiation to the gonads is 26 mrad, which is low. The failure rate of embolization of the testicular vein is between 1.25 and 4%.

Procedure Steps

1. Puncture the right common femoral vein after infiltrating 2% lidocaine solution with a 5F cobra or multipurpose catheter.
2. Look for the spermatic veins and perform phlebography. On the basis of the anatomy, decide whether to proceed with embolization.
3. Different materials including Ivalon, coils, gelfoam, sotradecol, detachable balloons, sclerosing agents, etc. can be used to embolize the spermatic vein. Coils are currently the most common.

Equipment List

1. Venous puncture needle, hydrophilic guidewires, introducer sheaths, guiding catheters, and different-shaped catheters.
2. Embolizing material: Mainly coils, slightly larger than the diameter of the spermatic vein (5–8 mm).

Further Reading

Al-Hwiesh AK, Abdul-Rahaman IS. Tunneled femoral vein catheterization for long term hemodialysis: a single center experience. Saudi J Kidney Dis Transpl 2007; 18(1): 37–42.

Bonvini RF, Rastan A, Sixt S, Noory E, Beschorner U, Leppanen O, March F, Schwarzwälder U, Bürgelin K, Zeller T. Percutaneous retrieval of intravascular and intracardiac foreign bodies with a dedicated three-dimensional snare: a 3 year single center experience. Catheter Cardiovasc Interv 2009; 74(6): 939–945.

Borrego-Utiel FJ, Pérez del Barrio P y col. Catéteres femorales como acceso vascular para hemodiálisis crónica en pacientes ambulatorios. Nefrologia 1996; 16(5): 432–438.

Chin D, Petersen B, Timmermans H, Rosch J. Stent-graft in the management of superior vena cava syndrome. Cardiovasc Intervent Radiol 1996; 19: 302–304.

Crotty KL, Orihuela E, Warren MM. Recent advances in the diagnosis and treatment of renal arteriovenous malformations and fistulas. J Urol 1993; 150(5 pt 1): 1355–1359.

Egglin TK, Dickey KW, Rosemblatt M, Pollak JS. Retrieval of intravascular foreign bodies: Experience in 32 cases. AJR Am J Roentgenol 1995; 164: 1259–1264.

Enden T, Klow NE, Sandvik L, et al Catheter-directed thrombolysis versus anticoagulant therapy alone in deep vein thrombosis: results of an open randomized, controlled trial reporting on short term patency. J Thromb Haemost 2009; 7(8): 1268–1275.

Kakkos SK, Haddad GK, Haddad JA, Scully MM. Secondary patency of thrombosed prosthetic vascular access grafts with aggressive surveillance, monitoring and endovascular management. Eur J Vasc Endovasc Surg 2008; 36: 356–365.

Kearon C, Kahn SR, Agnelli G, Goldhaber S, Raskob GE, Camerota AJ; American College of Chest Physicians. Antithrombotic therapy for venous thromboembolic disease. ACCP evidence-based clinical practice guidelines, 8th edn. Chest 2008; 133: 454S–545S.

Lai W-C, Fang J-T. Renal cyst mimicking arteriovenous malformation. Nephrol Dial Transplant 2006; 21(6): 1725–1726.

Lanciego C, Chacón JL, Julián A, Andrade J, López L, Martínez B, et al. Stenting as first option for endovascular treatment of malignant superior vena cava syndrome. AJR Am J Roentgenol 2001; 177: 585–593.

Maya ID, Allon M. Outcomes of tunneled femoral hemodialysis catheters: comparison with internal jugular vein catheters. Kidney Int 2005; 68(6): 2886–2889.

Molina JE, Hunter DW, Dietz CA. Protocols for Paget-Schroetter syndrome and late treatment of chronic subclavian vein obstruction. Ann Thorac Surg 2009; 87: 416–422.

Murphy EH, Davis CM, Journeycake JM, DeMuth RP, Arko FR. Symptomatic iliofemoral DVT after onset of oral contraceptive use in women with previously undiagnosed May-Thurner syndrome. J Vasc Surg 2009; 49(3): 697–703.

O'Sullivan GJ, Semba CP, Bittner CA, Kee ST, Razavi MK, Dake MD. Endovascular management of iliac vein compression (May-Thurner) syndrome. J Vasc Interv Radiol 2000; 11: 1297–1302.

Savader SJ, Treotola SO. Venous interventional radiology with clinical perspectives, 2nd edn. New York: Thieme; 1996.

Shah AD, Bajaklan DR, Olin JW, Lookstein RA. Power-pulse spray thrombectomy for the treatment of Paget-Schroetter syndrome. AJR Am J Roentgenol 2007; 188: 1215–1217.

Shebel ND, Whalen CC. Diagnosis and management of iliac veion compression syndrome. J Vasc Nurs 2005; 23: 10–17.

Trocciola SM, Chaer RA, Lin SC, et al. Embolization of renal artery aneurysm and arteriovenous fistula. A case report. Vasc Endovascular Surg 2005; 39: 525.

Turmel-Rodrigues L. Stenosis and thrombosis in hemodialysis fistulae and grafts: the radiologist's point of view. Nephrol Dial Transplant 2004; 19: 306–308.

Wang PC, Liang HL, Huang JS, et al. Percutaneous retrieval of dislodged central venous port catheter: experience of 25 patients in a single institute. Acta Radiol 2009; 50: 15–20.

Wilson LD, Detterbeck FC, Yahalom J. Superior vena cava syndrome with malignant causes. N Engl J Med 2007; 356: 1862–1869.

José J. Muñoz, José Rodriguez, Iván Artero, and Pedro J. Aranda

J.J. Muñoz and R. Ribes, *Learning Vascular and Interventional Radiology*, Learning Imaging,
DOI: 10.1007/978-3-540-87997-8_7, © Springer-Verlag Berlin Heidelberg 2010

Case 7.1

Aneurysm of the Ascending Aorta and Aortic Arch. Hybrid Treatment

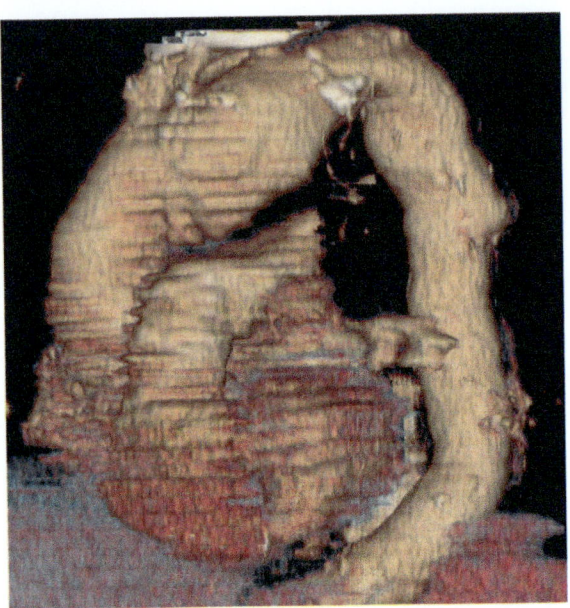

Fig. 7.1.1

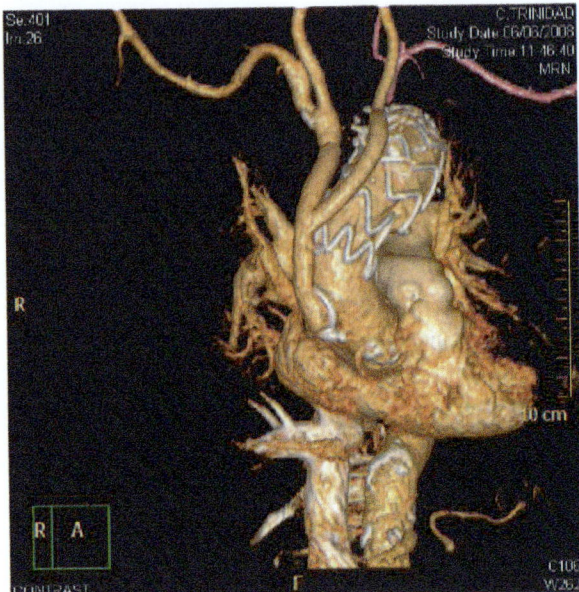

Fig. 7.1.2

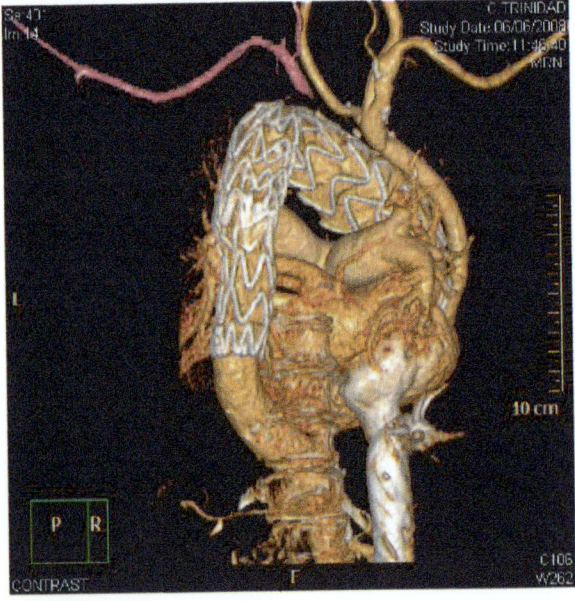

Fig. 7.1.3

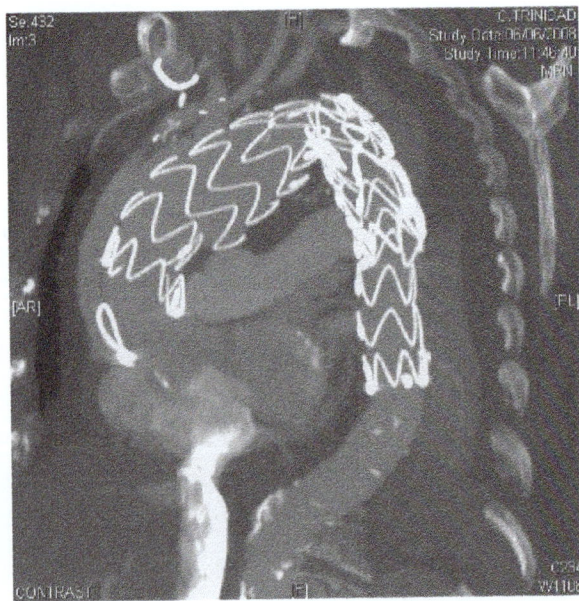

Fig. 7.1.4

Figure 7.1.1 Thoracic CT angiogram shows an aneurysm of the aortic arch involving the roots of the supraaortic trunk. The irregularity of the aortic wall extends to the proximal descending aorta. Some artifacts are present because the study was performed using helical CT

Figure 7.1.2 Volume-rendered thoracic CT angiogram obtained at an angle that allows the ascending aorta to be visualized. A Y-bypass joins the ascending aorta with the right brachiocephalic trunk and the left carotid artery. Late filling of the left subclavian artery through the ipsilateral vertebral artery is shown in red. The proximal tip of the stent-graft is only 1 cm from the anastomosis of the bypass

Figure 7.1.3 Posterior view volume-rendered CT angiogram shows the connection between the two stent-grafts with a 5-cm overlap. The proximal third of the distal stent-graft extends to the descending thoracic aorta

Figure 7.1.4 Parasagittal projection MPR CT angiogram shows the anterior situation of the bypass and the entire course of the two overlapping stent-grafts, with the exclusion of the aortic arch aneurysm

A 73-year-old female patient with a history of hypertension treated with two drugs, cholecystectomy, appendectomy, hiatal hernia, and dyslipemia presented at the emergency department with a 2-day history of central chest pain radiating to the shoulder and neck. Pulmonary thromboembolism was suspected but ruled out with lung scintigraphy. Pain ceased spontaneously and the patient's condition stabilized, so she was scheduled to undergo CT angiography on an outpatient basis. CT angiography showed an aneurysm of the ascending aorta and aortic arch measuring $77 \times 67 \times 60$ mm with a mural thrombus and a penetrating ulcer in the descending aorta (Fig. 7.1.1). The medical-surgical committee decided on hybrid treatment.

Comments

Aneurysms that affect the aortic arch represent a great challenge for endovascular treatment due to the curvature of the aorta and the variability in the position of the supra-aortic trunks. Thus, the procedure requires complex reconstruction techniques or personalized grafts to ensure adequate fixation and sealing without compromising the blood flow to the brain or upper limbs. Hybrid treatment is a feasible alternative that has lower morbidity and mortality than classical surgery.

Procedure Steps

1. Administer general anesthesia and perform midline sternotomy.
2. Effect an end-to-side bypass to the ascending aorta without extracorporeal circulation.
3. Place a Y-graft from ascending aorta, 2 cm distal the aortic valve, to the brachiocephalic trunk and the left carotid artery.
4. With a vascular micropuncture kit, place a 6F valved introducer sheath through the left brachial artery and pass a 260 cm long 0.035 in. Terumo guidewire and a 100 cm long 5F calibrated pigtail catheter for angiographic controls.
5. Insert a 6F introducer sheath through the left femoral artery.

6. Insert a multipurpose catheter through the introducer sheath and a 260 cm long 0.035 in. Terumo guidewire until the aortic arch.
7. Replace it with a 300 cm long superstiff 0.035 in. Lunderquist guidewire and pass a 36 × 36 × 150 mm straight Valiant (MEDTRONIC) endograft with a closed-web proximal configuration and place it in the aortic arch. Using an antegrade approach, pass a 46 × 46 × 200 mm straight Valiant (MEDTRONIC) endograft with FreeFlo proximal configuration to place it 1 cm from the anastomosis of the ascending aorta with an overlap of three rings on the distal endograft.
8. Check the results with angiography; in this case, the angiographic control showed a minimal late leak through the left subclavian artery and we decided to wait and see how it evolved.
9. Drain the cerebrospinal fluid through the upper spine, close in layers, and leave two mediastinal drains in place.

Follow-up CT angiography 5 days later showed patency of all supra-aortic vessels without evidence of leakage, patency of the left subclavian artery through the ipsilateral vertebral artery, patency of the endografts, and bilateral pleural effusion (Figs. 7.1.2–7.1.3). The patient evolved satisfactorily.

Equipment List

1. Material for midline sternotomy
2. 8 mm × 60 cm and 10 mm × 30 cm Dacron grafts (Hemashield)
3. Cerebrospinal fluid drainage
4. Valiant (MEDTRONIC) coated endografts (36 × 36 × 150 mm and 46 × 46 × 200 mm)
5. Aortic angioplasty balloon
6. 100 cm long multipurpose and pigtail catheters
7. 260 cm long 0.035 in. Terumo guidewire and 300 cm long 0.035 in. Lunderquist guidewire
8. Vascular micropuncture kit
9. Stopcocks, injection pump, nonionic iodinated contrast (320 mg I/mL)

Case 7.2
Endovascular Treatment of an Aortobronchial Fistula

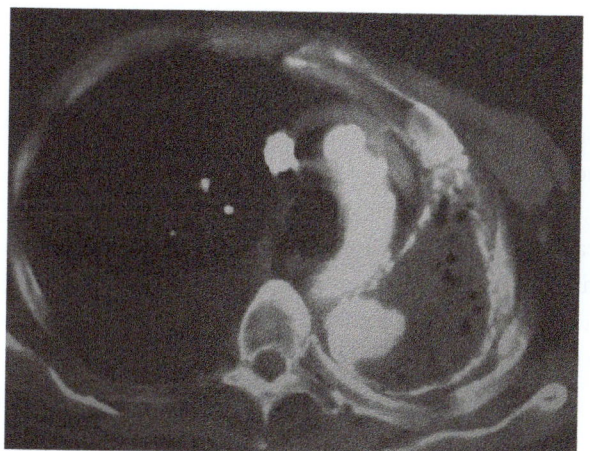

Fig. 7.2.1

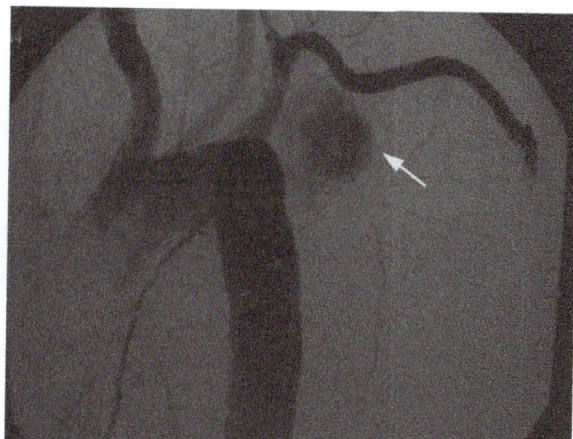

Fig. 7.2.2

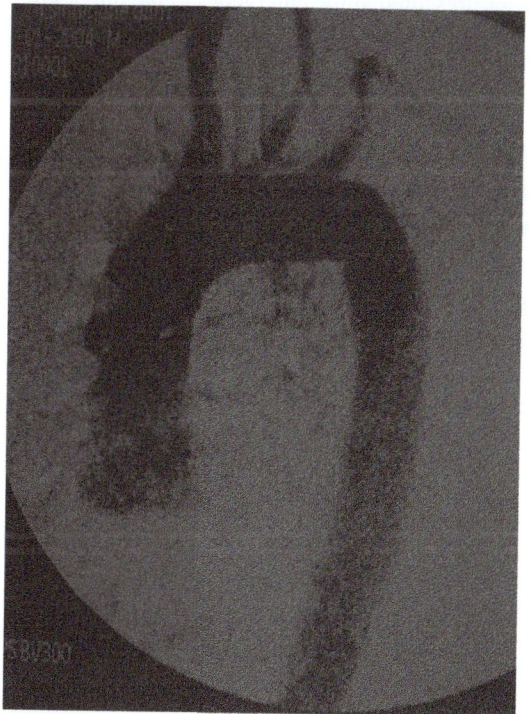

Fig. 7.2.3

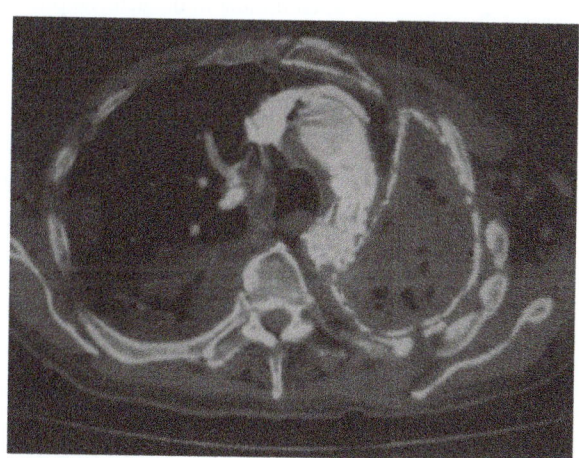

Fig. 7.2.4

Figure 7.2.1 Thoracic CT angiogram in a patient who had undergone left pneumonectomy shows a residual cavity with calcified walls and bubbles inside, probably due to superinfection, as well as an area with the density of fat, related to omental filling during pneumonectomy. The rounded image (*arrow*) with intense arterial phase enhancement suggests probable arterial vascular disease. Right pleural effusion with atelectasis due to compression of the right basal segments is also seen

Figure 7.2.2 Aortogram acquired through the femoral artery: a 5F pigtail catheter is in the aortic arch. There is a pseudoaneurysm of the proximal descending thoracic aorta (*arrow*) measuring 40 mm in diameter distal to the ostium of the left subclavian artery. Surgical clips from the previous thoracotomy. (**a**) Angiography of the thoracic aorta showed a pseudoaneurysm measuring 40 mm in diameter in the descending aorta 30 mm from the branching of the left subclavian artery. (**b**) The medical-surgical team decided on endovascular treatment of the pseudoaneurysm in the thoracic aorta

Figure 7.2.3 Intraoperative angiogram acquired with a portable Philips BV 300 plus fluoroscopy system through a pigtail catheter in the ascending aorta: no filling of the pseudoaneurysm is observed after the stent-graft is deployed

Figure 7.2.4 Postoperative thoracic CT angiogram shows the absence of pseudoaneurysmatic filling in the calcified cavity (compare with Fig. 7.2.1) and right pleural effusion

A 72-year-old male patient with a history of left pneumonectomy and posterior radiotherapy 12 years earlier for stage IIIA nonsmall-cell lung carcinoma, an abscess in the thoracotomy scar with empyema drained 4 years earlier, and a pleurocutaneous fistula and chronic bleeding embolized one year earlier presented at the emergency department after repeated episodes of bleeding from the fistula in the left hemithorax. He was admitted to the thoracic surgery ward, where he had several bleeding episodes that required red blood cell transfusion.

Chest CT showed a residual cavity after left pneumonectomy with calcified walls and bubbles inside, probably due to superinfection, and an area with the density of fat related to omental filling in the previous surgical intervention. A rounded image with intense contrast uptake in the arterial phase suggested arterial disease. He also had right pleural effusion with atelectasis due to the compression of the right lower segments.

Comments   Aortobronchial fistulas are rare and potentially life threatening. Classical treatment by open surgery led to high morbidity and mortality. Nowadays, endovascular treatment is the treatment of choice, especially in patients with high surgical risk. The endograft can become infected, but this occurs in a low percentage of patients. Close follow-up is necessary after treatment.

Procedure Steps

1. Administer general anesthesia. Approach through the left brachial artery with a Cook micropuncture kit and insert a 6F valved introducer sheath.
2. Insert a 100 cm long 5F pigtail catheter through the introducer sheath until the ascending aorta to obtain angiograms.
3. Once AP and 35° left oblique projections have been obtained, make a transversal incision in the right femoral artery and insert a 100 cm long 5F multipurpose catheter and a 260 cm long flexible 0.035 in. Terumo guidewire until the catheter reaches the ascending aorta.
4. Replace the Terumo guidewire with a 260 cm long extra-stiff 0.035 in. Amplatz guidewire, which should be left in the proximal ascending aorta.
5. Withdraw the multipurpose catheter and use the stiff guidewire to introduce 28 × 28 × 94 mm Talent stent-graft (MEDTRONIC) in the descending aorta, taking care not to obstruct the ostium of the left subclavian artery.
6. After placing the stent-graft, check to make sure that the aortic pseudoaneurysm does not fill or leak (Fig. 7.2.3).

Follow-up CT angiogram 4 days after the procedure shows the absence of pseudoaneurysmatic filling; the right pleural effusion persists (Fig. 7.2.4).

Equipment List

1. Cook micropuncture introducer set
2. 100 cm long 5F pigtail and multipurpose catheters
3. 260 cm long flexible Terumo 0.035 in. guidewire and 260 cm long extra-stiff 0.035 in. guidewire
4. 6F valved introducer sheaths, lengtheners, stopcocks, injection pump
5. Nonionic iodinated contrast material (320 mg I/mL)
6. 28 × 28 × 94 mm Talent stent-graft (MEDTRONIC)

Case 7.3
Stanford Type B Chronic Aortic Dissection Treated Endovascularly with a Stent-Graft

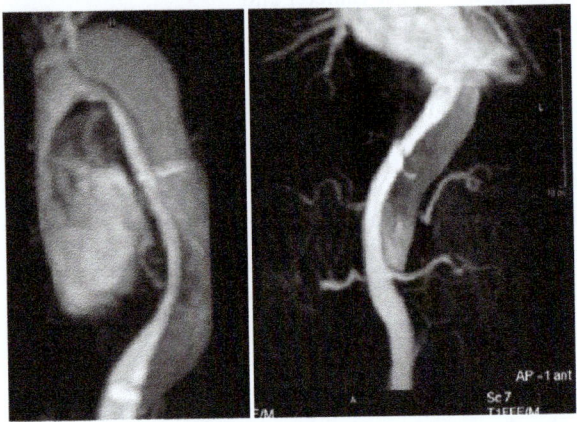

Fig. 7.3.1

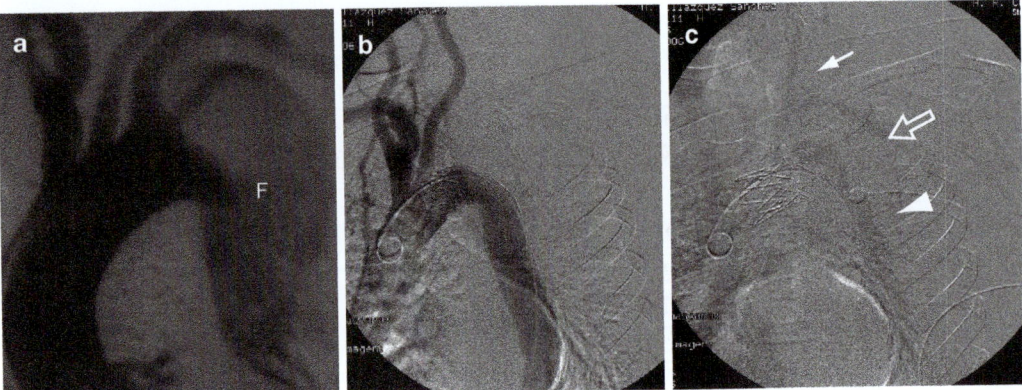

Fig. 7.3.2

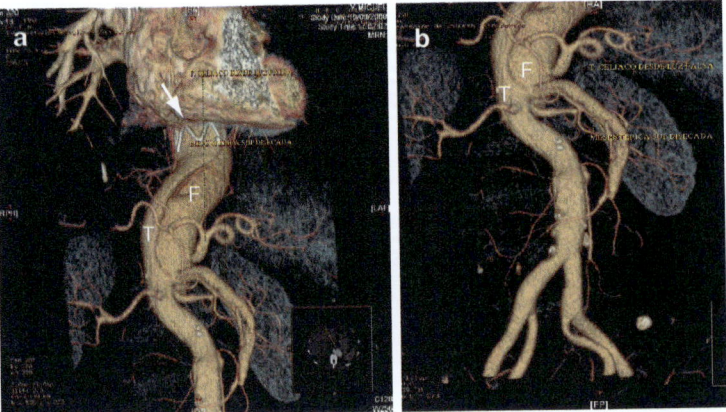

Fig. 7.3.3

Fig. 7.3.4

Figure 7.3.1 MR angiogram of the thoracic and abdominal aorta shows Stanford type B aortic dissection with primary intimal rupture immediately distal to the ostium of the left subclavian artery and distal extension to the level of the renal arteries

Figure 7.3.2 (a) Preoperative angiogram shows primary intimal tear with a contrast jet toward the false lumen (*F*). (b) Early-phase postoperative angiogram shows the absence of filling of the false lumen and of the left subclavian artery. (c) Late-phase postoperative angiogram shows retrograde filling of the left subclavian artery (*open arrow*) through the ipsilateral vertebral artery (*arrow*) and staining of the false lumen due to a retrograde leak distal to the stent (*arrow head*)

Figure 7.3.3 Volume-rendered 64-detector CT angiogram shows (a) the distal tip of the stent in the true lumen (*arrow*); the artery is dissected distal to the stent. (b) The dissection extends to the level of both renal arteries, which arise from the true lumen (*T*). The celiac trunk arises from the false lumen (*F*). The superior mesenteric artery is dissected

Figure 7.3.4 Sagittal MPR of a multislice CT angiogram of the thoracic and abdominal aorta shows the stent in the true lumen of the aorta, which has expanded. The diameter of the false lumen has decreased (*arrow*). The false lumen is partially thrombosed

A 44-year-old man with a history of hypertension refractory to treatment, no diabetes, ex-smoker (2 years before), with a family history of stroke (both parents), underwent CT angiography of the renal arteries to rule out renal causes of hypertension. He had moderate renal failure.

Abdominal CT angiography showed dissection of the abdominal aorta, so MR angiography was performed with intravenous gadolinium administration and thoracic slices. MR angiography showed a Stanford type B dissecting aortic aneurysm measuring 48.2 mm in maximum diameter extending from the ostium of the left subclavian artery to the level of the renal arteries. Despite the patient's age, the medical-surgical committee decided on endovascular treatment due to the size of the thoracic aorta and the high mortality associated with classical surgical treatment of this condition.

Comments

Stanford type B dissecting aortic aneurysms occur distal to the ostium of the left subclavian artery. In cases without complications, the treatment of choice is strict medical control of blood pressure. In cases with complications, the classical treatment is open surgery. Endovascular treatment is feasible and indicated in patients with complicated aortic dissection and high surgical risk. The mortality of untreated acute aortic dissection is 1–2% per hour. The operative mortality of acute aortic dissection treated with classical open surgery is 30%.

Procedure Steps

1. Administer general anesthesia. Approach through the left brachial artery with a Cook micropuncture kit and insert a 6F valved introducer sheath.
2. Introduce a 260 cm long flexible 0.035 in. Terumo guidewire through a 5F pigtail catheter through the left brachial artery and pull it through the left femoral artery (through and through procedure). Use transesophageal ultrasonography to check whether the guidewire has passed through the true lumen.

3. Use the flexible Terumo guidewire to introduce a multipurpose catheter to the ascending aorta through the femoral artery. Replace the Terumo guidewire with a 260 cm long extra-stiff 0.035 in. Amplatz guidewire.

4. Introduce a 100 cm long 5F pigtail catheter through the left brachial artery to the ascending aorta for angiographic control.

5. Perform right femoral arteriotomy and introduce a 30 × 28 × 200 mm Relay stent-graft (BOLTON) from the proximal area of the descending thoracic aorta until the distal third of the descending thoracic aorta, covering the primary intimal tear and the ostium of the left subclavian artery. Use transesophageal ultrasonographic guidance throughout the procedure.

6. Perform angiography to check that the stent-graft has been correctly placed; in this case, we observed it was correctly placed and the diameter of the true lumen was increased. We also observed a leak distal to the stent-graft with partial retrograde filling of the false lumen (Fig. 7.3.2).

The patient evolved satisfactorily, with decreased left radial pulse but without neurologic symptoms. His blood pressure is now 150/90.

Multidetector CT angiography confirmed the correct placement of the stent-graft in the true lumen and the increased diameter of the true lumen, as well as the distal leak in the infradiaphragmatic aorta with partial thrombosis of the false lumen (Figs. 7.3.3 and 7.3.4).

Equipment List

1. Cook micropuncture introducer set
2. 6F valved introducer sheaths
3. 100 cm long 5F pigtail and multipurpose catheters. Gadolinium
4. 260 cm long flexible Terumo 0.035 in. guidewire and 260 cm long 0.035 in. Amplatz guidewire
5. Surgical material for arteriotomy
6. 30 × 28 × 200 mm Relay aortic stent-graft (BOLTON – IZASA)
7. Transesophageal echography (TEE)

Case 7.4

Aneurysm of the Right Common Iliac Artery Treated with a Contralateral Aortomonoiliac Stent-Graft, Ipsilateral Vascular Plug, and Femorofemoral Bypass

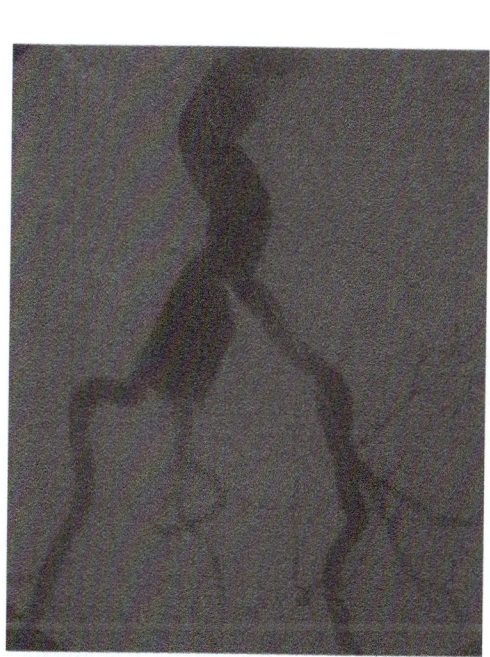

Fig. 7.4.1

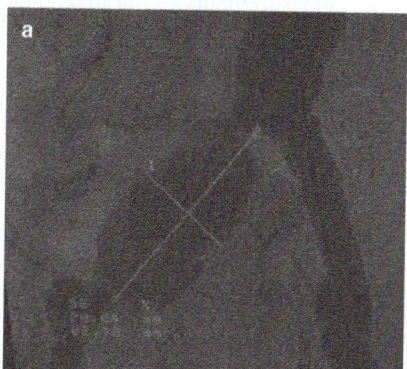

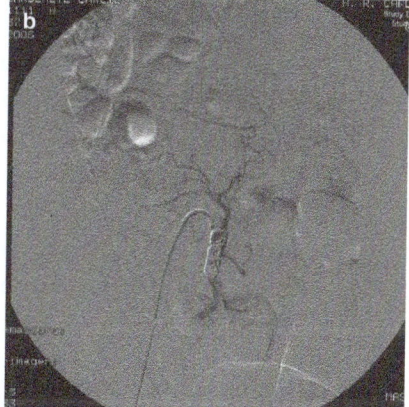

Fig. 7.4.2

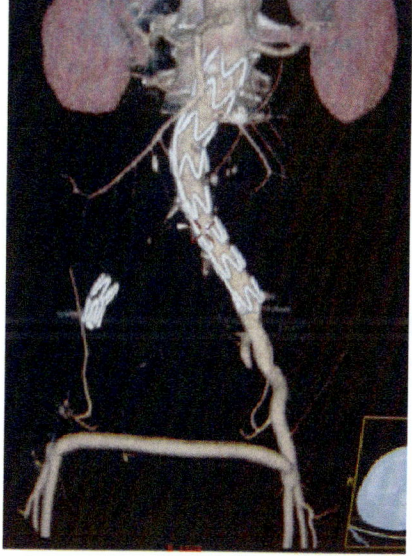

Fig. 7.4.3

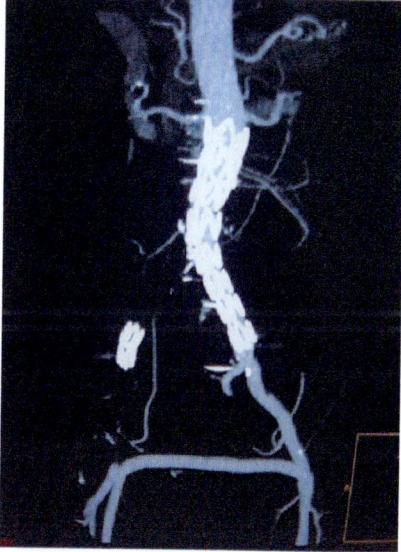

Fig. 7.4.4

Figure 7.4.1 Angiogram of the distal abdominal and pelvic aorta obtained with a 100 cm long 5F calibrated catheter introduced through the left femoral artery shows a straight stent placed in the distal aorta in a previous procedure and an aneurysm of the right common iliac artery measuring 40 × 62 mm that extends to the right iliac bifurcation

Figure 7.4.2 (a) Angiogram of the abdominal aorta and pelvic vessels centered on the aortoiliac sector shows the straight aortoaortic stent that extends to the aortic bifurcation. Measurements of the iliac aneurysm refer to the arterial lumen and do not measure the mural thrombosis of the aneurysm. (b) Simmons I catheter in the right hypogastric artery, which is embolized with coils before the aortic stent is deployed

Figure 7.4.3 Anterior-view volume-rendered multislice CT angiogram of the abdominal aorta and pelvic vessels shows the left aortoiliac stent extending from the level of the renal arteries to the left common iliac artery. The femorofemoral bypass is patent (BP). There is a metallic occluder in the right external iliac artery, which does not fill with contrast (*arrow*)

Figure 7.4.4 Coronal MPR of a multislice CT angiogram of the abdominal aorta and pelvic vessels shows the relation of the stent with the renal arteries in detail

A 62-year-old man with a history of colic nephritis and hepatitis C who had undergone urgent intervention for a ruptured aneurysm of the abdominal aorta 6 years before (20 mm straight Dacron aortoaortic stent placement) underwent follow-up multidetector CT angiography. A 40 × 62 mm aneurysm of the right common iliac artery was detected and the medical-surgical committee decided on elective endovascular intervention.

Aortoiliac angiography showed the aneurysm in the right common iliac artery (Figs. 7.4.1 and 7.4.2a) and the right hypogastric artery was embolized prior to stenting (Fig. 7.4.2b).

The patient evolved satisfactorily. Follow-up CT angiography 1 month later confirmed the exclusion of the aneurysm and the patency of the left iliac axis and of the femorofemoral bypass (Figs. 7.4.3 and 7.4.4).

Comments

Iliac artery aneurysms are detected in over 20% of patients with aneurysms of the abdominal aorta; the common and internal iliac arteries are the most frequently involved and elderly men are the most frequently affected patients. Isolated iliac aneurysms are much rarer and usually have an arteriosclerotic origin. Anastomotic pseudoaneurysms of the iliac arteries caused by surgery for occlusive aortic disease are more common, are often asymptomatic, and can be treated with stenting. Invasive treatment is recommended when they are larger than 30 mm. Endovascular treatment is becoming increasingly common because it results in less morbidity and mortality than classic open surgery.

Procedure Steps

1. Administer general anesthesia. Introduce a 100 cm long 5F pigtail catheter through the right femoral artery.
2. Place a Simmons I catheter in the right internal iliac artery.
3. Introduce a 2.7F Terumo microcatheter coaxially in the right internal iliac artery.

4. Embolize the internal iliac artery with microcoils (3×4, 4×5, 6×5, and 8×5 mm).

5. Introduce a multipurpose catheter through the left femoral artery and then change to a 260 cm long super-stiff 0.035 Amplatz guidewire.

6. Make an incision in the left femoral artery and introduce a $24 \times 14 \times 155$ mm Talent aortomonoiliac stent-graft (MEDTRONIC) under angiographic guidance using a 5F pigtail catheter through the right side.

7. Introduce a 260 cm long super-stiff 0.035 in. Amplatz guidewire through the right femoral artery.

8. Place the vascular plug (Occluder 14, MEDTRONIC) in the right external iliac artery.

9. Perform the femorofemoral bypass.

10. Check the patency of the left femoral axis and of the femorofemoral bypass.

1. 6F valved introducer sheaths, lengtheners, stopcocks, injection pump

2. Nonionic iodinated contrast material (320 mg I/mL)

3. 260 cm long flexible 0.035 in. Terumo guidewire and 260 cm long extra-stiff 0.035 in. Amplatz guidewire

4. 100 cm long 5F pigtail and multipurpose catheters

5. $24 \times 14 \times 155$ mm Talent aortomonoiliac stent-graft (MEDTRONIC)

6. 14 mm vascular plug (Occluder, MEDTRONIC)

7. 8 mm $\times$ 30 cm Dacron graft

Case 7.5

Acute Thoracic Aortic Syndrome Treated with a Stent-Graft

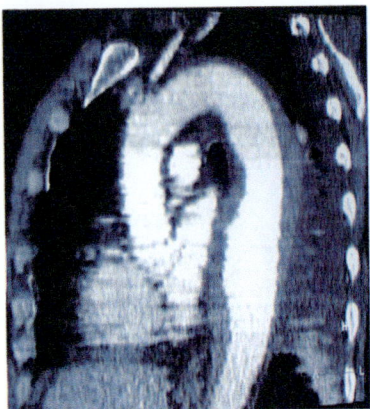

Fig. 7.5.1

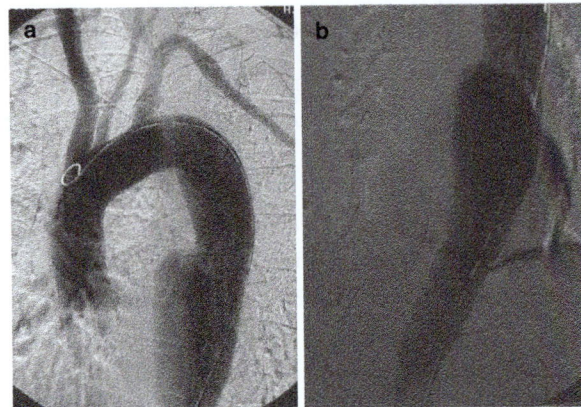

Fig. 7.5.2

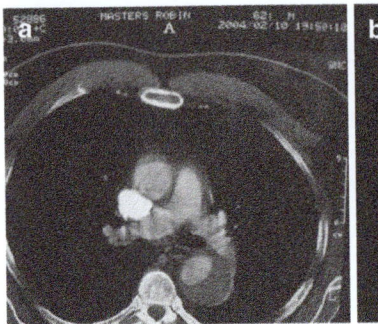

Fig. 7.5.3

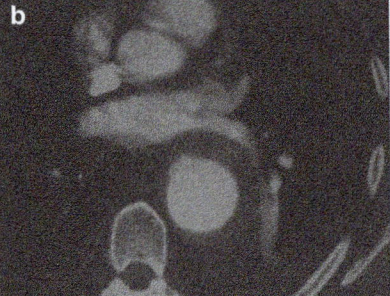

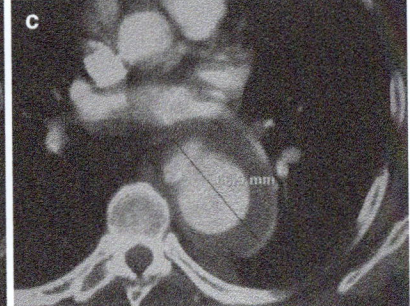

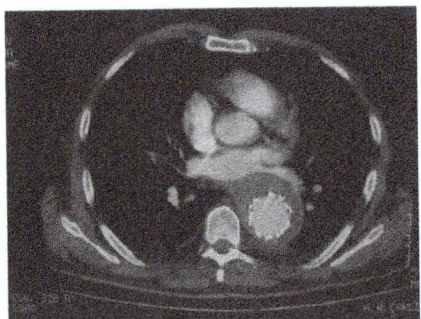

Fig. 7.5.4

Figure 7.5.1 Sagittal MIP reconstruction of a CT angiogram acquired with a helical scanner shows a type B intramural hematoma of the thoracic aorta. There is an aneurysmatic area in the proximal third of the descending thoracic aorta and left pleural effusion

Figure 7.5.2 (a) Thoracic aortogram obtained with a pigtail catheter in the ascending aorta shows an aneurysm in the descending aorta. (b) Aortogram of the descending thoracic aorta obtained with a catheter in the aortic arch shows the extension of the aneurysm to the diaphragmatic zone

Figure 7.5.3 (a) Axial CT angiogram acquired with a helical scanner at the level of the left atrium shows an intramural hematoma in the descending aorta. A glove-finger-like prolongation in the aortic lumen suggestive of a penetrating ulcer of the aorta is barely perceptible in the 11 o'clock position (arrow). (b) CT angiogram obtained with a helical scanner 2 weeks later shows that the aortic ulcer has grown larger. The patient's pain was not alleviated with the standard treatment

Figure 7.5.4 Helical CT angiogram of the descending aorta at the level of the left atrium shows the dynamic evolution of the acute aortic syndrome in this patient from an intramural hematoma (1) to the insinuation of aortic ulceration (2) to an established penetrating aortic ulcer (3) and finally to the follow-up after placing two coated stents

A 62-year-old male patient with a history of hypertension but no other risk factors presented at the emergency department after sudden onset chest and upper back pain at rest that was refractory to treatment with analgesics. A cardiac origin was ruled out and thoracic CT angiography showed a type B intramural aortic hematoma in the distal aortic arch and descending thoracic aorta Fig. 7.5.1, suggestive of acute aortic syndrome.

At first, the patient underwent medical treatment and blood pressure control; his condition improved and the pain disappeared.

Preoperative angiography showed an aneurysm in the descending thoracic aorta (Fig. 7.5.2a, b).

One week later, after he had another episode of chest pain, CT angiography showed a penetrating ulcer of the aorta (Fig. 7.5.3a, b) in the middle third of the descending aorta. One week later, another CT angiogram showed that the penetrating ulcer and intramural hematoma in the aorta had increased in size.

The medical-surgical committee opted for endovascular stenting. Follow-up imaging 1 month after the procedure showed favorable evolution of the lesions (Fig. 7.5.4).

Comments

Acute aortic syndrome was first described by Vilacosta et al. It comprises various entities that can cause each other, for example: classical aortic dissection, intramural hematoma, and acute penetrating ulcer.

Treatment is generally the same as for classical aortic dissection.

In our patient, the dynamics of the aortic disease and the development of a painful extensive intramural hematoma made endovascular treatment the best choice. Nevertheless, further studies are needed to help select patients appropriately.

Procedure Steps

1. Administer general anesthesia. Approach through the left brachial artery using an arterial micropuncture set and insert a 5F valved introducer sheath.
2. Introduce a 90 cm long 5F pigtail catheter to the ascending aorta.
3. Perform transversal arteriotomy in the right femoral artery.
4. Place a 6F valved introducer sheath in the right femoral artery.
5. Pass a 260 cm long 0.035 in. Terumo guidewire and 100 cm long 5F multipurpose catheter through the right femoral artery to the ascending aorta.
6. Pass a 300 cm long 0.035 in. Lunderquist guidewire through it to the ascending aorta. Pass the Talent stent ($40 \times 40 \times 114$ mm) delivery system (MEDTRONIC) using a superstiff guidewire.
7. Place a second, distal Talent stent ($42 \times 38 \times 110$ mm) (MEDTRONIC) to the diaphragmatic region.
8. Balloon the stents in their tips and in the area where they overlap.
9. Obtain a final angiogram through a 5F pigtail catheter in the ascending aorta to check the results.

Equipment List

1. 5F and 6F valved introducer sheaths
2. Nonionic iodinated contrast material (320 mg I/mL), stopcocks, injection pump
3. 100 cm long 5F pigtail and multipurpose catheters
4. 260 cm long 0.035 in. Terumo guidewire and 300 cm long 0.035 in. superstiff Lunderquist guidewire
5. Femoral arteriotomy set
6. $40 \times 40 \times 114$ mm Talent stent (MEDTRONIC) with a $42 \times 38 \times 110$ mm distal extension
7. Reliant aortic remodeling balloon (MEDTRONIC)

Case 7.6

Traumatic Dissection of the Descending Aorta Treated in the Acute Phase with a Stent-Graft

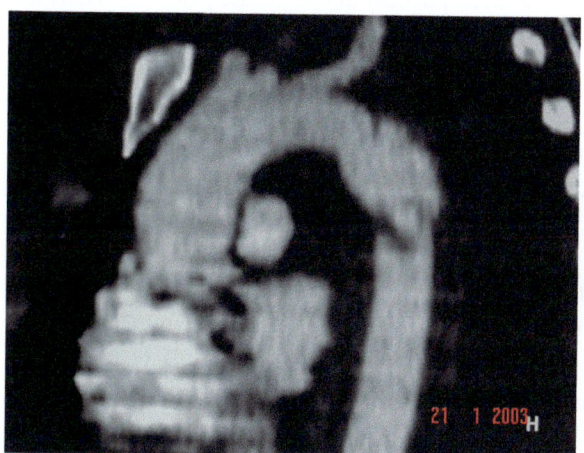

Fig. 7.6.1

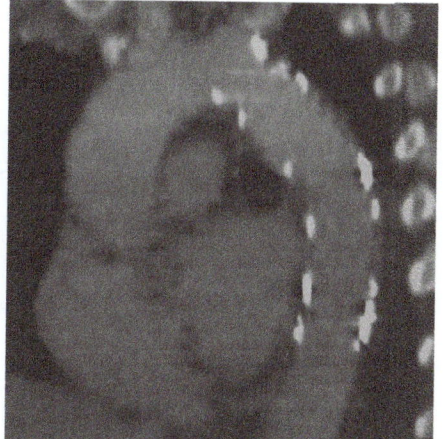

Fig. 7.6.2

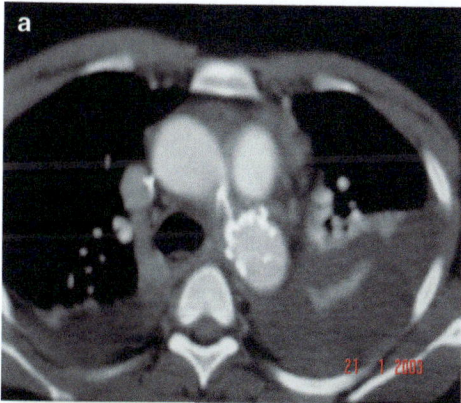

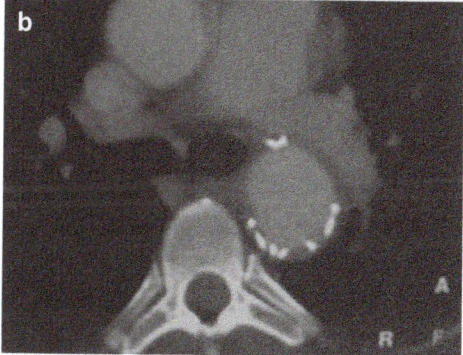

Fig. 7.6.3

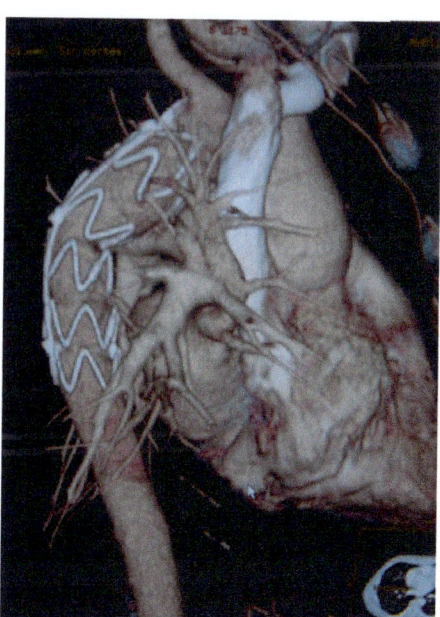

Fig. 7.6.4

Figure 7.6.1 Sagittal MIP of a CT angiogram acquired with a helical scanner shows a complex traumatic aortic dissection of the proximal third of the descending thoracic aorta at the level of the aortic isthmus

Figure 7.6.2 Sagittal MIP of a CT angiogram acquired with a helical scanner shows that the stent has been deployed in the correct position, conserving the left subclavian artery (*arrow*) with the expansion of the aortic lumen

Figure 7.6.3 (**a**) Axial CT angiogram acquired with a helical scanner at the level of the carina shows a posterior leak through the stent, possibly due to porosity (*arrow*). There are bilateral pleural effusion and a mediastinal hematoma with the displacement of the mediastinum to the right. (**b**) Follow-up 1 year later shows that the leak is no longer evident and the aortic lumen has expanded

Figure 7.6.4 Sagittal volume-rendered CT angiogram acquired on a multidetector scanner 6 years after the procedure shows the stent in the correct position

A 31-year-old man involved in an automobile accident was brought to the emergency department by ambulance; he was conscious (Glasgow scale 15). Physical and CT examination found:

1. Traumatic brain injury. Conscious, oriented. Scalp injury; posttraumatic amnesia; pupils equal, round, and reactive to light. CT: slight frontal parenchymal atrophy
2. Thoracic trauma. Parasternal hematoma due to hitting the steering wheel.
   Thoracic CT angiography: large mediastinal hematoma with the image of an aortic flap in the region of the aortic isthmus suggestive of nonocclusive thrombosis of the descending aorta, left pleural effusion, and minimal pericardial effusion (Fig. 7.6.1).
3. Abdominal trauma.
   Abdominal CT angiography: small hepatic laceration with a slight amount of free peritoneal fluid.
   Two RBC units were transfused in the referring hospital and the patient was transferred to our center for treatment of the aortic lesions.
   The multidisciplinary emergency team decided on endovascular treatment of the descending aorta.

Comments   Traumatic lesions of the thoracic aorta tend to occur at the level of the aortic isthmus and are associated to high morbidity and mortality. These patients often have lesions in other locations (abdomen, brain, etc.) and treatment of the aortic lesions is often delayed. Endovascular treatment is becoming increasingly more common because recent studies have shown its feasibility and lower morbidity and mortality compared to classical treatment. The optimal time for this treatment is yet to be determined.

Procedure Steps   1. Administer general anesthesia. Approach through the left brachial artery using an arterial micropuncture set and insert a 5F valved introducer sheath.
2. Introduce a 90 cm long 5F pigtail catheter to the ascending aorta.

3. Perform transversal arteriotomy in the right femoral artery.

4. Place a 6F valved introducer sheath in the right femoral artery.

5. Pass a 260 cm long 0.035 in. Terumo guidewire and 100 cm long 5F multipurpose catheter through the right femoral artery to the ascending aorta.

6. Pass a 300 cm long 0.035 in. super-stiff Lunderquist guidewire through it to the ascending aorta.

7. Pass the Talent stent ($30 \times 30 \times 101$ mm) delivery system (MEDTRONIC) using a super-stiff guidewire.

8. Use a balloon to expand both ends of the stent (Reliant, MEDTRONIC).

9. Check the results with an angiogram obtained through a 5F pigtail catheter situated in the ascending aorta.

10. Follow-up CT angiography (Fig. 7.6.2) shows the correct placement of the stent-graft and slight leakage of contrast material in the center of the stent-graft (arrow) (Fig. 7.6.3a), which we assume is due to porosity (type IV leak). No signs of this leakage were seen on long-term follow-up images (Figs. 7.6.3b and 7.6.4).

The patient evolved satisfactorily.

Equipment List

1. 5F and 6F valved introducer sheaths

2. Nonionic iodinated contrast material (320 mg I/mL), stopcocks

3. 90 cm long 5F pigtail catheter and 100 cm long multipurpose catheter

4. 260 cm long 0.035 in. Terumo guidewire and 300 cm long 0.035 in. superstiff Lunderquist guidewire

5. Femoral arteriotomy set

6. $30 \times 30 \times 101$ mm Talent stent (MEDTRONIC)

7. Reliant aortic remodeling balloon (MEDTRONIC)

Case 7.7
■
Endovascular Treatment of Rupture of the Thoracic Aorta in the Acute Phase Using a Stent-Graft

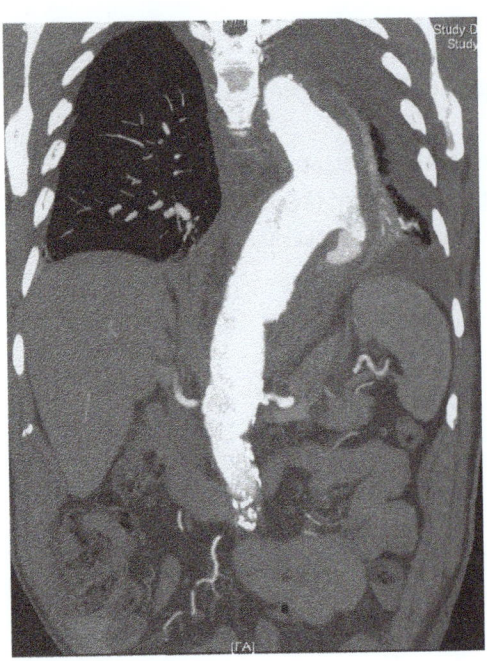

Fig. 7.7.1

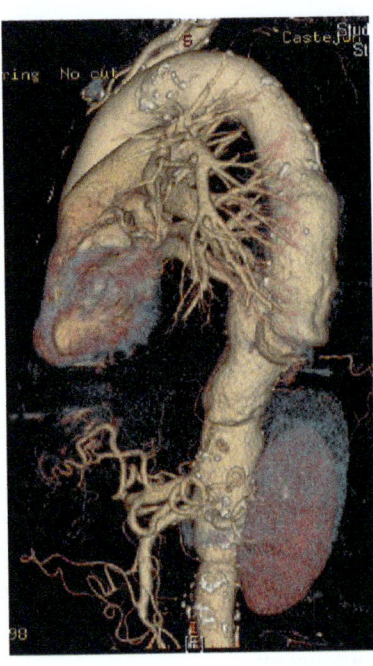

Fig. 7.7.2

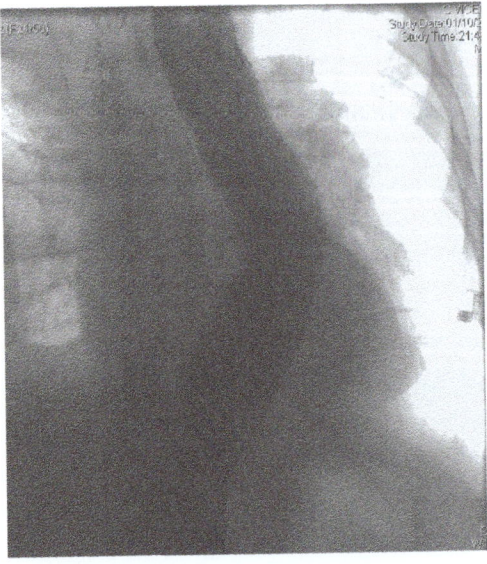

Fig. 7.7.3

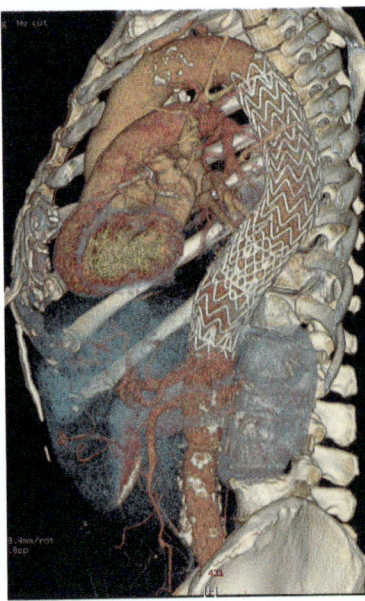

Fig. 7.7.4

Figure 7.7.1 Coronal MIP CT angiogram of the thoracoabdominal aorta shows an aneurysm of the thoracoabdominal aorta with an image suggestive of aortic tear (*arrow*). Note the hemomediastinum and massive hemothorax

Figure 7.7.2 Posterolateral view volume-rendered CT angiogram of the thoracoabdominal aorta shows an aneurysm in the descending thoracic aorta that starts in the proximal third and extends nearly to the celiac trunk

Figure 7.7.3 Intraoperative thoracoabdominal aortogram after the placement of two coated stents. No extravasation of contrast material outside the aortic lumen is seen

Figure 7.7.4 Lateral view volume-rendered CT angiogram of the thoracoabdominal aorta after treatment with coated stents shows the stents extending from the proximal descending thoracic aorta to the celiac trunk; there is a 5 cm overlap between the two stents

A 69-year-old male patient with a history of medically treated hypertension, type II diabetes, dyslipemia, and gout, who was treated for an aneurysm of the abdominal aorta 7 years before, presented with oppressive pain in the chest and between the shoulder blades at rest that was exacerbated by walking. He also had profuse sweating, nausea, vomiting, and sudden shortness of breath. He had no fever, expectoration, or cough. No ECG alterations or markers of myocardial damage were present. He was admitted to the ward and his general condition deteriorated, so he was admitted to the ICU.

He was conscious, oriented, and anxious, as well as well nourished and hydrated. Percussion was regular, but his skin was pallid and he had slight tachypnea and dyspnea.

His blood pressure was 117/95; his heart rate was 107 bpm, and he had moderate jugular vein distention.

Cardiac auscultation: rhythmic, without murmurs or rubs; muffled tones.

Lung auscultation: slight hypoventilation in both bases with a left predominance.

Abdomen: soft, depressible, somewhat painful in the epigastric region, without rebound or guarding, preserved peristalsis. Midline laparotomy scar.

Lower limbs: peripheral pulses present and symmetric, without edema.

Thoracoabdominal CT angiography showed a ruptured aneurysm in the descending thoracic aorta with a large mediastinal hematoma and bilateral pleural effusion (with more fluid on the left side) (Figs. 7.7.1 and 7.7.2).

Endovascular treatment was considered the first choice. The patient had several cardiac arrests that responded to resuscitation. His posterior evolution was satisfactory without evidence of stroke or paraplegia.

Comments

Aortic rupture is the final outcome in the natural history of aortic aneurysms; it is associated to high mortality and is more common in cases of dissecting aneurysm.

Since Dake first used a coated stent to treat an aneurysm of thoracic aorta in a human in 1994, endovascular treatment for this condition has undergone tremendous development. Today, endovascular treatment can be considered the treatment of choice for aortic rupture, as mortality is lower than in open surgery.

Procedure Steps

1. Administer general anesthesia. Approach through the left brachial artery using an arterial micropuncture set and insert a 5F valved introducer sheath.
2. Introduce a 90 cm long 5F pigtail catheter to the ascending aorta.
3. Perform transversal arteriotomy in the right femoral artery.
4. Place a 6F valved introducer sheath in the right femoral artery.
5. Pass a 260 cm long 0.035 in. Terumo guidewire and 100 cm long 5F multipurpose catheter through the right femoral artery to the ascending aorta.
6. Pass a 300 cm long 0.035 in. super-stiff Lunderquist guidewire through it to the ascending aorta.
7. Pass the Excluder stent (42 × 42 × 150 mm) delivery system and another one measuring 45 × 45 × 100 mm (GORE) using a super-stiff guidewire.
8. Use a balloon to expand both ends of the stent and the overlapping area (Trilobe, GORE).
9. Check the results with an angiogram obtained through a 5F pigtail catheter situated in the ascending aorta (Fig. 7.7.3).
10. Use multidetector CT angiography (Fig. 7.7.4) to reconfirm the correct placement of the stent-graft.

Equipment List

1. 5F and 6F valved introducer sheaths
2. Nonionic iodinated contrast material (320 mg I/mL), stopcocks, injection pump
3. 90 cm long 5F pigtail catheter and 100 cm long multipurpose catheter
4. 260 cm long 0.035 in. Terumo guidewire and 300 cm long 0.035 in. superstiff Lunderquist guidewire
5. Femoral arteriotomy set
6. Two Excluder stents (42 × 42 × 150 and 45 × 45 × 100 mm) (GORE)
7. Trilobe remodeling balloon (GORE)

Case 7.8

■

Penetrating Ulcer of the Descending Thoracic Aorta: Endovascular Treatment with an Aortobifemoral Graft

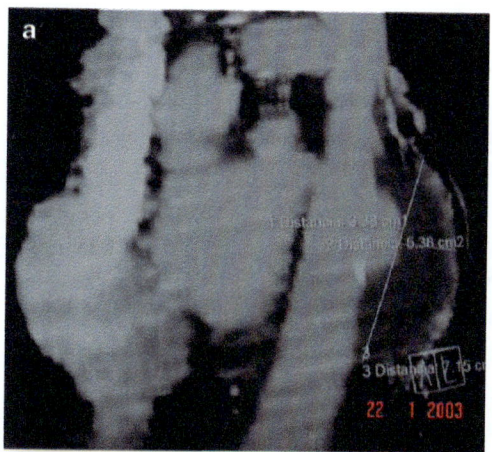

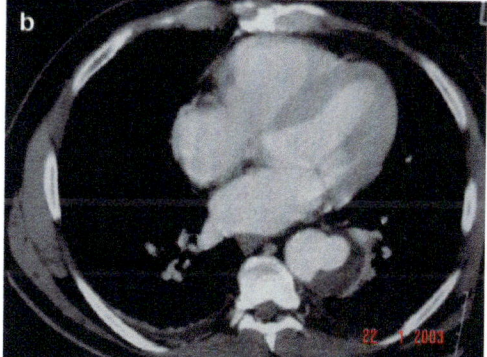

Fig. 7.8.1

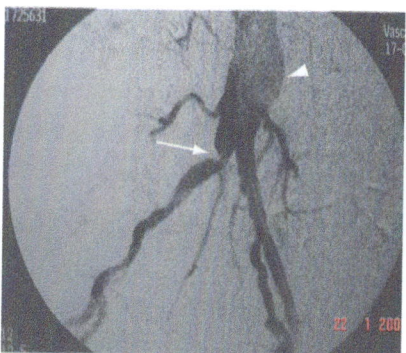

Fig. 7.8.2

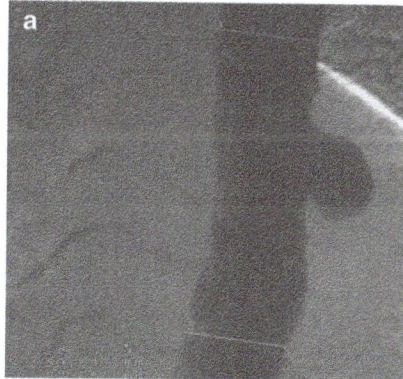

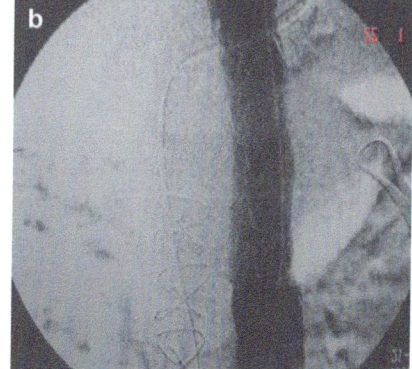

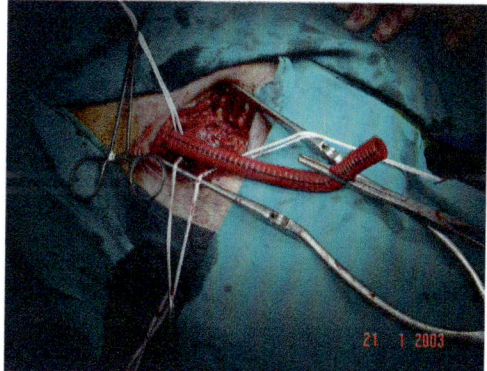

Fig. 7.8.3

Fig. 7.8.4

Figure 7.8.1 Coronal (**a**) and axial (**b**) CT angiograms at the level of the descending thoracic aorta shows an aortic ulcer with an eccentric saccular aneurysm in the distal third of the descending aorta

Figure 7.8.4a Intraoperative aortogram of the descending thoracic aorta shows an aortic ulcer and measurements of the healthy aorta above and below the lesion

Figure 7.8.3 Intraoperative angiogram of the aortoiliac sector (*right image*) shows severe stenosis of the right common iliac artery (*arrow*). The left iliac artery was also unsuitable for the introduction of the stent. There is an aneurysm of the abdominal aorta (*arrow head*)

Figure 7.8.3 An aortobifemoral bypass was placed and the thoracic stent was introduced through the right branch of the aortobifemoral bypass (*left image*)

Figure 7.8.4b Intraoperative arteriogram after stent placement shows the absence of ulcer filling. Compare this image with the aortogram obtained before stent placement (**a**)

A hypertensive 67-year-old man with a history of ischemic heart disease and acute myocardial infarction treated with a double coronary bypass in another hospital 1 year earlier presented after the onset of acute chest pain after a coughing attack and syncope leading to a fall. A second, less intense episode occurred, and the patient was admitted to another hospital, where CT angiography showed an aneurysm of the thoracic aorta and slight gastric bleeding. Gastroscopy showed esophagitis, hiatal hernia, and an inactive duodenal ulcer.

Five days later, CT angiography at our hospital confirmed a saccular aneurysm of the descending thoracic aorta with an image suggestive of a penetrating aortic ulcer. Moreover, we observed an aneurysm of the abdominal aorta measuring 55 mm that did not involve the iliac arteries. The medical-surgical committee considered that endovascular treatment was the best option.

We attempted to implant a stent-graft through the femoral artery, but it was impossible to advance through both iliac arteries due to bilateral iliac stenosis that had not been adequately evaluated.

Four days later, he underwent surgical treatment for the aneurysm of the abdominal aorta with an 18×9 mm Dacron aortobifemoral graft. Before suturing the right femoral branch of the graft, we implanted a $36 \times 36 \times 114$ mm Talent stent-graft (MEDTRONIC) to treat the saccular aneurysm of the descending thoracic aorta. The final results were good.

The patient evolved satisfactorily without paraplegia or other complications.

Comments   An acute penetrating ulcer forms part of the acute aortic syndrome. Its natural history can include an intramural hematoma, aortic dissection, or saccular aneurysm with possible rupture. An acute penetrating ulcer with pain that is refractory to treatment is considered by some to be a surgical emergency. Treatment with a stent-graft is a new alternative to classical treatment with open surgery and has lower morbidity and mortality. In our case, the patient also had an aneurysm of the abdominal aorta with poor vascular access through the iliac arteries, so we treated the acute penetrating ulcer of the descending aorta through the aortobifemoral graft.

1. Administer general anesthesia. Perform upper and lower midline laparotomy.
2. Perform bilateral femoral arteriotomy.
3. Perform aneurysmorrhaphy and place an 18 × 9 mm Dacron graft.
4. Insert a 6F valved introducer sheath in the left brachial artery.
5. Insert a 100 cm long 5F pigtail catheter in the descending thoracic aorta to enable angiographic control.
6. Insert a 6F valved introducer sheath through the right branch of the Dacron graft.
7. Insert a 260 cm long 0.035 in. Terumo guidewire to the aortic arch.
8. Insert a 100 cm long 5F multipurpose catheter and introduce a 260 cm long super-stiff 0.035 in. Amplatz guidewire.
9. Use this stiff guidewire to introduce a 36 × 36 × 114 mm Talent stent delivery system (MEDTRONIC) into the descending thoracic aorta.
10. Release the stent-graft, check to make sure it is correctly positioned, and check the right femoral anastomosis of the Dacron graft.

1. 6F valved introducer sheaths
2. Vascular micropuncture kit
3. Stopcocks, injection pump
4. Nonionic iodinated contrast material (320 mg I/mL)
5. 100 cm long 5F pigtail catheter and 100 cm long 5F multipurpose catheter
6. 260 cm long 0.035 in. Terumo guidewire and 260 cm long 0.035 in. super-stiff Amplatz guidewire
7. 36 × 36 × 114 mm Talent stent-graft (MEDTRONIC)
8. 18 × 9 mm Dacron graft for the aortobifemoral bypass

Case 7.9

Endovascular Treatment of an Infrarenal Aneurysm of the Abdominal Aorta with a Bifurcated Stent-Graft

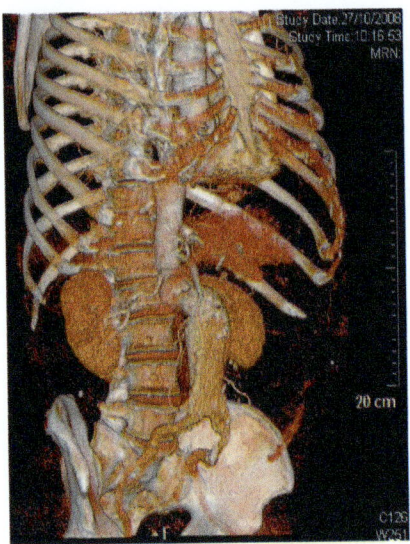

Fig. 7.9.1

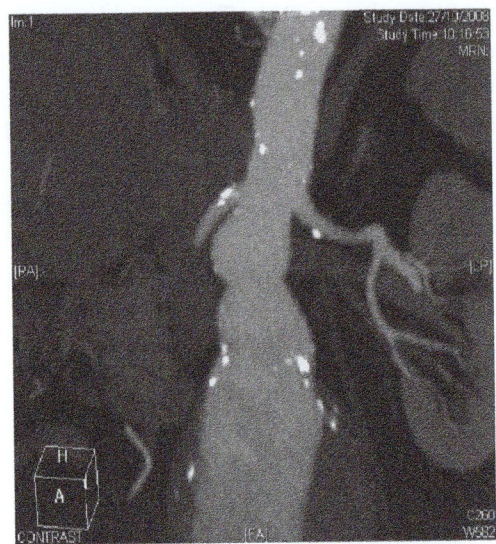

Fig. 7.9.2

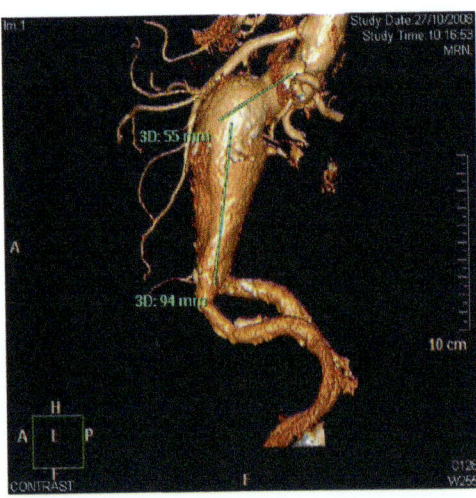

Fig. 7.9.3

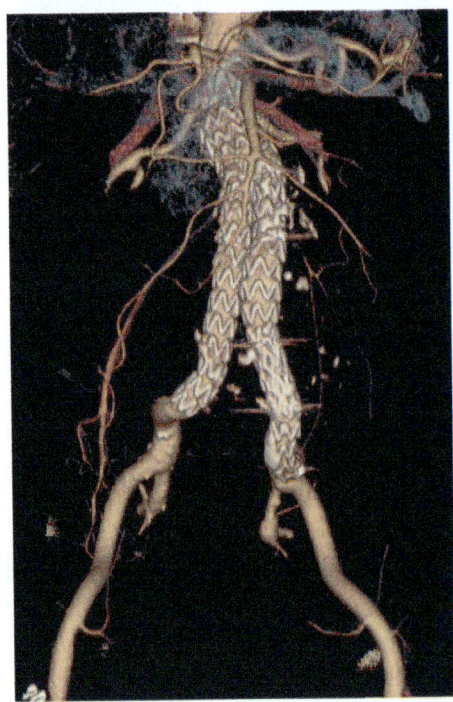

Fig. 7.9.4

Figure 7.9.1 Volume-rendered thoracoabdominal CT angiogram shows an infrarenal aneurysm of the abdominal aorta (AAA) with a conical neck angled forward. The AAA extends to the aortic bifurcation

Figure 7.9.2 Coronal MPR of an abdominal CT angiogram shows an AAA with a conical neck and some calcification but no evidence of thrombosis. The relation of the AAA with the renal arteries is depicted in detail

Figure 7.9.3 Volume-rendered abdominal CT angiogram provides a lateral view of the AAA, showing the anterior angling of the neck of the AAA and the elongation of both iliac arteries

Figure 7.9.4 Volume-rendered abdominal CT angiogram after stenting shows the correct placement of the stent, with suprarenal extension and coverage to the common iliac arteries. No leaks are seen in the follow-up image

An infrarenal aneurysm of the abdominal aorta was incidentally discovered in a routine abdominal US examination in an 80-year-old man with a history of hypertension, severe COPD, cataracts, hydrocele, and prostate cancer in remission with hormone therapy. The aneurysm was confirmed at multidetector CT angiography (Figs. 7.9.1–7.9.3): its maximum diameter was 85 mm, its neck was angled, conical, and free of thrombi.

The medical-surgical committee decided on endovascular treatment due to the patient's age and concomitant disease.

Follow-up multidetector CT angiography 3 days after the intervention showed the correct placement of the stent-graft without evidence of leakage.

Comments

Endovascular treatment of aneurysms of the abdominal aorta was first carried out in humans by Parodi et al. in 1991. Larger and larger series of patients have benefited from this treatment, and randomized trials have shown lower short-term morbidity and mortality for endovascular treatment compared to open surgery. Nevertheless, more follow-up studies are necessary, and for the time being, the long-term morbidity and mortality of the two approaches appear to be similar.

Procedure Steps

1. Administer general anesthesia and perform bilateral femoral arteriotomy.
2. Insert a valved 6F introducer sheath through the left femoral artery.
3. Introduce a 5F multipurpose catheter using a 260 cm long 0.035 in. Terumo guidewire.
4. Replace the multipurpose catheter with a 100 cm long 5F pigtail catheter.
5. Insert a 6F valved introducer sheath through the right femoral artery.
6. Pass a multipurpose catheter and 260 cm long 0.035 in. Terumo guidewire through the right femoral artery. Replace the guidewire with a 300 cm long super-stiff 0.035 in. Lunderquist guidewire.
7. Introduce the 28 × 13 × 170 mm Endurant stent-graft (MEDTRONIC) through the right femoral artery, with the main body of the stent-graft until its placement at the level of the renal arteries.

8. Obtain an angiogram through the pigtail catheter to check placement and mark the renal arteries.
9. Unfold the main body of the stent-graft and its right branch.
10. Approach the left part of the main body and pass a guidewire through the left femoral artery and through the left part of the main body of the stent-graft.
11. Place the left branch of the $16 \times 13 \times 120$ mm stent-graft and a $16 \times 13 \times 80$ mm left extension.
12. Inflate a stent-graft balloon catheter (RELIANT) at the level of the renal arteries and overlapping sites.
13. Check the results by angiography.
14. Close the arteriotomies.

Equipment List

1. 6F valved introducer sheaths
2. Stopcocks, injection pump
3. Nonionic iodinated contrast material (320 mg I/mL)
4. 100 cm long 5F pigtail catheter and 100 cm long 5F multipurpose catheter
5. 260 cm long 0.035 in. Terumo guidewire and 300 cm long 0.035 in. super-stiff Lunderquist guidewire
6. Material for femoral arteriotomy
7. $28 \times 13 \times 170$ mm Endurant bifurcated stent-graft
8. Extension limbs $16 \times 13 \times 120$ and $16 \times 13 \times 80$ mm for the left side
9. Aortic remodeling balloon

Case 7.10

■

Treatment of an Aneurysm of the Abdominal Aorta with a Stent-Graft: Type II Leak (Endoleak)

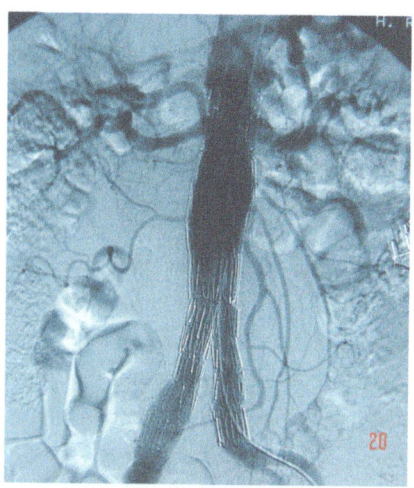

Fig. 7.10.1

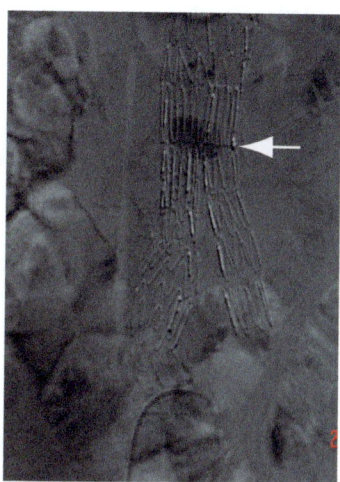

Fig. 7.10.2

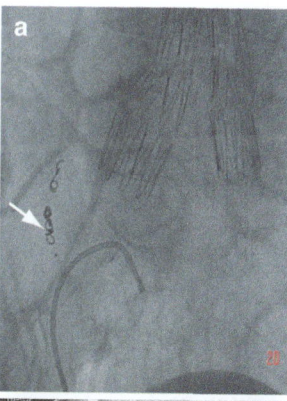

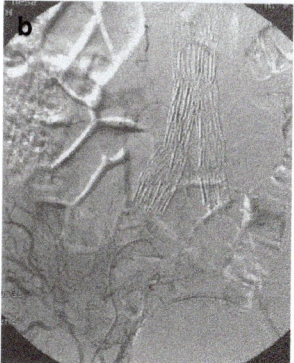

Fig. 7.10.3

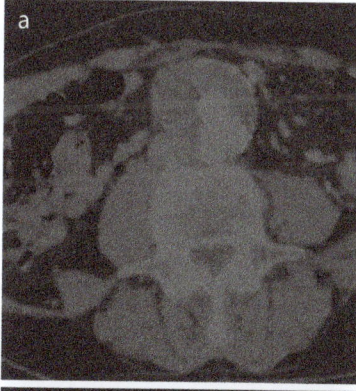

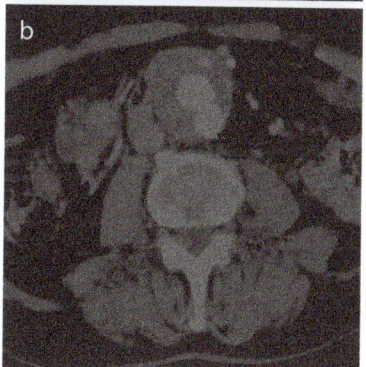

Fig. 7.10.4

Figure 7.10.1 Angiogram of the abdominal aorta after deployment of a bifurcated covered stent with suprarenal coverage. No leaks are seen in the early arterial phase

Figure 7.10.2 Late-phase angiogram of the abdominal aorta after deployment of the bifurcated stent. A type II leak through the iliolumbar branches is shown as a rounded area superposed on the stent (*arrow*)

Figure 7.10.3 (**a**) A 2.7F microcatheter (*arrow*) introduced through a cobra catheter (*triangle*) in the right hypogastric artery has enabled metallic coils measuring 2×3 and 3×4 mm to be placed (*thick blue arrow*). (**b**) No late filling from the leak is observed after coil placement

Figure 7.10.4 (**a**) Arterial phase intravenous contrast-enhanced abdominal CT after deployment of an abdominal stent shows a type II leak with filling of collateral vessels at the posterior level (*black arrow*). (**b**) Abdominal CT after embolization of the collateral branches with coils shows that the leak has resolved

An 81-year-old man with hypertension (treated with 50 mg oral captopril every 8h), benign prostatic hypertrophy, cholecystectomy, tonsillectomy, and hip fracture underwent CT angiography to follow up an infrarenal aneurysm of the abdominal aorta detected during an abdominal US examination performed for nonspecific digestive complaints 4 years before. The aneurysm measured $63 \times 50 \times 50$ mm and had a mural thrombus, so the medical-surgical team decided on endovascular treatment.

A type II leak developed, with filling of the aneurysmatic sac through the iliolumbar arteries on the right side; these arteries are branches of the right hypogastric artery (Figs. 7.10.1 and 7.10.2).

We embolized the iliolumbar arteries and achieved total occlusion. The final check showed that the aneurysmatic sac no longer filled (Fig. 7.10.3a, b)

Follow-up CT angiography showed the resolution of the leak (Fig. 7.10.4a, b).

Comments Endovascular treatment of abdominal aortic aneurysms with coated stents was first reported by Parodi in 1991. This technique has proven feasible and effective in both the short and long term, and is therefore being indicated in more and more situations. However, one of the major limitations of this technique is leaks. Five kinds of leaks can occur: TYPE I: proximal or distal leak; TYPE II: due to collateral vessels, generally lumbar arteries; TYPE III: due to a defect in the materials that the stent is made of; TYPE IV: due to porosity; TYPE V: due to endotension.

The treatment of type II leaks can range from watchful waiting in cases where the aneurysmatic sac does not enlarge to embolization of the arteries responsible or to direct percutaneous treatment of the aneurysmatic sac by introducing thrombin or other embolizing materials.

Procedure Steps 1. Administer general anesthesia and perform bilateral femoral arteriotomy.
2. Insert a 6F valved introducer sheath through the left femoral artery.

3. Introduce a 100 cm long 5F multipurpose catheter using a 260 cm long 0.035 in. Terumo guidewire to L1.

4. Replace the multipurpose catheter with a 100 cm long 5F pigtail catheter.

5. Insert a 260 cm long stiff 0.035 in. Amplatz guidewire through the right femoral artery.

6. Introduce the stent-graft, containing its main body, through the right femoral artery, until it is released below the renal arteries. Then, place a right iliac extension limb.

7. Pass a 260 cm long stiff 0.035 in. Amplatz guidewire through the left femoral artery.

8. Place a left iliac extension limb.

9. Use a balloon to expand the stent at the level of the neck of the aneurysm and where the stents overlap. Check the results with angiography obtained through a pigtail catheter situated at L1.

10. Embolize the iliolumbar branches of the right hypogastric artery using a 2.7F microcatheter and 2×3 and 3×4 mm microcoils.

Equipment List

1. 6F valved introducer sheaths. Stopcocks, injection pump
2. Nonionic iodinated contrast material (329 mg I/mL)
3. 100 cm long 5F pigtail catheter and 100 cm long 5F multipurpose catheter
4. 260 cm long 0.035 in. Terumo guidewire and 260 cm long 0.035 in. super-stiff Amplatz guidewire
5. Material for femoral arteriotomy
6. Bifurcated coated stent
7. Aortic remodeling balloons
8. 2.7F Progreat microcatheter
9. 2×3 and 3×4 mm microcoils

Further Reading

Bean MJ, Johnson PT, Roseborough GS, Black JH, Fishman EK. Thoracic aortic stent-grafts: utility of multidetector CT for pre- and postprocedure evaluation. Radiographics. 2008;28(7):1835–1851 (review)

Bergqvist D, Björck M, Nyman R. Secondary aortoenteric fistula after endovascular aortic interventions: a systematic literature review. J Vasc Interv Radiol. 2008;19(2 Pt 1):163–165 (review)

Brown LC, Greenhalgh RM, Kwong GP, Powell JT, Thompson SG, Wyatt MG. Secondary interventions and mortality following endovascular aortic aneurysm repair: device-specific results from the UK EVAR trials. Eur J Vasc Endovasc Surg. 2007;34(3):281–290

Chuter TA. Fenestrated and branched stent-grafts for thoracoabdominal, pararenal and juxtarenal aortic aneurysm repair. Semin Vasc Surg. 2007;20(2):90–96 (review)

Chuter TA, Schneider DB. Endovascular repair of the aortic arch. Perspect Vasc Surg Endovasc Ther. 2007;19(2):188–192 (review)

Cochennec F, Gazaigne L, Lesprit P, Desgranges P, Allaire E, Becquemin JP. Aortoiliac aneurysms infected by Campylobacter fetus. J Vasc Surg. 2008;48(4):815–820 (review)

Corbett TJ, Callanan A, Morris LG, Doyle BJ, Grace PA, Kavanagh EG, McGloughlin TM. A review of the in vivo and in vitro biomechanical behavior and performance of postoperative abdominal aortic aneurysms and implanted stent-grafts. J Endovasc Ther. 2008;15(4):468–484 (review)

Dake MD, Miller DC, Semba CP, Mitchell RS, Walker PJ, Liddell RP. Transluminal placement of endovascular stent-grafts for the treatment of descending thoracic aortic aneurysms. N Engl J Med. 1994;331(26):1729–1734

Davey P, Peaston R, Rose JD, Jackson RA, Wyatt MG. Impact on renal function after endovascular aneurysm repair with uncovered supra-renal fixation assessed by serum cystatin C. Eur J Vasc Endovasc Surg. 2008;35(4):439–445

Donas KP, Czerny M, Guber I, Teufelsbauer H, Nanobachvili J. Hybrid open-endovascular repair for thoracoabdominal aortic aneurysms: current status and level of evidence. Eur J Vasc Endovasc Surg. 2007;34(5):528–533 (review)

Gawenda M, Brunkwall J. When is safe to cover the left subclavian and celiac arteries. Part II: celiac artery. J Cardiovasc Surg (Torino). 2008;49(4):479–482 (review)

Greenberg RK, Lytle B. Endovascular repair of thoracoabdominal aneurysms. Circulation. 2008;117(17):2288–2296 (review)

Hoang JK, Martinez S, Hurwitz LM. MDCT angiography of thoracic aorta endovascular stent-grafts: pearls and pitfalls. AJR Am J Roentgenol. 2009;192(2):515–524 (review)

Karmy-Jones R, Simeone A, Meissner M, Granvall B, Nicholls S. Descending thoracic aortic dissections. Surg Clin North Am. 2007;87(5):1047–1086, viii–ix (review)

Nienaber CA, Kische S, Ince H. Thoracic aortic stent-graft devices: problems, failure modes, and applicability. Semin Vasc Surg. 2007;20(2):81–89 (review)

Parker JD, Golledge J. Outcome of endovascular treatment of acute type B aortic dissection. Ann Thorac Surg. 2008;86(5):1707–1712 (review)

Parodi JC. Endovascular repair of abdominal aortic aneurysms and other arterial lesions. J Vasc Surg. 1995;21(4):549–555; discussion 556–567

Razavi MK, Razavi MD. Stent-graft treatment of mycotic aneurysms: a review of the current literature. J Vasc Interv Radiol. 2008;19(6 Suppl):S51–S56 (review)

Ricotta JJ II, Oderich GS. Fenestrated and branched stent-grafts. Perspect Vasc Surg Endovasc Ther. 2008;20(2):174–187; discussion 188–189 (review)

Rose J. Stent-grafts for unruptured abdominal aortic aneurysms: current status. Cardiovasc Intervent Radiol. 2006;29(3):332–343 (review)

Rousseau H, Marcheix B, Chabbert V, Dambrin C, Cron C, Leobon B, Conil C, Massabuau P, Otal P, Joffre F. [Endografts (or stent-grafts) and diseases of the descending thoracic aorta]. Arch Mal Coeur Vaiss. 2006;99(12):1215–1224 (review, French)

Sun Z, Stevenson G. Transrenal fixation of aortic stent-grafts: short- to midterm effects on renal function–a systematic review. Radiology. 2006;240(1):65–72 (review)

Svensson LG, Kouchoukos NT, Miller DC, Bavaria JE, Coselli JS, Curi MA, Eggebrecht H, Elefteriades JA, Erbel R, Gleason TG, Lytle BW, Mitchell RS, Nienaber CA, Roselli EE, Safi HJ, Shemin RJ, Sicard GA, Sundt TM III, Szeto WY, Wheatley GH III; Society of Thoracic Surgeons Endovascular Surgery Task Force. Expert consensus document on the treatment of descending thoracic aortic disease using endovascular stent-grafts. Ann Thorac Surg. 2008;85(1 Suppl):S1–S41

Westaby S, Bertoni GB. Fifty years of thoracic aortic surgery: lessons learned and future directions. Ann Thorac Surg. 2007;83(2):S832–S834; discussion S846–S850 (review)

Xenos ES, Abedi NN, Davenport DL, Minion DJ, Hamdallah O, Sorial EE, Endean ED. Meta-analysis of endovascular vs open repair for traumatic descending thoracic aortic rupture. J Vasc Surg. 2008;48(5):1343–1351 (review)

Percutaneous Drainage of Abdominal Fluid Collections

8

José Rodríguez, Iván Artero, and José J. Muñoz

J.J. Muñoz and R. Ribes, *Learning Vascular and Interventional Radiology*, Learning Imaging,
DOI: 10.1007/978-3-540-87997-8_8, © Springer-Verlag Berlin Heidelberg 2010

Case 8.1

■

Liver Abscess Percutaneous Drainage

Figure 8.1.1 Abdominal CT showing a 5 cm collection in the left liver lobe with an air-fluid level

Figure 8.1.2 US image shows the needle tract into the collection

Figure 8.1.3 US image shows the catheter inside the collection

Figure 8.1.4 Follow-up CT showing the tip of the catheter inside the collection

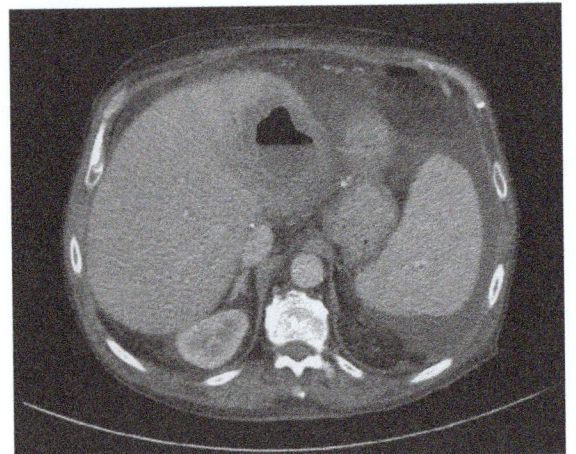

Fig. 8.1.1

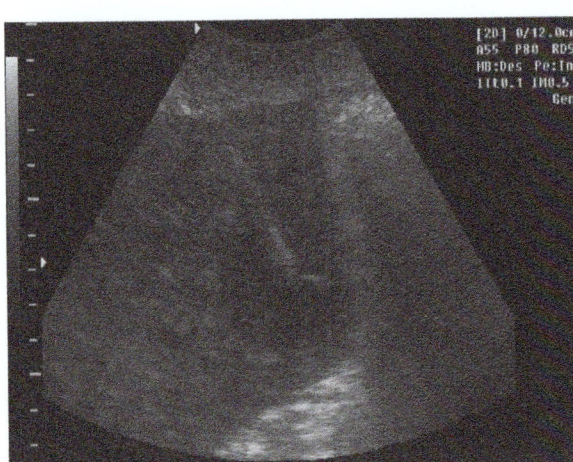

Fig. 8.1.2

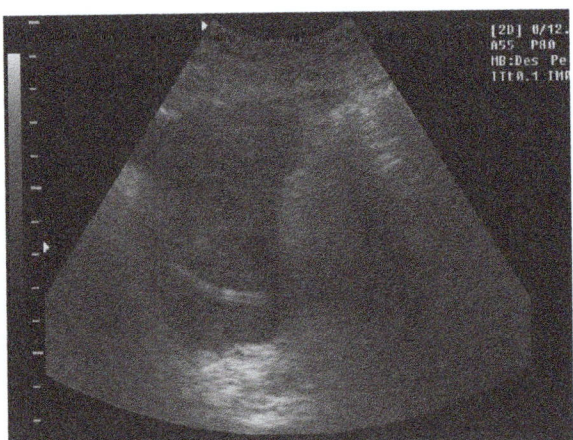

Fig. 8.1.3

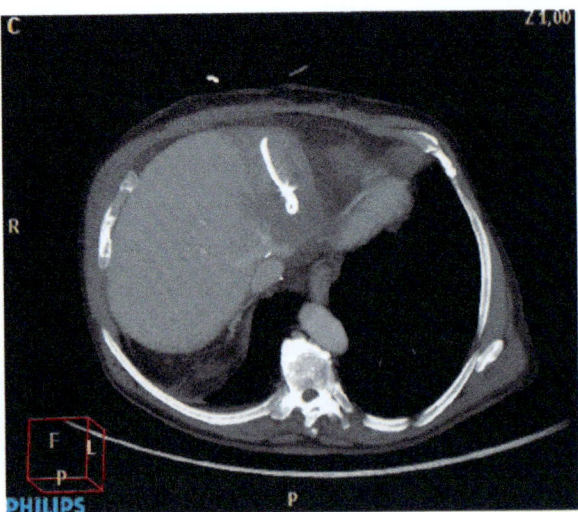

Fig. 8.1.4

A 67-year-old man with a liver transplant 1 year before developed stenosis of the biliary anastomosis that required stent placement by ERCP.

He was admitted for cholangitis, and the stent was removed.

He was readmitted for fever without an apparent focus of infection. Abdominal CT showed a gas-containing collection in the left liver lobe.

Purulent content was aspirated from the collection and an 8.5 F catheter was left in place for drainage.

Comments

In recent decades, the treatment of liver abscesses has changed to a nonsurgical approach. Likewise, the mean age of patients with liver abscesses has increased progressively.

Most liver abscesses are pyogenic in origin and occur secondary to portal dissemination of gastrointestinal disease (mainly, diverticular, inflammatory, or malignant disease) or secondary to biliary tract disease.

After the acute episode resolves, it is important to determine the cause of the abscess.

The diagnosis can be reached via CT or US; both techniques provide information about the size and location of the abscess and make it possible to select the approach to percutaneous treatment and the image method to guide it.

Abscesses located near the diaphragm are more difficult to treat and involve the risk of puncturing the pleura.

In the present case, after we were unable to perform the procedure under US guidance, we successfully resolved the episode under CT guidance.

Cultures of the aspirate enabled more specific antibiotic treatment.

The time to clinical improvement varies.

Catheters should be washed often. Cases with thick contents or septa may require larger bore catheters, multiple catheters, and/or fibrinolytics.

As a rule of thumb, we withdraw the catheters when the output is less than 10cc/day, and the disappearance of the collection is confirmed by imaging.

Equipment List

- 18 G needle
- Curved tip stiff 0.035" Amplatz guidewire
- 6 and 9 F dilators
- 8.5 F multipurpose drainage catheter

Procedure Steps

- Perform US examination and choose access route, measuring the depth and angle of entry.
- Instill local anesthetic (lidocaine 2%) at the entry site and make a 3 mm scalpel incision.
- Insert the 18 G needle under real-time US guidance.
- After correct placement within the collection, aspirate specimens for cultures.
- Introduce the stiff 0.035" guidewire and withdraw the needle.
- Progressively dilate the needle tract using the dilators over the guidewire.
- Introduce the catheter over the guidewire. Fix the catheter in place.
- Connect the catheter to the bag.

Case 8.2

■

Percutaneous Cholecystostomy

Figure 8.2.1 Abdominal CT showing the distended gallbladder with thickened walls due to acute cholecystitis

Figure 8.2.2 US shows the transhepatic needle tract into the gallbladder; the dependent contents of the gallbladder are echogenic

Figure 8.2.3 US shows the catheter inside the gallbladder

Figure 8.2.4 Follow-up study including administration of contrast material through the cholecystostomy catheter shows the patency of the cystic duct and the flow of contrast through the common bile duct into the duodenum

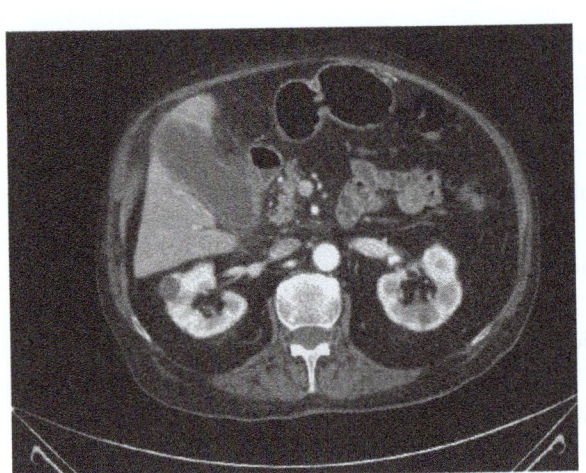

Fig. 8.2.1

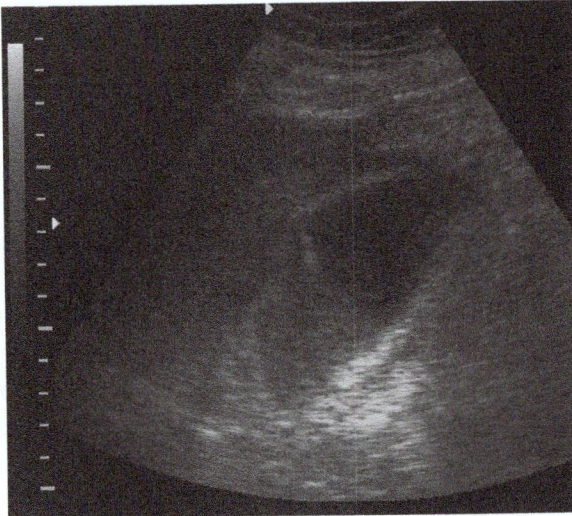

Fig. 8.2.2

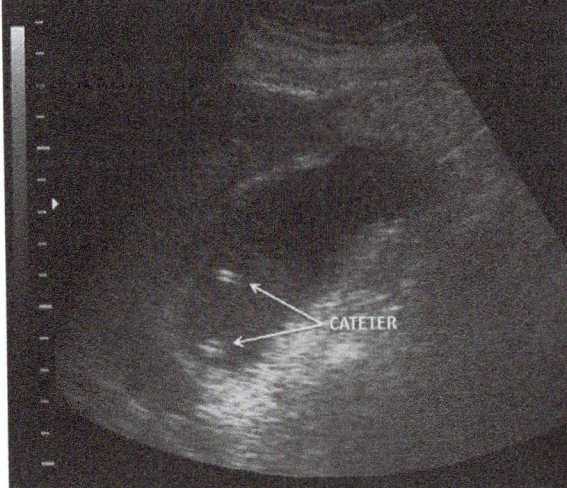

Fig. 8.2.3

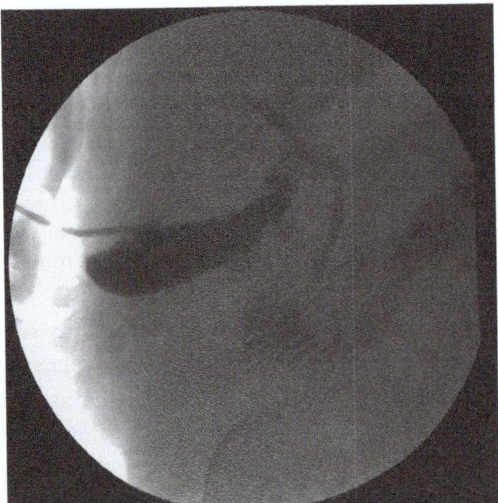

Fig. 8.2.4

A 76-year-old man with heart failure and COPD presented with fever and pain in the epigastric and right hypochondrial regions.

US diagnosed acute cholecystitis after identifying gallbladder distention, gallbladder wall thickening, and positive Murphy sign.

Surgery was ruled out due to the patient's comorbidities, septic state, and anesthetic risk (ASA IV).

We performed percutaneous cholecystostomy, aspirating turbid bile for cultures.

The patient's clinical condition and blood test results improved after 48 h.

Follow-up demonstrated the patency of the cystic duct, and the catheter was withdrawn.

The patient was discharged without surgery.

No recurrence was observed during 14 months' follow-up.

Open or laparoscopic cholecystectomy is the treatment of choice for acute cholecystitis, whether due to gallstones or otherwise.

However, morbidity and mortality increase substantially in critical patients or those with high surgical risk.

In these patients, cholecystostomy is an alternative to surgery. The mortality rates for cholecystostomy range from 0.1 to 3%, and many authors consider it the treatment of choice for all patients.

Cholecystostomy makes it possible to culture the contents of the gallbladder and thus to define a more efficacious antibiotic treatment.

Patients' clinical condition and blood test results improve in 24–48 h, enabling elective surgery with lower morbidity and mortality after resolution of the acute episode.

Nevertheless, not all patients are candidates for surgery; in these cases, drainage and antibiotics are the definitive treatment, with a recurrence of cholecystitis in 5–25%.

The procedure is performed under local anesthesia, usually under US guidance. Whenever possible, the transhepatic approach through the right liver lobe should be used instead of the transperitoneal approach; this reduces the risk of biliary peritonitis due to an intraperitoneal biliary fistula as well as the risk of lesion to the right colic flexure.

After clinical improvement, injecting contrast material through the catheter confirmed the patency of the cystic duct and detected gallstones in the common bile duct, so ERCP was indicated.

Interventional Procedure

Equipment List

- 18 G needle
- Curved tip stiff 0.035" Amplatz guidewire
- 6 and 9 F dilators
- 8.5 F multipurpose drainage catheter

Procedure Steps	• Perform US examination and choose access route, preferably transhepatic, measuring the depth and angle of entry. • Instill local anesthetic (lidocaine 2%) at the entry site and make a 3 mm scalpel incision. • Under real-time US guidance, insert the 18 G needle at the established angle to the determined depth. • After correct placement within the collection, aspirate specimens for cultures. • Introduce the stiff 0.035" guidewire and withdraw the needle. • Progressively dilate the needle tract using the dilators over the guidewire. • Introduce the catheter over the guidewire. Fix the catheter in place. • Connect the catheter to the bag.

Case 8.3
■
Postoperative Retroperitoneal Collection

Figure 8.3.1 Abdominal CT shows a retroperitoneal collection with air-fluid level displacing a small bowel loop. Note the absence of an anterior or lateral window for puncture

Figure 8.3.2 Confirmation of the position of the 18 G needle after a translumbar approach with the patient in the prone position. The tip of the needle is a few centimeters from the collection; the collection can be reached by advancing the needle

Figure 8.3.3 Confirmation of catheter placement within the collection

Figure 8.3.4 Follow-up CT shows that the collection has virtually disappeared

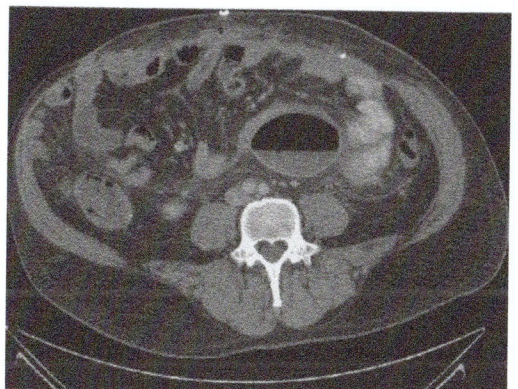

Fig. 8.3.1

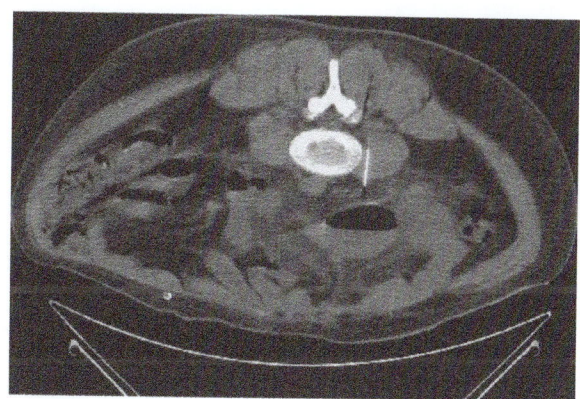

Fig. 8.3.2

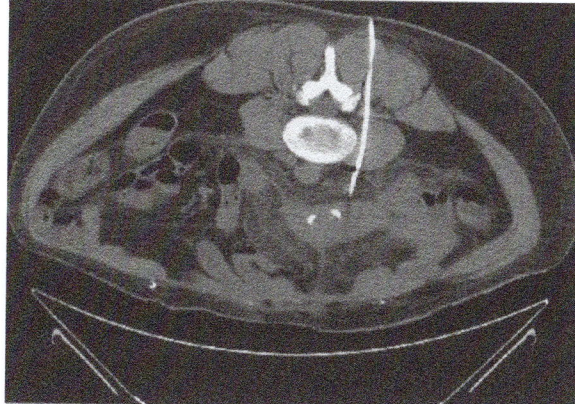

Fig. 8.3.3

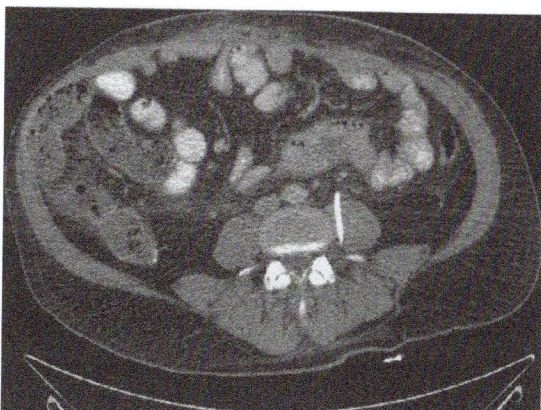

Fig. 8.3.4

A 42-year-old man treated 16 months earlier for fecal peritonitis secondary to foreign body perforation of the colon with a terminal colostomy in left iliac fossa was admitted for restoration of intestinal transit with a side-to-side colorectal anastomosis.

In the postoperative period, he presented fever and a small leak in the anastomosis. CT showed a retroperitoneal collection.

The collection was catheterized using a CT-guided translumbar approach; purulent contents were aspirated, and a drainage catheter was left in place.

Follow-up studies showed a significant reduction in the size of the collection, and the drainage catheter was withdrawn.

Comments

Intraabdominal collections are relatively common after surgery.

The type of collection varies and may include hematomas, seromas, abscesses, bilomas, or urinomas, depending on the type of surgery.

The presence of a collection does not necessarily call for its drainage. Drainage is necessary only when infection is suspected or the collection causes symptoms by compression.

Nevertheless, in cases with associated fever, puncture is indicated to determine the contents of the collection and to decide whether to leave a drainage catheter.

Retroperitoneal collections usually require CT-guided translumbar access; however, large collections near the abdominal wall sometimes allow US-guided anterior or lateral access.

Catheters are withdrawn after clinical improvement and output less than 10 cc/day.

Interventional Procedure

Equipment List

- 18 G needle
- Curved tip stiff 0.035" Amplatz guidewire
- 6 and 9 F dilators
- 8.5 F multipurpose drainage catheter

Procedure Steps

- Perform CT examination with the patient in the prone position and mark the theoretical point of access.
- Select the appropriate slice for access; measure the depth and angle of entry. Mark the access site on the skin.
- Instill local anesthetic (lidocaine 2%) at the entry site and make a 3 mm scalpel incision.
- Insert the 18 G needle at the established angle to the determined depth.
- Confirm the position of the needle by CT.
- Introduce the stiff 0.035" guidewire and withdraw the needle.
- Progressively dilate the needle tract using the dilators over the guidewire.
- Introduce the catheter over the guidewire. Fix the catheter in place.
- Confirm the position of the catheter by CT.
- Connect the catheter to the bag.

Case 8.4

Collections in the Psoas Muscle

Figure 8.4.1 Confirmation of the position of the drainage catheter after puncture of the right psoas

Figure 8.4.2 Follow-up image shows the practical disappearance of the collection. Note the collection in the left psoas

Figure 8.4.3 Slice selected for access to the collection in the left psoas, with measurements of the depth and angle of entry

Figure 8.4.4 Confirmation of the position of the drainage catheter after puncture of the left psoas

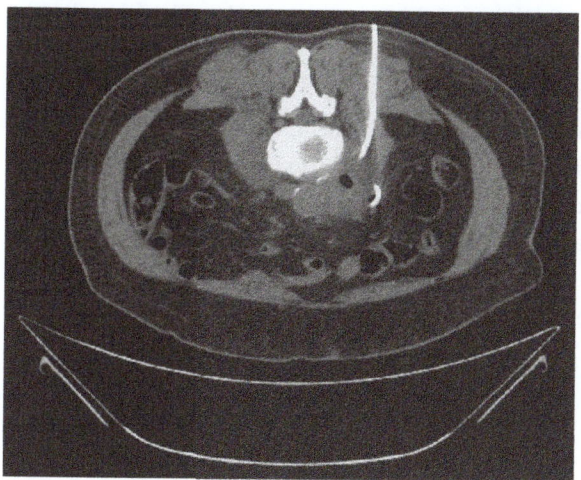

Fig. 8.4.1

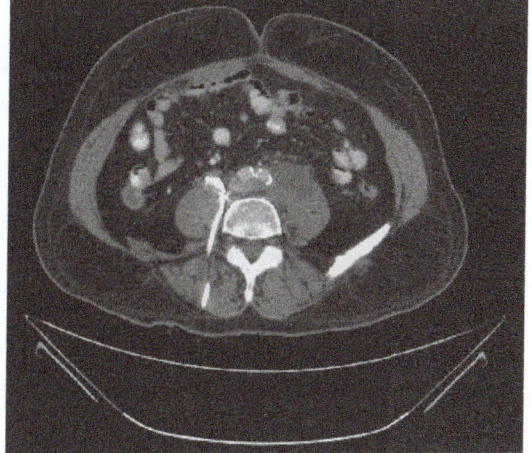

Fig. 8.4.2

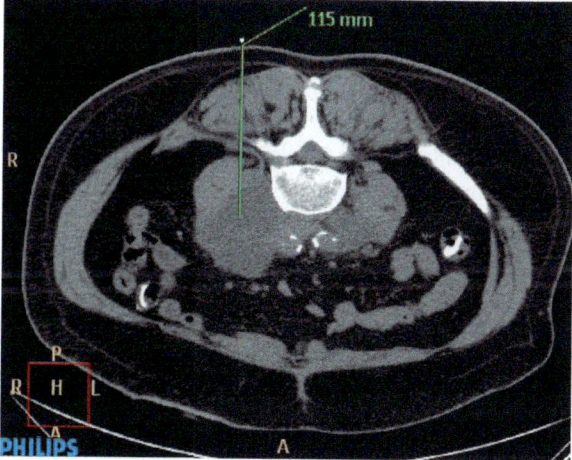

Fig. 8.4.3

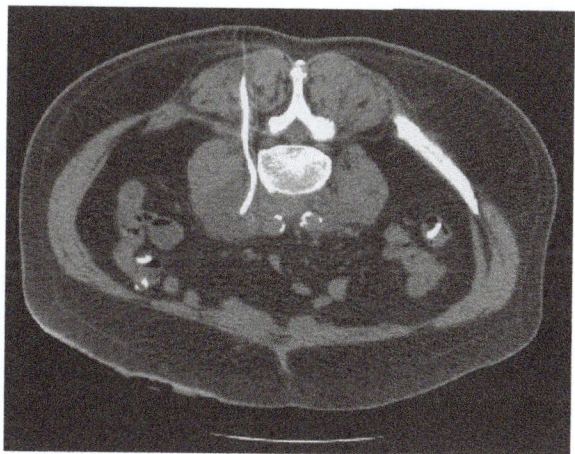

Fig. 8.4.4

A 63-year-old man treated for bladder cancer with radical cystoprostatectomy and Bricker-type ileal conduit urinary diversion plus bilateral iliac lymph node resection was admitted for right leg pain and later left leg pain. He had no fever or other symptoms.

Abdominal CT showed collections in both psoas.

The collection in the right psoas was drained; and analysis of the specimen showed transudates, and an infectious origin was ruled out.

When symptoms appeared in the left leg, the collection in the left psoas was drained, and analysis of the specimen yielded identical results.

Symptoms disappeared and the collections decreased in size, so the drainages were withdrawn.

Comments

The iliopsoas compartment extends from T12 to the lesser trochanter of the femur. Its close relation to the retroperitoneal organs, pelvis, and thigh means it can be affected by diverse processes.

Iliopsoas compartment involvement in tuberculosis from a spondylotic focus has been widely reported, and percutaneous drainage with antibiotic therapy is the treatment of choice.

In the present case, the collection was iatrogenic secondary to radical cystoprostatectomy with bilateral iliac lymph node resection leading to lymphocele formation in both psoas.

These collections require drainage only in cases with pain or functional impotence of the lower limbs.

CT-guided translumbar access enables safe and accurate needle and catheter insertion, minimizing complications.

Interventional Procedure

Equipment List

- 18 G needle
- Curved tip stiff 0.035" Amplatz guidewire
- 6 and 9 F dilators
- 8.5 F multipurpose drainage catheter

Procedure Steps

- Perform CT examination with the patient in the prone position and mark the theoretical point of access.
- Select the appropriate slice for access; measure the depth and angle of entry. Mark the access site on the skin.
- Instill local anesthetic (lidocaine 2%) at the entry site and make a 3 mm scalpel incision.
- Insert the 18 G needle at the established angle to the determined depth.
- Confirm the position of the needle by CT.
- After ensuring correct needle placement, aspirate a specimen for analysis and cultures.
- Introduce the stiff 0.035" guidewire and withdraw the needle.
- Progressively dilate the needle tract using the dilators over the guidewire.
- Introduce the catheter over the guidewire. Fix the catheter in place.
- Confirm the position of the catheter by CT.
- Connect the catheter to the bag.

Figure 8.5.1 US showing the collection in the surgical bed

Figure 8.5.2 Image showing the guidewire inside the collection

Figure 8.5.3 Follow-up US image showing the catheter inside the collection

Figure 8.5.4 Cholangio-MRI reconstruction showing the catheter in the liver parenchyma and absence of the collection. There was no evidence of biliary leaks

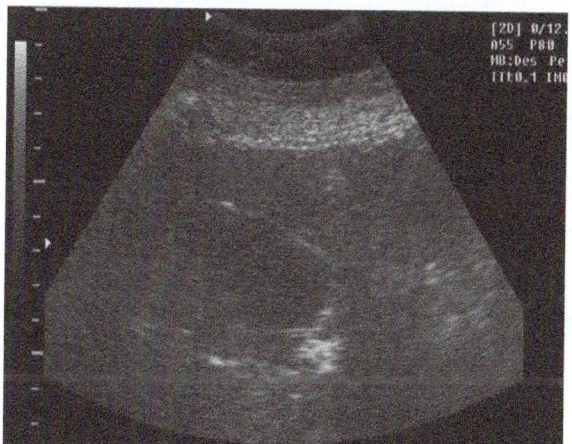

Fig. 8.5.1

Fig. 8.5.2

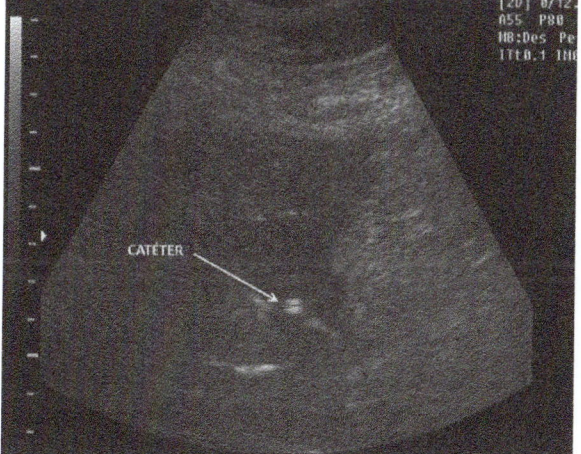

Fig. 8.5.3

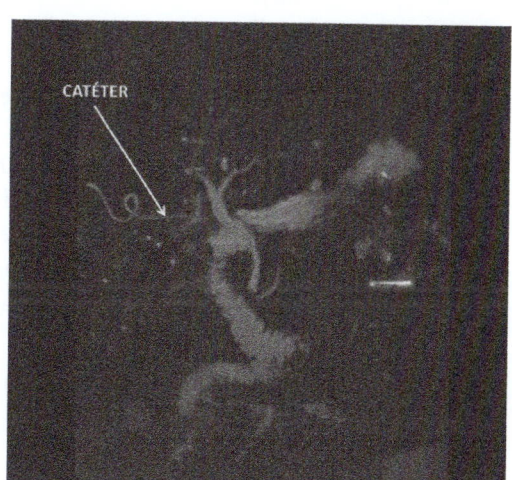

Fig. 8.5.4

A 33-year-old woman with a history of symptomatic cholelithiasis presented with abdominal pain and was diagnosed with cholecystitis.

Laparoscopic cholecystectomy was performed without incidents.

In the postoperative period, a collection was observed in the surgical bed.

The collection was drained; aspiration yielded serous-sanguineous fluid followed by bilious fluid.

Despite scant output, the fistula did not disappear, so a stent was placed by ERCP. After the fistula closed, the stent was removed on an outpatient basis.

Comments

Given the number of gallbladder interventions, postoperative complications of gallbladder surgery are relatively common.

In most cases, the patient is referred for a collection in the surgical bed. The collection may correspond to a hematoma, abscess, or biloma due to a biliary fistula.

Small collections without clinical signs of infection should not be drained, although puncture-aspiration is often performed to confirm the nature of the collection.

In cases with suspected infection, a drainage catheter should be left in place.

Depending on the output, it may be necessary to isolate the fistula in cases with bile leaks. In the present case, this was accomplished by ERCP stent placement; however, surgical repair is sometimes necessary.

When these options are not viable, percutaneous biliary drainage may be necessary.

Interventional Procedure Equipment List

- 18 G needle
- Curved tip stiff 0.035" Amplatz guidewire
- 6 and 9 F dilators
- 8.5 F multipurpose drainage catheter

Procedure Steps

- Perform US examination and choose access route, measuring the depth and angle of entry.
- Instill local anesthetic (lidocaine 2%) at the entry site and make a 3 mm scalpel incision.
- Under real-time US guidance, insert the 18 G needle at the established angle to the determined depth.
- After correct placement within the collection, aspirate specimens for cultures.
- Introduce the stiff 0.035" guidewire and withdraw the needle.
- Progressively dilate the needle tract using the dilators over the guidewire.
- Introduce the catheter over the guidewire. Fix the catheter in place.
- Connect the catheter to the bag.

Figure 8.6.1 Hepatic collection with an air-fluid level adjacent to the diaphragm

Figure 8.6.2 Topogram with a radiopaque marker in the axillary midline to locate the access site. Note the gas below the right diaphragm, indicative of an abscess

Figure 8.6.3 Confirmation of correct catheter placement by introducing contrast material: the contrast mixes with the contents of the collection

Figure 8.6.4 Follow-up US shows the virtual disappearance of the collection

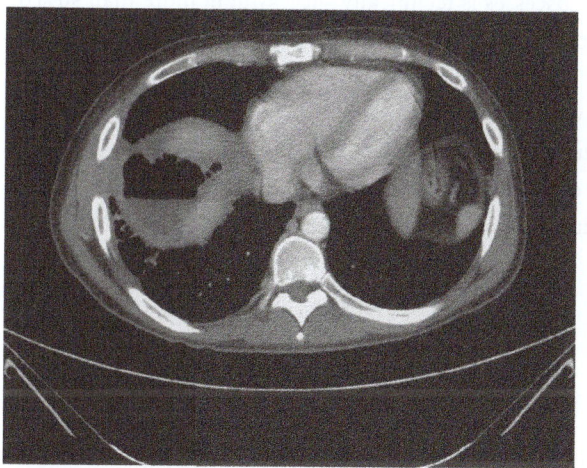

Fig. 8.6.1

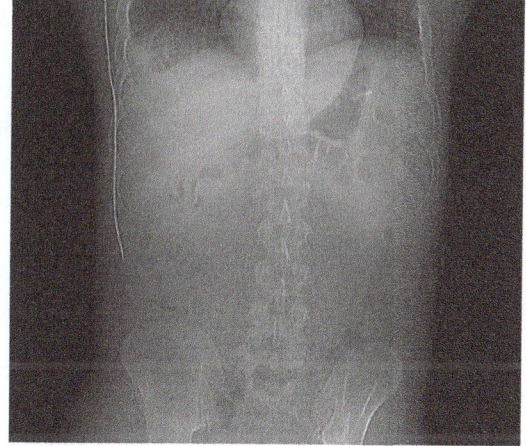

Fig. 8.6.2

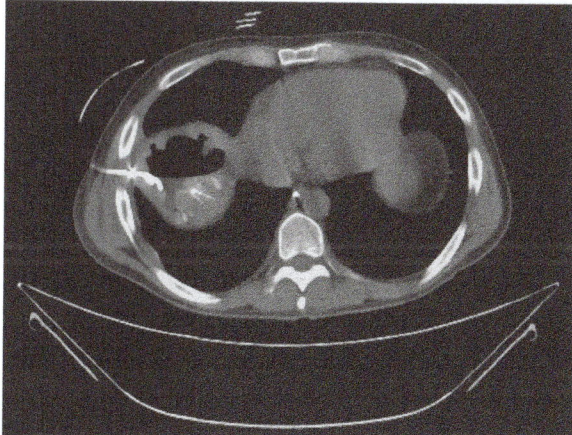

Fig. 8.6.3

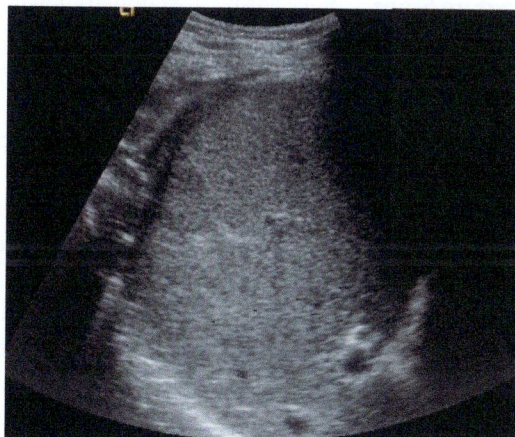

Fig. 8.6.4

A 32-year-old man underwent right hemicolectomy for Crohn's disease; recovery was slow, and 4 months later, he was admitted for abdominal pain, abdominal wall tumefaction, and fever. Empirical antibiotic treatment was initiated.

Plain-film chest X-rays showed gas below the right diaphragm. Abdominal CT showed a gas collection measuring 8×2 cm below the right diaphragm.

Attempts to drain the collection under US guidance were unsuccessful. CT-guided drainage achieved purulent aspirate for cultures.

The patient's condition improved, and follow-up images prior to discharge showed a thick-walled virtual cavity with output less than 10 cc/day, so the drainage catheter was withdrawn.

Comments

Abdominal or pelvic abscesses often develop in patients with Crohn's disease after fistulization and contained perforation of the inflamed intestinal loops.

The most frequent locations are the lower right quadrant, lower left quadrant, and the psoas.

Percutaneous drainage of these abscesses is technically successful in more than 90% of cases, with adequate drainage regardless of its location; however, the recurrence rate is high (35%).

Between 70 and 90% of patients with Crohn's disease will require surgery, and more than 30% will require more than one surgical intervention.

In many cases, drainage cannot obviate eventual surgery, although it does help ensure a cleaner surgical field and thus reduces the difficulty, complications, and morbidity of the intervention.

Interventional Procedure

Equipment List

- 18 G needle
- Curved tip stiff 0.035" Amplatz guidewire
- 6 and 9 F dilators
- 8.5 F multipurpose drainage catheter

Procedure Steps

- Perform CT examination with the patient in the prone position and mark the theoretical point of access.
- Select the appropriate slice for access; measure the depth and angle of entry. Mark the access site on the skin.
- Instill local anesthetic (lidocaine 2%) at the entry site and make a 3 mm scalpel incision.
- Insert the 18 G needle at the established angle to the determined depth.
- Confirm the position of the needle by CT.
- After ensuring correct needle placement, aspirate a specimen for analysis and cultures.
- Introduce the stiff 0.035" guidewire and withdraw the needle.
- Progressively dilate the needle tract using the dilators over the guidewire.
- Introduce the catheter over the guidewire. Fix the catheter in place.
- Confirm the position of the catheter by CT.
- Connect the catheter to the bag.

<table>
<tr>
<td>

Case 8.7

■

Urinoma

</td>
<td>

Figure 8.7.1 Doppler US shows a collection measuring 50 × 23 mm at the level of the hilum of the renal graft in the right iliac fossa

Figure 8.7.2 Pulsed Doppler US shows systolic velocities greater than 100 cm/sec

Figure 8.7.3 CT image showing the guidewire inside the collection through the narrow window between the renal graft and the bladder

Figure 8.7.4 Disappearance of the collection after aspiration of its contents

</td>
</tr>
</table>

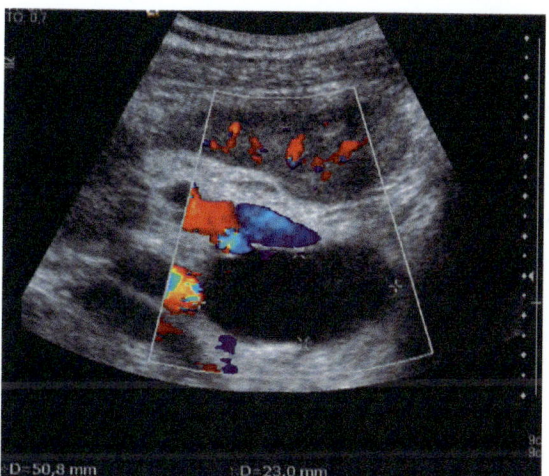

Fig. 8.7.1

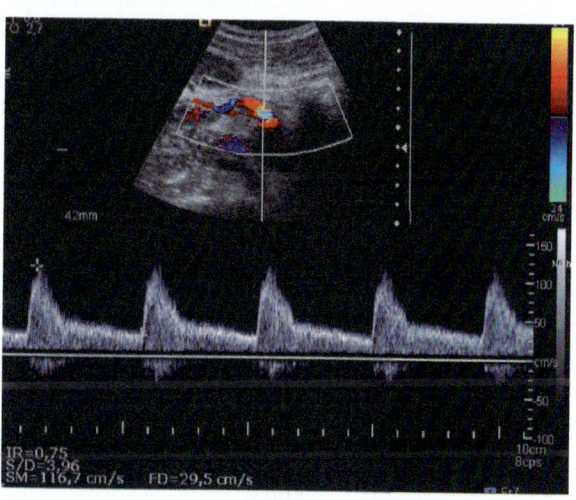

Fig. 8.7.2

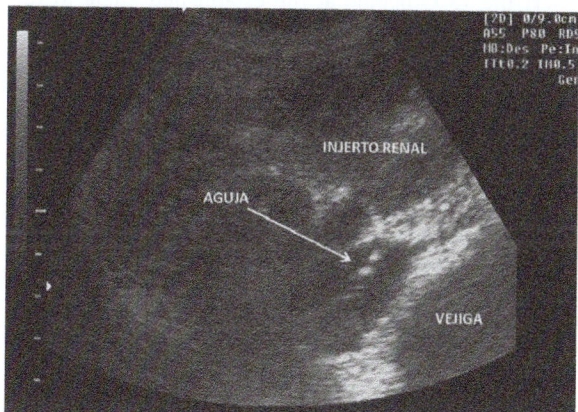

Fig. 8.7.3

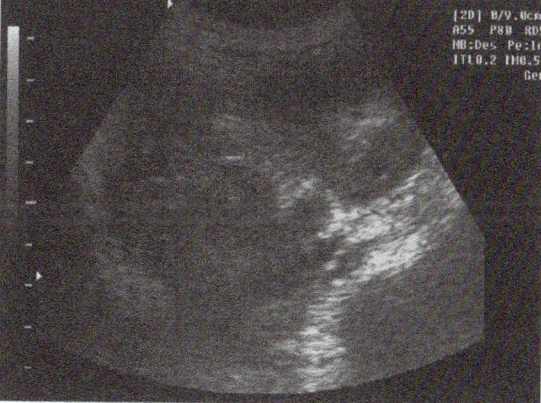

Fig. 8.7.4

Six months after kidney transplantation, a 56-year old male patient presented a perirenal collection that compressed the hilum of the graft, causing extremely high-velocity arterial flow. The contents of the collection were aspirated, and it was not necessary to leave a drainage catheter in place.

Follow-up US showed the disappearance of the collection and the normalization of arterial flow.

Analysis of the aspirate showed the collection was a urinoma.

Comments

Urinary leaks and urinomas can have a variety of causes, including trauma; most leaks and urinomas at the level of the ureters are iatrogenic in origin. Leaks and urinomas occasionally go undetected and can cause delayed complications.

Urinomas secondary to ureteral lesions can be treated by drainage, although they sometimes require nephrostomy and/or nephroureteral catheter placement for 4–6 weeks to enable the leak to resolve.

In cases of total rupture, nephrostomy would be necessary or, in inoperable patients, the ureter would have to be embolized.

The approach used for percutaneous drainage will depend on the location of the lesion and on whether CT or US is used to guide the procedure.

In the present case, although the collection was small, it was necessary to drain it because of its effects on flow through the graft.

The location of the collection left a very small US window between the bladder and the transplanted kidney.

Interventional Procedure

Equipment List

- 18 G needle

Procedure Steps

- Perform US examination and choose access route, measuring the depth and angle of entry.
- Instill local anesthetic (lidocaine 2%) at the entry site and make a 3 mm scalpel incision.
- Under real-time US guidance, insert the 18 G needle at the established angle to the determined depth.
- After correct placement within the collection, aspirate specimens for cultures.
- Confirm the disappearance of the collection.

Case 8.8
■

**Transgluteal
Drainage**

Figure 8.8.1 Patient in the lateral decubitus position with a radiopaque marker in the intergluteal line. Presacral collection with an air-fluid level. Surgical drainage between bowel loops

Figure 8.8.2 Confirmation of the needle inside the collection

Figure 8.8.3 Disappearance of the collection: the catheter is shown in a virtual cavity

Figure 8.8.4 Follow-up several months later shows the absence of the collection

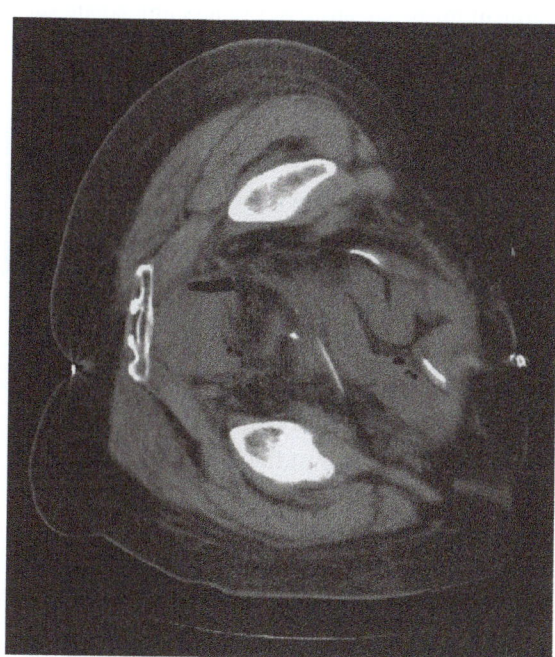

Fig. 8.8.1

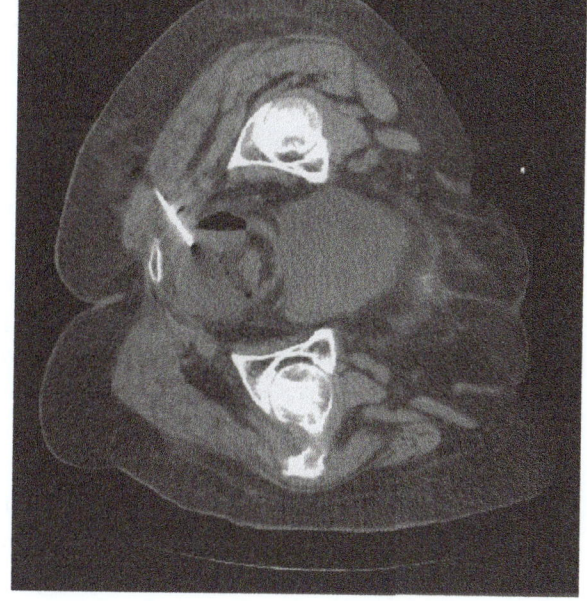

Fig. 8.8.2

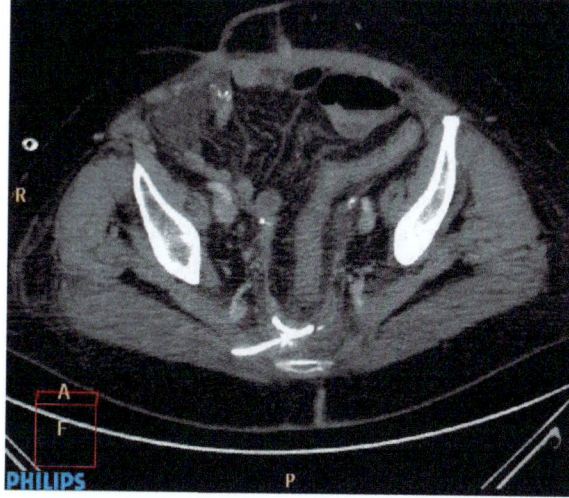

Fig. 8.8.3

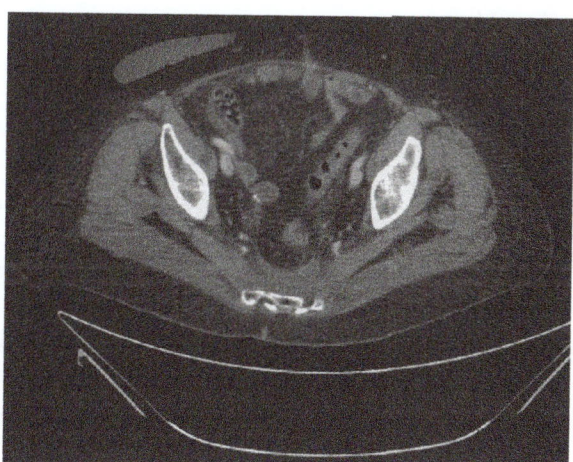

Fig. 8.8.4

A 72-year-old woman underwent surgery for rectal cancer, and a protective ileostomy was created. She had a fever, ileus, and bilious vomiting in the postoperative period.

CT showed a presacral collection posterior to the sutures of the rectal stump.

The collection was drained under CT guidance, and a 10.2 F catheter was left in place; the purulent aspirate was cultured.

Follow-up CT 12 days later showed no collection, and the catheter was withdrawn.

Comments

Percutaneous drainage is the usual treatment for pelvic abscesses unless immediate surgery is indicated.

The presence of multiple structures makes it challenging to plan a safe access.

In most cases, a US-guided anterior approach is not possible due to the interposition of bowel loops, bladder, etc.

CT-guided transgluteal access makes it possible to avoid these structures through a safe approach.

Thorough knowledge of pelvic anatomy will enable lesions to structures to be avoided and will reduce the risk of complications.

The ideal access route will be through the sacrospinous ligament, as close to the sacrum as possible to avoid crossing the piriformis muscle, which is situated cephalad to the ligament whenever possible, so we will use the angling of the gantry if necessary.

The sacral plexus and the gluteal arteries and veins flow at the level of the piriformis muscle, increasing the risk of hemorrhagic complications or nerve lesions if access is through the muscle.

Likewise, peri and postprocedural pain is greater when the piriformis muscle is crossed.

Catheter care and withdrawal are the same as in other cases.

Interventional Procedure Equipment List

- 18 G needle
- Curved tip stiff 0.035" Amplatz guidewire
- 6, 8, and 10 F dilators
- 10.2 F multipurpose drainage catheter

Procedure Steps

- Perform CT examination with the patient in the lateral decubitus position with a marker on the intergluteal line.
- Select the appropriate slice for access; measure the depth and angle of entry. Mark the access site on the skin.
- Instill local anesthetic (lidocaine 2%) at the entry site and make a 3 mm scalpel incision.
- Insert the 18 G needle at the established angle to the determined depth.
- Confirm the position of the needle by CT.
- After ensuring correct needle placement, aspirate a specimen for analysis and cultures.
- Introduce the stiff 0.035" guidewire and withdraw the needle.
- Progressively dilate the needle tract using the dilators over the guidewire.
- Introduce the catheter over the guidewire. Fix the catheter in place.
- Confirm the position of the catheter by CT.
- Connect the catheter to the bag.

Case 8.9
Peripancreatic Collection

Figure 8.9.1 Slice selected to determine the approach: a radiopaque marker is on the skin

Figure 8.9.2 Confirmation of needle placement inside the collection

Figure 8.9.3 Confirmation of catheter positioning within the collection

Figure 8.9.4 Follow-up CT showing that the collection has disappeared

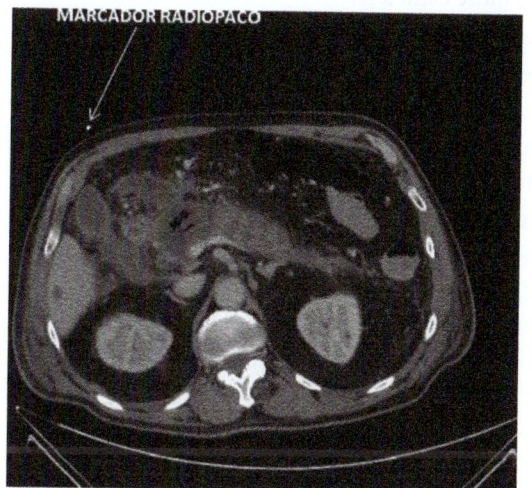

Fig. 8.9.1

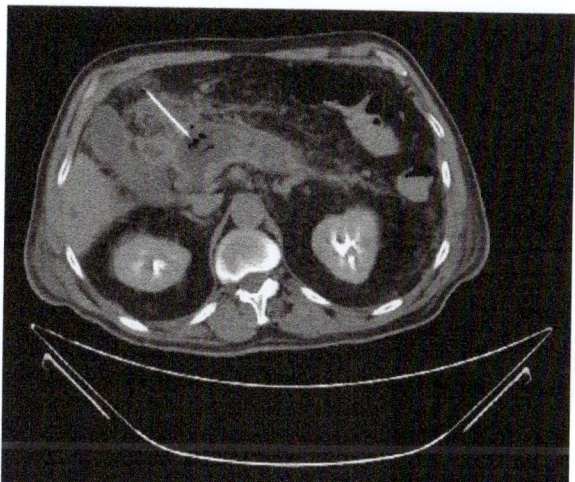

Fig. 8.9.2

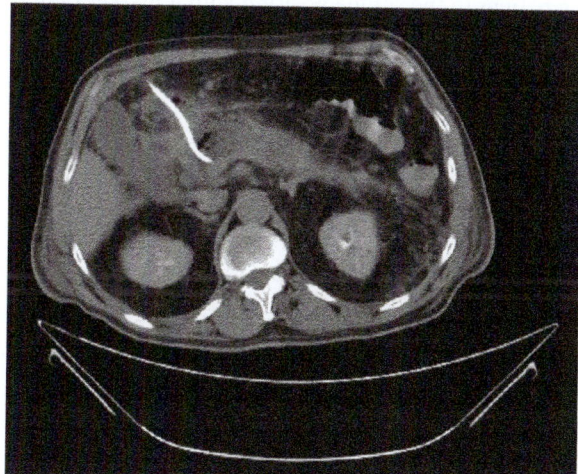

Fig. 8.9.3

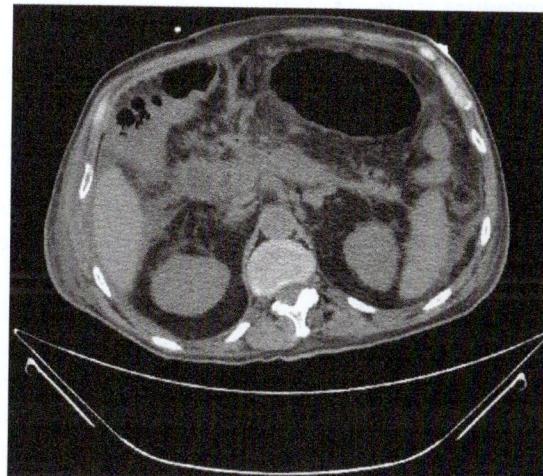

Fig. 8.9.4

An 80-year-old woman was admitted for acute necrotic pancreatitis with poor evolution, respiratory distress, and persistent ileus.

CT showed a collection containing gas at the level of the pancreatic head.

Drainage resulted in clinical improvement, and CT before discharge showed the collection had decreased in size.

Comments

The course of acute pancreatitis can be unpredictable, and treatment is mainly supportive.

However, local complications require invasive treatment and the direct involvement of interventional radiologists.

Pancreatic necrosis implies a worse prognosis if it is extensive or if a superinfection develops. CT-guided aspiration makes it possible to take a specimen for culturing and to leave a drainage catheter in place if necessary.

Abscesses must be drained with one or more catheters.

Pseudocysts should be evacuated when they are symptomatic, when superinfections develop, or when they persist. Sometimes catheters must be left in place for more than 5 weeks when the pseudocyst communicates with pancreatic ducts.

CT guidance is required in most cases, although US guidance can be used in some cases with large pseudocysts adjacent to the abdominal wall.

The access route will depend on the location of the collection: collections near the head of the pancreas require an approach through the gastrocolic ligament whereas collections near the body or tail require an approach through the left anterior pararenal space.

Interventional Procedure Equipment List

- 18 G needle
- Curved tip stiff 0.035" Amplatz guidewire
- 6 and 9 F dilators
- 8.5 F multipurpose drainage catheter

Procedure Steps

- Perform CT examination with the patient in the supine position with a marker on the presumed area of access.
- Select the appropriate slice for access; measure the depth and angle of entry. Mark the access site on the skin.
- Instill local anesthetic (lidocaine 2%) at the entry site and make a 3 mm scalpel incision.
- Insert the 18 G needle at the established angle to the determined depth.
- Confirm the position of the needle by CT.
- After ensuring correct needle placement, aspirate a specimen for analysis and cultures.
- Introduce the stiff 0.035" guidewire and withdraw the needle.
- Progressively dilate the needle tract using the dilators over the guidewire.
- Introduce the catheter over the guidewire. Fix the catheter in place.
- Confirm the position of the catheter by CT.
- Connect the catheter to the bag.

Case 8.10

■

Pleural Drainage

Figure 8.10.1 Plain-film chest X-ray showing bilateral pleural effusion, greater on the left side

Figure 8.10.2 US shows free effusion without septa

Figure 8.10.3 The guidewire in the pleural cavity after US-guided puncture

Figure 8.10.4 Follow-up US shows the effusion has resolved. The catheter is seen in the pleural cavity. Note the wall thickening

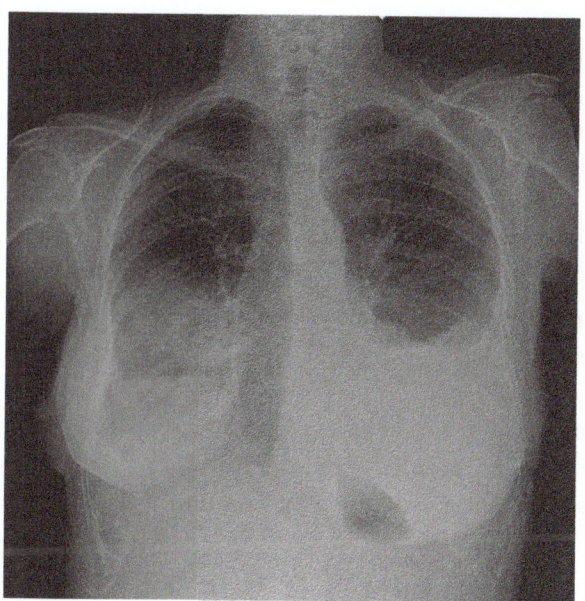

Fig. 8.10.1

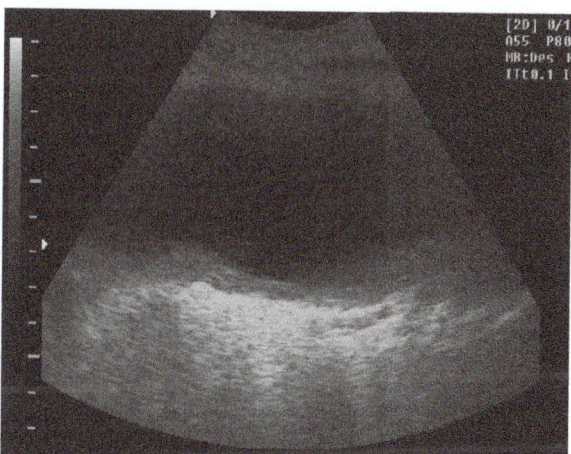

Fig. 8.10.2

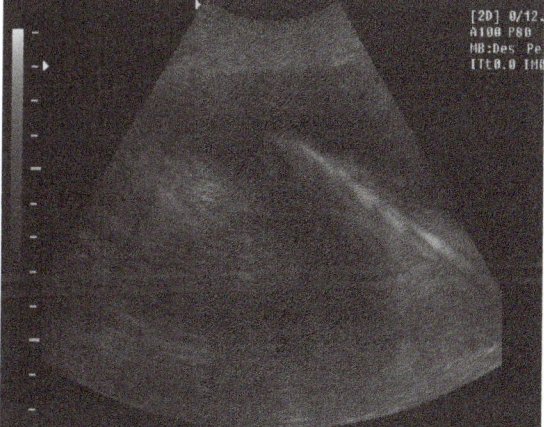

Fig. 8.10.3

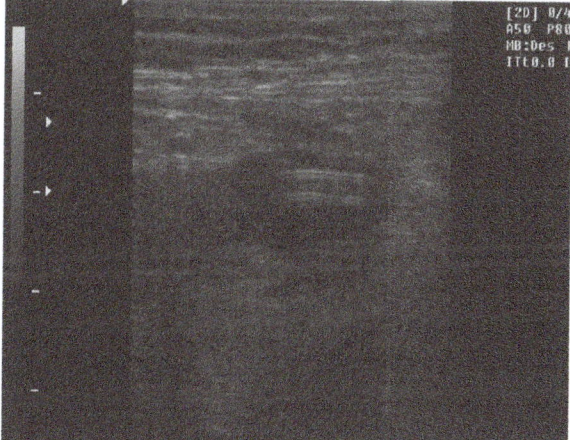

Fig. 8.10.4

A 66-year-old woman with a breast implant after surgery for a carcinoma in her right breast developed bone and pleural metastases with bilateral pleural effusion requiring repeated thoracocentesis to relieve respiratory symptoms.

A drainage catheter was placed in the left pleura, where effusion was more abundant.

The patient died before pleurodesis could be performed.

Comments

Pleural effusions have diverse origins, from empyemas, parapneumonic effusions, malignant effusions, or even hemothorax.

When appropriately indicated, all these types of effusion can be drained percutaneously.

In the vast majority of cases, US guidance suffices; CT guidance is used only in exceptional cases, especially in loculated collections associated to consolidation of the underlying parenchyma.

In patients with suspected infection, diagnostic thoracocentesis is performed first, and then a drainage catheter is implanted if infection is confirmed.

In free collections, the steepest area is approached normally from the level of the medial or posterior axillary line over the upper margin of the rib to avoid damage to the intercostal nerves and vessels.

The location of loculated collections will determine the approach used, and the catheter should be left in the steepest part. In most cases, catheters ranging in size from 8 to 12 F will be sufficient and will be better tolerated than thicker catheters.

Empyemas should be drained early, in the acute phase (1–4 weeks), to obtain a good outcome and avoid the formation of septa.

Many cases with effusions of malignant origin require repeated thoracocentesis for drainage; so drainage catheters are often implanted. After catheter placement, the contents are aspirated; however, no more than 1–1.5 L should be drained to avoid pulmonary edema due to re-expansion. After this, the catheter should be connected to an aspiration system. Once the effusion has disappeared and the lung has re-expanded, chemical pleurodesis should be performed.

If drainage output decreases but the amount of effusion on plain-film X-rays does not decrease, it is likely that debris, septa, or loculations are present. In these cases, the instillation of fibrinolytic drugs is useful. We use 100,000 UI urokinase in 100 mL saline solution through the catheter and clamp it for 2 h, having the patient change position. Finally, the contents are aspirated.

Interventional Procedure Equipment List

- 18 G needle
- Curved tip stiff 0.035" Amplatz guidewire
- 6 and 9 F dilators
- 8.5 F multipurpose drainage catheter

- Perform US examination and choose access route to the steepest zone, measuring the depth and angle of entry.
- Instill local anesthetic (lidocaine 2%) at the entry site and make a 3 mm scalpel incision.
- Under real-time US guidance, insert the 18 G needle over the upper portion of the rib at the established angle to the determined depth.
- After correct placement within the collection, aspirate specimens for cultures.
- Introduce the stiff 0.035" guidewire and withdraw the needle.
- Progressively dilate the needle tract using the dilators over the guidewire.
- Introduce the catheter over the guidewire. Fix the catheter in place.
- Connect the catheter to the aspiration system.

Further Reading

Arnaud JP, Pessaux P. Percutaneous cholecystostomy for high-risk acute cholecystitis patients. South Med J 2008; 101(6):577

Beland MD, Gervais DA, Levis DA, Hahn PF, Arellano RS, Mueller PR. Complex abdominal and pelvic abscesses: efficacy of adjunctive tissue-type plasminogen activator for drainage. Radiology 2008; 247(2):567–573. Epub 2008 Mar 27

Dinç H, Ahmeto lu A, Baykal S, Sari A, Sayil O, Gümele HR. Image-guided percutaneous drainage of tuberculous iliopsoas and spondylodiskitic abscesses: midterm results. Radiology 2002; 225(2):353–358

Gervais DA, Hahn PF, O'Neill MJ, Mueller PR. Percutaneous abscess drainage in Crohn disease: technical success and short- and long-term outcomes during 14 years. Radiology 2002; 222(3):645–651

Griniatsos J, Petrou A, Pappas P, Revenas K, Karavokyros I, Michail OP, Tsigris C, Giannopoulos A, Felekouras E. Percutaneous cholecystostomy without interval cholecystectomy as definitive treatment of acute cholecystitis in elderly and critically ill patients. South Med J 2008; 101(6):586–590

Harisinghani MG, Gervais DA, Hahn PF, Cho CH, Jhaveri K, Varghese J, Mueller PR. CT-guided transgluteal drainage of deep pelvic abscesses: indications, technique, procedure-related complications, and clinical outcome. Radiographics 2002; 22(6):1353–1367. Review

Kim JK, Jeong YY, Kim YH, Kim YC, Kang HK, Choi HS. Postoperative pelvic lymphocele: treatment with simple percutaneous catheter drainage. Radiology 1999; 212(2):390–394

Klein JS, Schultz S, Heffner JE. Interventional radiology of the chest: image-guided percutaneous drainage of pleural effusions, lung abscess, and pneumothorax. AJR Am J Roentgenol 1995; 164(3):581–588. Review

Lee MJ, Wittich GR, Mueller PR. Percutaneous intervention in acute pancreatitis. Radiographics 1998; 18(3):711–724; discussion 728. Review. Erratum in: Radiographics 1998; 18(5):1336

Maher MM, Kealey S, McNamara A, O'Laoide R, Gibney RG, Malone DE. Management of visceral interventional radiology catheters: a troubleshooting guide for interventional radiologists. Radiographics 2002; 22(2):305–322. Review

Mohsen AH, Green ST, Read RC, McKendrick MW. Liver abscess in adults: ten years experience in a UK centre. QJM 2002; 95(12):797–802

Moulton JS. Image-guided management of complicated pleural fluid collections. Radiol Clin North Am 2000; 38(2):345–374. Review

Shankar S, vanSonnenberg E, Silverman SG, Tuncali K, Banks PA. Imaging and percutaneous management of acute complicated pancreatitis. Cardiovasc Intervent Radiol 2004; 27(6):567–580. Epub 2004 Aug 12. Review

Titton RL, Gervais DA, Hahn PF, Harisinghani MG, Arellano RS, Mueller PR. Urine leaks and urinomas: diagnosis and imaging-guided intervention. Radiographics 2003; 23(5):1133–1147. Review

vanSonnenberg E, Wittich GR, Goodacre BW, Casola G, D'Agostino HB. Percutaneous abscess drainage: update. World J Surg 2001; 25(3):362–369; discussion 370–372. Epub 2001 Apr 11. Review

Biliary Interventions and Treatment of Focal Hepatic Lesions

9

Carlos Lanciego and Lorenzo García

J.J. Muñoz and R. Ribes, *Learning Vascular and Interventional Radiology*, Learning Imaging,
DOI: 10.1007/978-3-540-87997-8_9, © Springer-Verlag Berlin Heidelberg 2010

Case 9.1

Percutaneous External Biliary Drainage

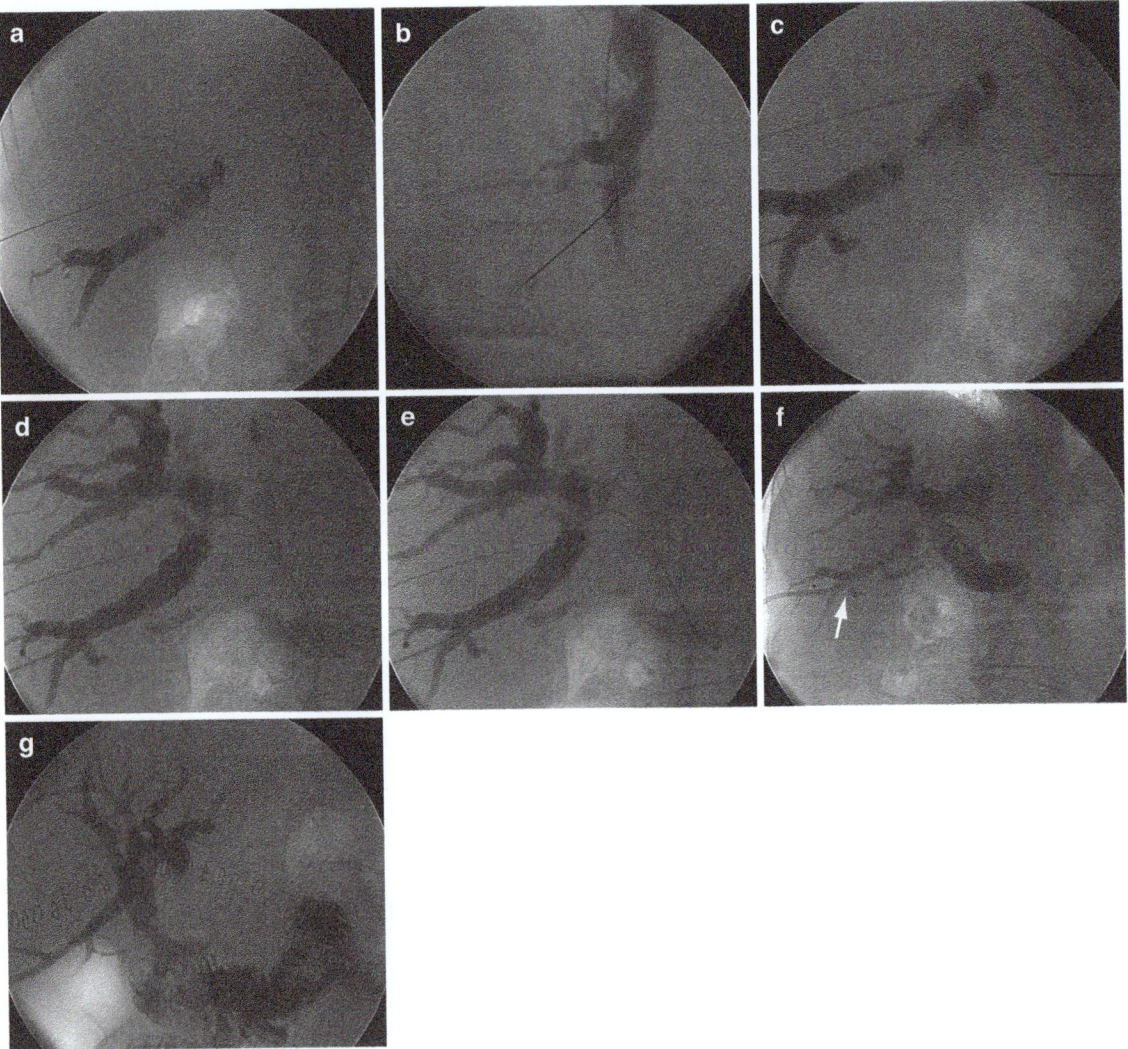

Fig. 9.1.1

Figure 9.1.1 (**a**) Fine-needle transhepatic cholangiography, PA projection. (**b**) Choosing the point of access for the second puncture, lateral projection. Passing the 0.018 in. guidewire. (**c**) Advancing the unipuncture system, maintaining the metallic component in the point of access to the biliary canaliculus. (**d**) Passing to the main biliary tract with a hydrophilic guidew1ire and multipurpose catheter. (**e**) Passing the drainage catheter over the stiff guidewire (Amplatz). (**f**) Definitive situation of the drainage catheter and cholangiography through it (point of entrance to the intrahepatic bile duct: (*arrow*). (**g**) Postoperative cholangiography through the biliary drainage catheter, which was withdrawn after the correct functioning of the biliodigestive anastomosis was confirmed

A 76-year-old-male patient as admitted with a 4-day history of jaundice, choluria, and acholia. Abdominal US and CT showed dilation of the intrahepatic and extrahepatic biliary tracts and of the duct of Wirsung secondary to a 2.5×2-cm mass in the head of the pancreas. The patient was a candidate for surgical treatment of the pancreatic neoplasm and was scheduled to undergo percutaneous external biliary drainage prior to surgery. Fourteen days after biliary drainage, he underwent surgery and the external drainage catheter was left in place. Fifteen days later, after follow-up cholangiography confirmed the correct functioning of the bilioenteric anastomosis and ruled out alterations of the intrahepatic biliary tract, the external drainage catheter was withdrawn.

Comments

Percutaneous external biliary drainage is the fastest, safest, most efficacious, and most economical way to drain bile, which is often infected, in patients with biliary tract obstruction.

It may be the only procedure performed (e.g., for acute cholangitis that responds poorly to conservative medical treatment) or may be performed as a first intervention to enable posterior interventional procedures in cases of choledocholithiasis or biliopancreatic neoplasms.

The possibility of performing percutaneous biliary drainage 24 h a day is especially important in cases of severe acute cholangitis that does not respond adequately to antibiotic treatment. Percutaneous external biliary drainage may be the only treatment option in these patients, and many would not survive delays in the procedure. The procedure consists of placing a catheter in the biliary tract proximal to the obstruction to enable bile to drain to the exterior. It is generally performed as a scheduled procedure in patients with obstruction due to neoplasm and in those scheduled to undergo posterior surgery. It is generally performed as an urgent procedure in patients with severe acute cholangitis and in those in whom endoscopic biliary drainage fails.

Procedure Steps

1. Prepare the patient: coagulation tests, antibiotic prophylaxis, thorough examination of the clinical history, and available imaging tests.
2. Use the double-puncture technique. For the first puncture, use a fine needle (21G–23G) and lateral access, choosing the puncture site between the midline and posterior axillary lines under fluoroscopic guidance (avoiding the interpositioning of the costophrenic sinus and hepatic flexure of the colon).

3. Access the peripheral bile duct, using an angle of at least 90° and keeping the distance between the point of entry on the skin to a minimum.
4. For the second puncture, with a C-arm arc in the lateral position and an intensifier by your side, mark the puncture site on the skin. The needle can be advanced in the lateral position with the help of a mosquito clamp to avoid radiation to your hand. Once the selected bile duct has been punctured, place the C-arm in the PA position again, and if necessary, withdraw the fine needle until its tip is in the lumen of the duct.
5. Next, pass a 0.018-in. guide as distal as possible, even to the common biliary duct.
6. Introduce a unipuncture system over the 0.018 in. guidewire all together until the bile duct and only its plastic parts thereafter. A shapeable catheter and a hydrophilic guidewire may be necessary to reach the bile duct where you want to place the drain. Next, replace the hydrophilic guidewire with a stiff guidewire and slide the drainage catheter over it (always with retaining systems on its tip).
7. Once the drainage catheter has been correctly positioned, aspirate as much bile as possible and withdraw the needle used for the first puncture.
8. Make sure the drainage catheter is large enough (generally 8.5F) and that it runs as far as possible into the biliary tract to ensure stability.

Equipment

1. Two 22G needles.
2. 0.018 in. guidewire.
3. Unipuncture system.
4. 0.035 in. guidewire.
5. 4F–5F multipurpose catheter.
6. 0.035 stiff guidewire (Amplatz).
7. 8F biliary drainage catheter.

Case 9.2
■
Complications of Percutaneous Biliary Drainage: Hemobilia

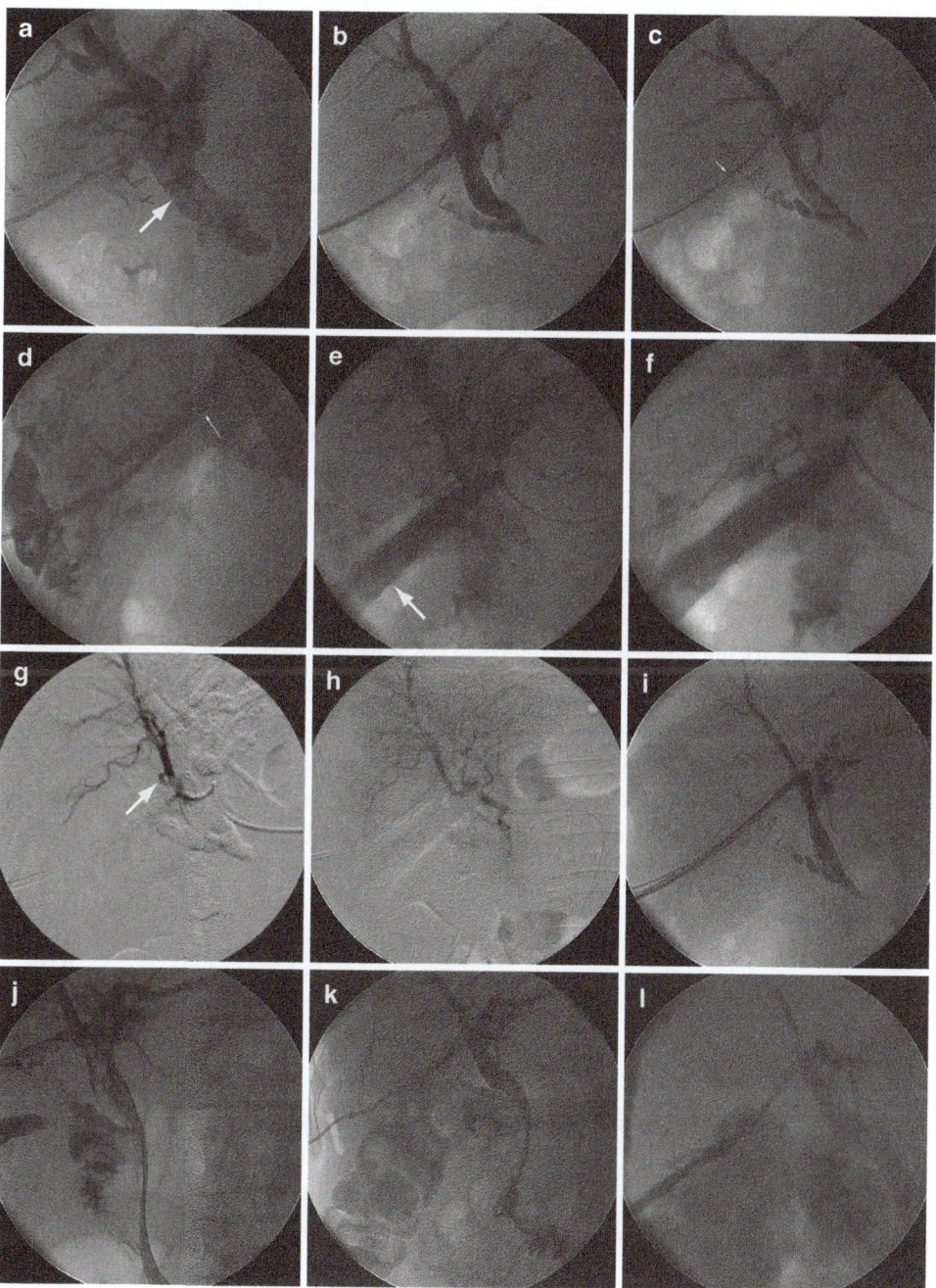

Fig. 9.2.1

Figure 9.2.1 Arterial bleeding into the biliary tree: (**a**) external biliary drainage; filling defects corresponding to hemobilia at the end of the procedure (*arrows*). (**b**) Cholangiogram 48 h after the procedure. (**c**) Rapid, massive washout of contrast material from the biliary tract when the drainage catheter is withdrawn over the 0.035 in. guidewire (starting at the point marked with the *arrow*). (**d**) Replacement of the drainage catheter with a vascular introducer sheath and injection of contrast material through the hepatic tract, opacifying the arterial branches that depend on the right hepatic artery. (**e**) Hepatic angiogram showing a pseudoaneurysm adjacent to the access to the intrahepatic biliary tract. Subhepatic hematoma (*arrow*). (**f**) Selective catheterization of the right hepatic artery and the damaged branch. (**g**) Selective embolization of the damaged artery (*arrow*) using PVA (350–500 micras) particles. (**h**) Hepatic angiogram after embolization. (**i**) Cholangiogram 4 days after the procedure shows the absence of washout after the drainage catheter is withdrawn. (**j**) Implantation of the biliary stent. (**k**) Control 24 h after implantation shows the correct functioning of the stent. (**l**) Withdrawal of the external biliary drainage catheter and embolization of the hepatic tract using 0.035 in. coils

A 68-year-old-man with a history of chronic alcoholism and insulin-dependent diabetes mellitus was referred to the emergency department with abdominal pain, jaundice, and laboratory findings indicative of cytolysis and cholestasis. Imaging studies showed a mass in the head of the pancreas with signs of vascular infiltration and secondary dilation of the intra and extrahepatic biliary tract. Cytology confirmed the diagnosis of a tumor in the head of the pancreas and surgical treatment was ruled out.

We performed percutaneous external bile drainage using the double-puncture technique, accessing the bile tract through the segmental duct of liver segment V (acceptable access). After placing the drainage catheter in the main biliary tract, we appreciated scant, self-limiting hemobilia, and the patient was scheduled for biliary stenting 48 h later.

The initial cholangiogram showed small clots in the main biliary tract. We injected contrast material through the drainage catheter to opacify the biliary tract completely and then withdrew the catheter slowly over a guidewire. We observed massive, rapid washout of contrast material suggestive of arterial bleeding into the biliary tree.

Comments   The most common complications of percutaneous biliary drainage are hemorrhages, and arterial hemorrhage is the most serious of these. If the technique and access to the biliary tract are right, most bleeding originates from the manipulation of guidewires and catheters or in lesions to small venous vessels, and these will be self-limiting and without clinical significance.

Hemobilia caused by vascular lesions are more serious, especially when caused by damage to arterial vessels, which can be life-threatening. The likelihood and severity of hemobilia due to vascular lesions are directly related to the access to the biliary tract. The more peripheral the access, the lesser the probability of a vascular lesion and the less severe it is likely to be.

Biliary access can be classified in function of the risk of vascular lesion as:
- Ideal: Subsegmental ducts; considered to carry minimal risk.
- Acceptable: Segmental ducts.
- Dangerous: Central ducts (anterior or posterior segmental ducts).
- Prohibited: Common hepatic duct; placing a drainage catheter in this location is not justifiable under any circumstance.

Procedure Steps

1. Replace the drainage catheter with an introducer sheath and inject contrast material into the tract near the access to the bile duct; this should opacify the damaged segmental hepatic artery.
2. Obtain a hepatic angiogram to confirm the findings.
3. Selectively embolize the damaged vessels through a microcatheter with permanent PVA (350–500 micras) particles.
4. Four days later, after confirming the complete resolution of hemobilia, implant a stent for palliative treatment of the biliary obstruction and leave an external drainage catheter in place.
5. Forty-eight hours after stent implantation, obtain a cholangiogram to check the adequate expansion of the stent and complete resolution of the hemobilia; withdraw the external drainage catheter and embolize the hepatic tract with 0.035 in. fibered coils.

Equipment

1. Two 22G needles
2. 0.018 in. guidewire
3. Unipuncture system
4. 0.035 in. hydrophilic and stiff guidewires
5. 4F–5F multipurpose, Simmons, and cobra catheters
6. 8F biliary drainage catheter
7. Hydrophilic microcatheter
8. PVA particles (350–500 micras)
9. Biliary stent
10. 10.0.035 in. fibered metallic coils

Case 9.3
Percutaneous Treatment of Multiple Choledocholithiasis

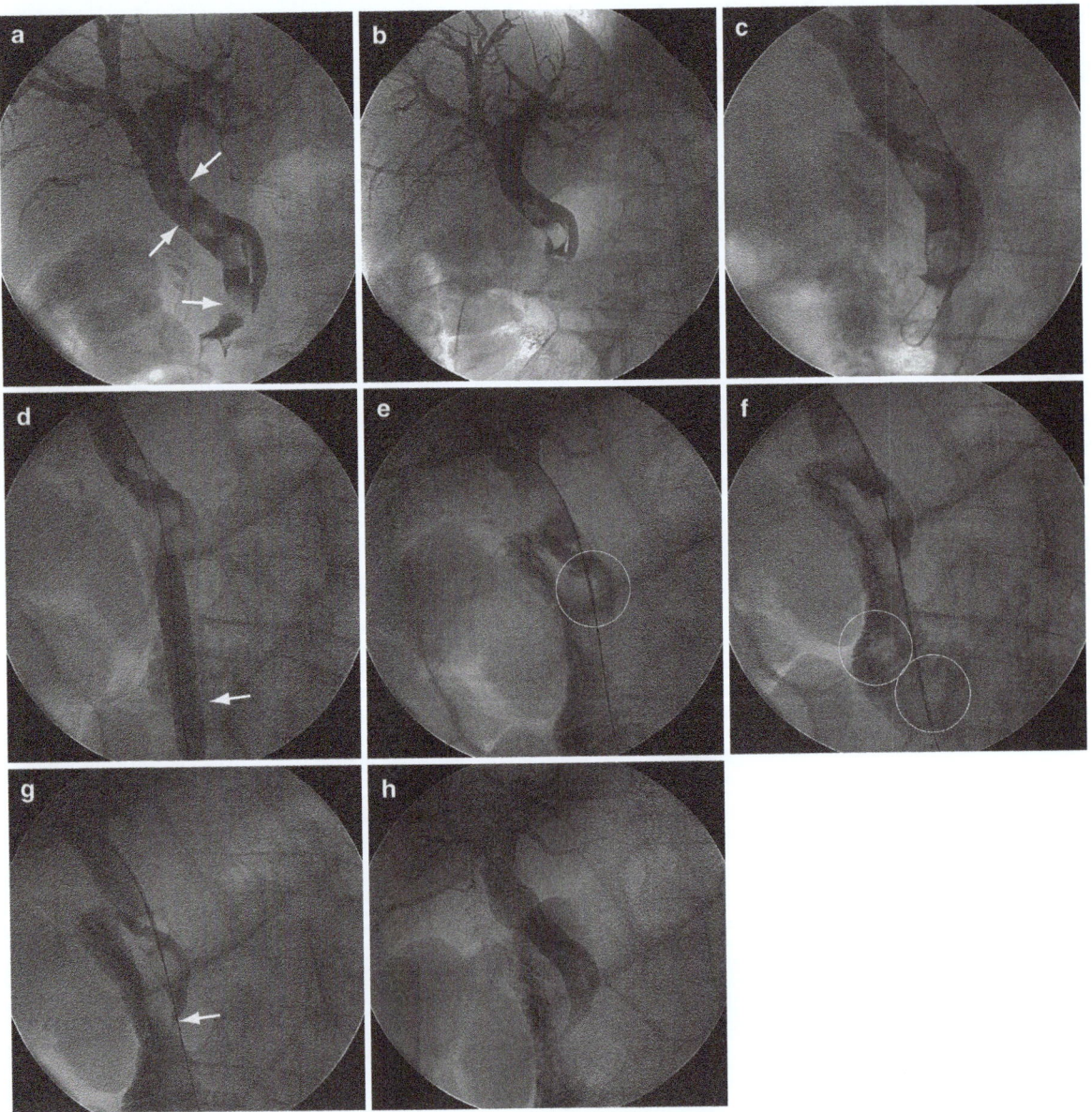

Fig. 9.3.1

Figure 9.3.1 (**a**) Fine-needle transhepatic cholangiography shows a large number of stones lodged in the main biliary tract (*arrows*) and selection of the intrahepatic biliary radical to be accessed; (**b**) external biliary drainage; (**c**) measuring the size of the stones with a calibrated catheter; (**d**) papilloplasty with a 12-mm high-pressure catheter-balloon (*arrow*); the stones should remain above the catheter (*circle*) to avoid becoming lodged in the wall of the bile duct; (**e**) Fogarty catheter placed between the stones to expel them one by one to the duodenum (*circle*); (**f**) catheter and one of the stones in the duodenum (*circles*); (**g**) relation between the Fogarty catheter (*arrow*) and the last stone before it was expelled to the duodenum; (**h**) final cholangiographic check shows the main biliary track is free of stones

A 68-year-old-woman was admitted with slight fever and obstructive jaundice, together with mild discomfort in her right hypochondrium. She had a history of repeated episodes of acute cholangitis that ceased with medical treatment.

Emergency abdominal ultrasonography showed marked dilation of the intra and extrahepatic biliary tract and images suggestive of bile stones in the main biliary tract. Percutaneous external biliary drainage corroborated the ultrasonographic findings.

Once the symptoms of acute cholangitis were resolved, different treatment options for her choledocholithiasis were reviewed. Surgery was ruled out, leaving endoscopic papillotomy and expulsion of the stones to the duodenum.

The medical-surgical committee decided on interventional treatment because a percutaneous biliary drainage catheter was already in place and the stones were the right size to be expelled to the duodenum. The patient provided her informed consent to undergo the procedure.

Comments

Choledocholithiasis has been treated percutaneously for many years, and various alternative treatments have been developed. The first methods to be used were chemicals (basically methyl tert-butyl ether) to dissolve the stones (no longer in use) and extracting stones to the exterior in a similar way to that used with residual bile stones. This method was difficult to carry out because in most cases the size of the stones required large transhepatic tracts to be made, which resulted in problems like prior fragmentation of the stones and excessive time to allow the tract to mature.

Nowadays, percutaneous treatment usually involves expelling gallstones to the duodenum. This is a perfectly valid alternative that has clear advantages over other invasive techniques like surgery or endoscopic papillotomy. In summary, this technique (a) is fast, safe, and economical; (b) it is unlikely to leave residual stones, and if residual stones are left, the solution is easy because the main biliary tract can be accessed again and the procedure can be repeated without dilating the papilla again; (c) with certain limitations, which on the other hand are rare, the number of stones or their situation (main biliary tract or intrahepatic tracts) are hurdles that can be overcome, as we can, in principle, access any part of the biliary tree; (d) neither general anesthesia nor deep sedation is necessary, although the collaboration of an anesthesiologist is advisable to avoid the pain involved in sphincteroplasty.

Procedure Steps

1. If complete obstruction is seen when contrast material is passed to the duodenum (as in this case), first dislodge the most distal stones by sliding guidewires and catheters between the stone and the wall of the common bile duct. This will enable you to precisely define the number of stones before proceeding.
2. Once all of the stones have been dislodged, the next step is to perform papilloplasty with a high-pressure balloon that has a diameter equal to or slightly larger than the stones to be expelled. Use a mixture of contrast material and saline solution to dilate the balloon and a manometer to control the pressure.
3. Expel the stones to the duodenum, using a double-lumen Fogarty balloon.
4. Leave a external percutaneous biliary drainage catheter in place for 48 h after the procedure, until a final check will determine if any stones are present and the catheter can be withdrawn. In the unlikely case that residual stones are present, use a Fogarty catheter to expel them. It will not be necessary to perform papilloplasty again.

Equipment

(1) The equipment described in case 1 for percutaneous external biliary drainage; (2) calibrated catheter; (3) high-pressure balloon catheter; (4) double-lumen Fogarty balloon catheter.

Case 9.4

Percutaneous Treatment of Residual Biliary Lithiasis

Figure 9.4.1 (**a**) Cholangiogram obtained through a T-tube shows residual lithiasis (*arrow*); the entrance to the main biliary tract is perpendicular; (**b**) withdrawing the T-tube and passing the guidewire; (**c**) papilloplasty with a high-pressure catheter-balloon; the stones are situated above the catheter to avoid damaging the wall of the common bile duct (*arrow*); (**d**) inflated Fogarty catheter situated above

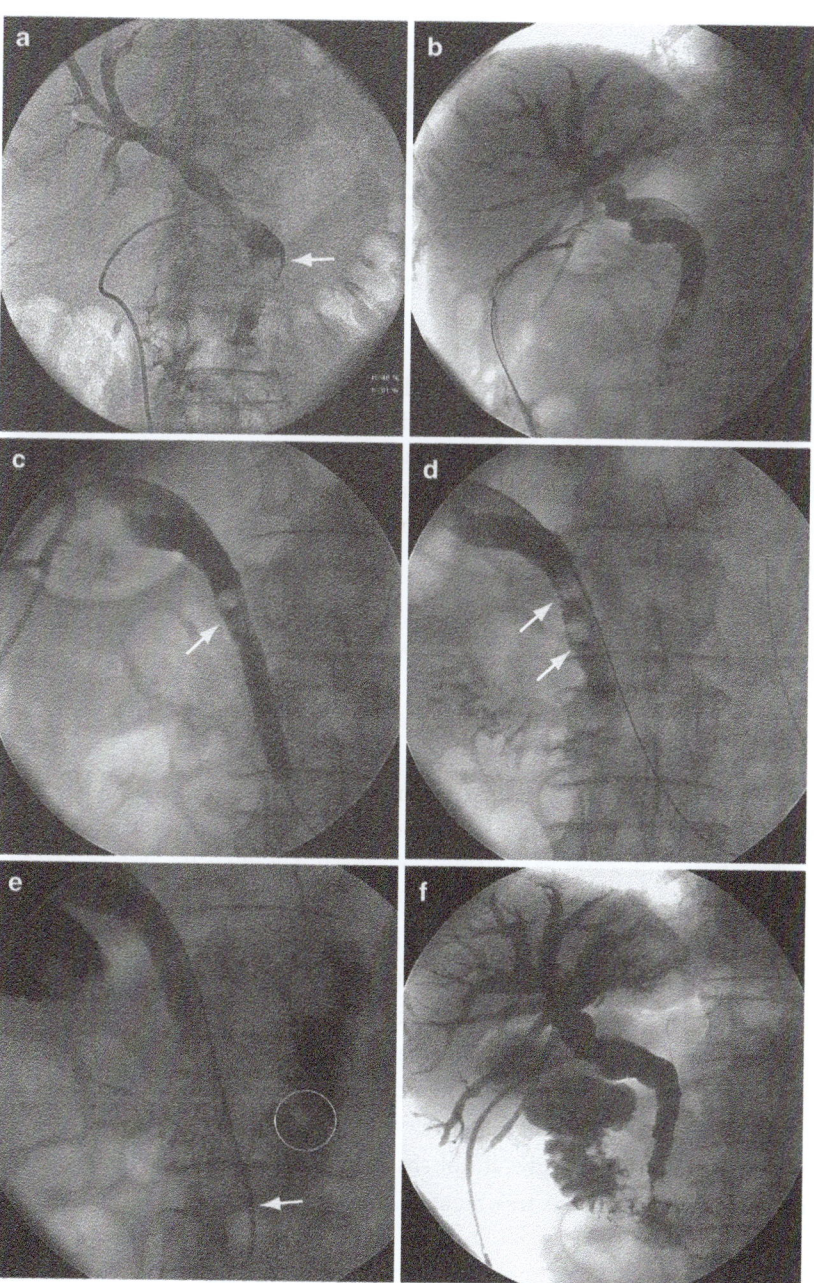

Fig. 9.4.1

the stones (*arrows*); (e) Fogarty catheter (*arrow*) and stone expelled to the duodenum (*circle*); (f) final-check cholangiogram obtained through a biliary drainage catheter situated in the main biliary tract through the percutaneous tract of the T-tube

A 47-year-old-woman was referred from another hospital where she had undergone surgery 4 weeks prior for multiple stones in the common bile duct. Follow-up cholangiography performed through a T-tube 1 week after surgery showed a residual stone measuring approximately 1 cm in diameter, and percutaneous treatment was indicated.

Comments

After surgery, about 5–8% of patients have residual lithiasis.

The advantages of percutaneous vs. endoscopic treatment have been debated for years. The advantages of each treatment are summarized below:

● *Percutaneous treatment*: This approach takes advantage of the tract from the T-tube, which allows easy access to the rest of the biliary tree. The major drawback is that it takes 4 weeks for the tract to mature. The percutaneous approach enables two technical modalities: (a) Direct extraction of the stones, and (b) expulsion of the stones to the duodenum. We believe the second approach is clearly better.
● *Endoscopic treatment*: The main advantage of this approach is that it is not necessary to wait. Its main drawback is the difficulties involved in extracting stones situated above the T-tube and biliary contamination (which can be severe) in cases in which all the residual stones are not extracted and in which no biliary drainage (nasobiliary or plastic prosthesis) is left in place.

Hemobilia is the most common complication; acute pancreatitis is an uncommon complication.

Procedure Steps

Whether the stones can be expelled to the duodenum depends on their size and shape. Moreover, in these cases, another factor, which depends on the surgeon, is the appropriate placement of the T-tube, with a straight pathway running as directly to the skin as possible and entering the main biliary tract at an angle as close to 90° as possible. The technical steps are identical to those described in Case 3; as mentioned above, the technical success of percutaneous treatment in residual lithiasis led to the use of this technique for treating native lithiasis. The only difference is that the stones might be situated above or below the T-tube, although they are usually below. If they are situated above the T-tube, they can be easily brought down by placing catheters above them and injecting contrast material with pressure or using Fogarty-type balloon catheters.

The correct placement of the T-tube, if not absolutely essential, is of primary importance for the success of percutaneous treatment.

Equipment

The same equipment described in case 3, except those used for percutaneous biliary drainage.

Case 9.5

Balloon Dilation of Stenosis of a Biliodigestive Anastomosis

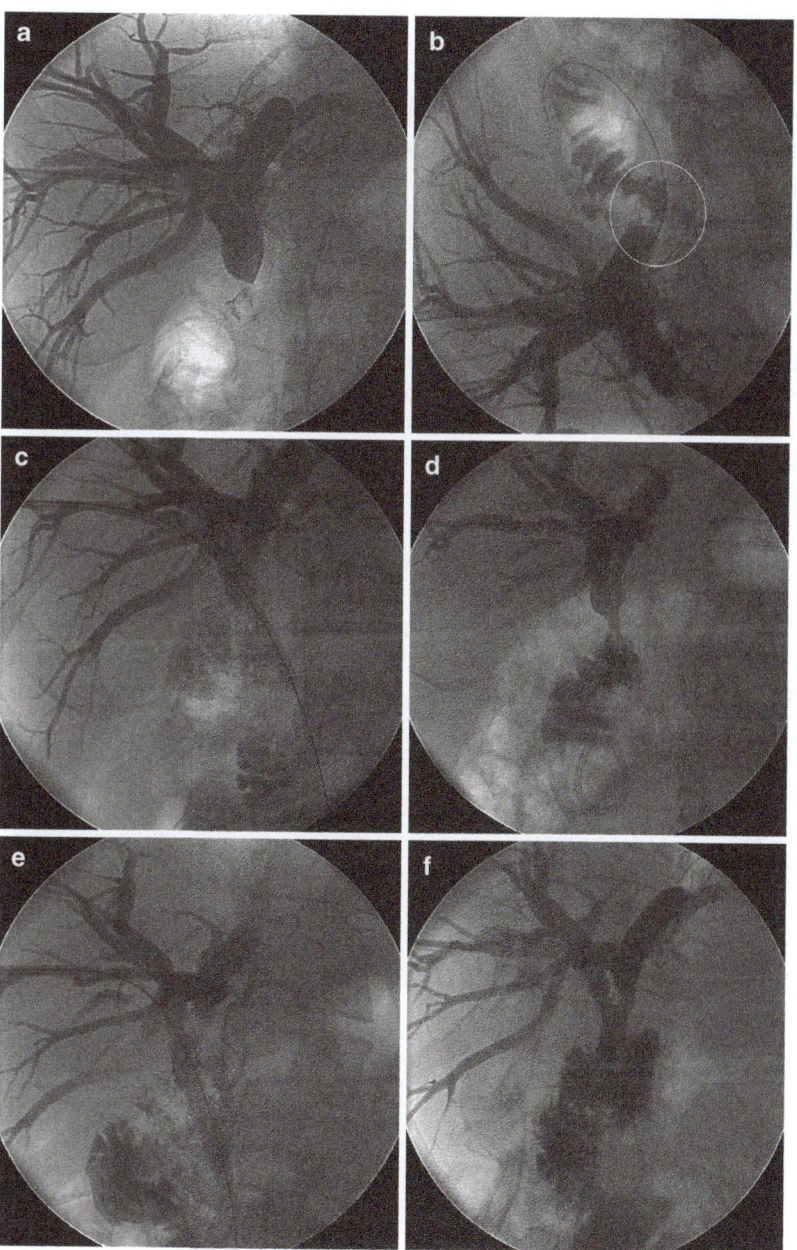

Fig. 9.5.1

Figure 9.5.1 (**a**) Severe stenosis and the tip of the multipurpose catheter in the lesion. (**b**) Introducing the hydrophilic guidewire and catheter to the intestinal loop (*circle*). Introducer sheath. (**c**) Dilation using a balloon catheter. (**d**) Good outcome at the end of the first intervention and placement of an internal–external biliary drainage catheter. (**e**) Two weeks later: a restenosis was dilated. (**f**) Excellent final outcome

A 63-year-old-man in whom a Roux-en-Y anastomosis was affected to treat a tumor in the ampulla of Vater 1 year earlier was readmitted with a 1-week history of intense jaundice and pruritus. Cholangiography showed severe stenosis of the surgical anastomosis.

Comments

The pneumatic dilation of the biliary tract after surgery can be reattempted on several occasions. In this patient, an internal–external drainage catheter was left in place for 2 weeks after the first pneumatic dilation, when restenosis was seen. The excellent behavior of the lesion in the weeks following a second dilation enabled us to withdraw the biliary drainage.

Procedure Steps

1. Perform an initial biliary drainage.
2. Use a 7F or 8F introducer sheath with a hydrophilic guidewire and multipurpose catheter to advance through the stenosis to the intestinal loop.
3. Replace the hydrophilic guidewire with an extra-stiff or working guidewire, over which the stenosis will be dilated with a high-pressure balloon catheter: observe how the notch disappears.
4. Leave an internal–external biliary drainage catheter in place for 2 or 3 weeks. Check the response to treatment by cholangiography (only with the introducer sheath and guidewire). If the results are good, leave an external biliary catheter in place and close it for a few days. If the results are still good, withdraw the catheter definitively. If not, dilate the stenosis again in the same way. If the results are still poor, consider another surgical intervention.

Equipment

(1) Biliary drainage set; (2) 7F–8F introducer sheath; (3) 0.035 in. hydrophilic and extra-stiff guidewires; (4) 90 cm long 5F multipurpose catheter; (5) high-pressure balloon catheter.

Case 9.6

Iatrogenic or Postsurgical Biliary Fistula

Figure 9.6.1 (**a-c**) Percutaneous colangiography showing a biliocolonic fistula and a severe stenosis of the common bile duct. Notice the presence of contrast material in the colon. (**d**) A 10F internal-external biliary drainage catheter was placed in the biliary system

A 59-year-old-man presented jaundice and dilation of the intrahepatic biliary tract with a biloma in the vesicular bed after undergoing laparoscopic cholecystectomy converted to open surgery after complications 2 weeks before.

Comments

Benign disease of the biliary tract is usually iatrogenic. Although surgical treatment should first be considered, percutaneous procedures can yield good results in selected cases, especially those with stenosis of the biliodigestive anastomosis.

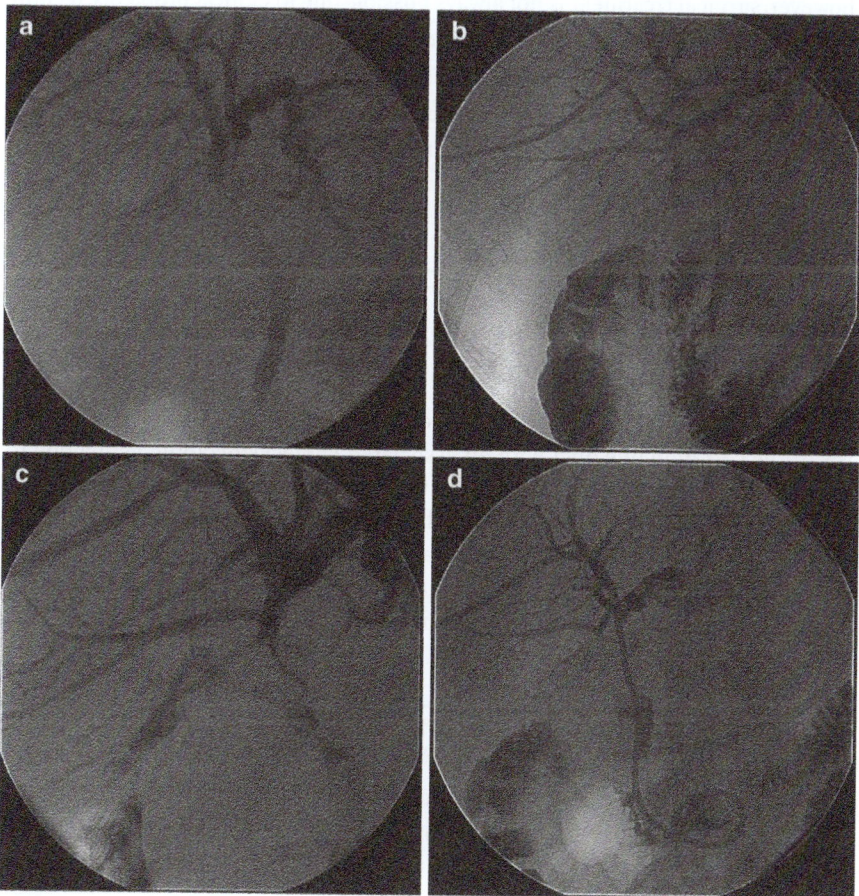

Fig. 9.6.1

One of the most important aspects is early diagnosis and treatment. Ideally, intraoperative cholangiography should be performed to diagnose and surgically treat these complications in the same surgical act. However, this is generally not the case, and both leaks and benign stenoses are not diagnosed until weeks or months after surgery.

● Bile leaks

If the amount is small, they usually close after percutaneous biliary drainage.

● Laceration of the biliary tract

Laceration is usually diagnosed with noninvasive techniques (US, CT, MRI) 3–7 days after the intervention. These patients usually present jaundice, fever, and bile in drainage tubes. Cholangiography can show the site and severity of the lesion more accurately and can be used for planning treatment. Surgery should be reserved for cases in which percutaneous treatment is not possible.

● Benign stenosis of the biliary tract

Benign stenosis of the biliary tract is usually a consequence of iatrogenic laceration that does not cause symptoms until scarring produces fibrosis and stenosis of the bile duct (main biliary tract) or at the level of the biliodigestive anastomosis causing biliary stasis. The most appropriate treatment option is surgery, which gives good results (10–30% restenosis); however, surgical treatment is not always possible due to clinical problems, technical impossibility, advanced age, and refusal to undergo surgery and these cases are usually treated percutaneously. Percutaneous treatment is contraindicated when stenosis is due to complete obstruction due to silk sutures or staples.

Stenosis can occur at the level of the biliodigestive anastomosis or in the main bile tract.

There are two percutaneous procedures:
1. Pneumatic dilation with a high-pressure catheter
2. Placing a biliary prosthesis

Procedure Steps

1. Perform percutaneous right biliary drainage and check for the presence of severe stenosis of the common bile duct with an associated cholecystocolonic fistula due to laceration of the extrahepatic biliary tract during surgery.
2. With the help of a hydrophilic guidewire and multipurpose catheter, access the distal common bile duct and the duodenum and place an internal–external biliary drainage catheter to act as a tutor of the biliary tract and help close the leak in the following weeks, as occurred in this case. However, if the section is complete or if the leak does not resolve, surgical reintervention is usually necessary.

Equipment

(1) 150 cm long 0.035 in. Teflon exchange guidewires; (2) 7F or 8F introducer sheath; (3) 40 cm long multipurpose catheter; (4) 150 cm long 0.035 in. hydrophilic guidewire; (5) 145 cm long extra-stiff guidewire; (6) 40 cm long variable caliber (6–8 mm) angioplasty balloon catheter; (7) 6F–8.5F external biliary drainage catheter; (8) 8.5F internal–external biliary drainage catheter; (9) Manometer

Case 9.7
Transpapillary Stenting

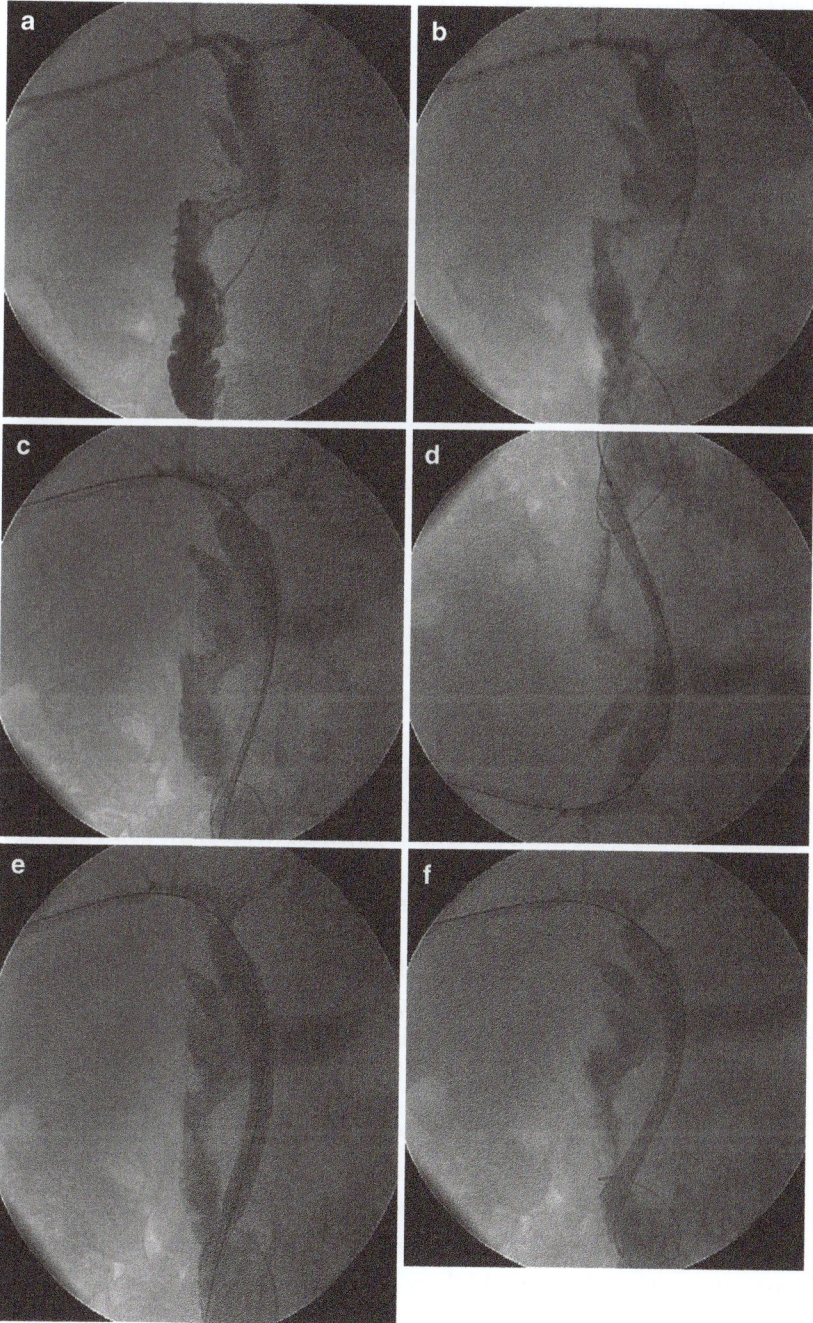

Fig. 9.7.1

Figure 9.7.1 (**a**) Stenosis of the distal common bile duct with a 4F multipurpose catheter through it; (**b**) calibrated catheter over a stiff guidewire; (**c**) initial deployment of the metallic Wallstent; (**d–e**) dilation of the entire length of the stent using a high-pressure catheter; (**f**) situation, expansion, and ideal functioning of the stent

A 74-year-old-man presented obstructive jaundice due to a tumor in the head of the pancreas that occluded the distal common bile duct. Surgery was considered unviable due to vascular infiltration, so a stent was placed for palliative treatment.

Comments

Malignant disease affecting the biliary tract usually manifests with symptoms of obstructive jaundice caused by compression or even invalidation of the lumen of the bile ducts. Depending on the location of the stenosis, we refer to distal lesions (lesions that involve the papilla and/or common bile duct near it) or proximal lesions (lesions that involve the common hepatic duct and its hilar subdivision – Klatskin tumors, classified from BI to BIV on the Bismuth classification).

For the percutaneous management of these patients, we recommend external biliary drainage and then placing a metallic stent a few days later in a second act to gather time for reaching an agreement with the referring physician about stent placement (remember that the stent will only be placed if surgical resection with the intent to cure is ruled out). An additional benefit of waiting a few days after drainage is that the patient will be in better condition and the biliary tract will be decompressed.

The next four cases show different situations that are often encountered in daily practice; we discuss the management of each case and the importance of using the right strategy to ensure success in this type of palliative procedures.

Procedure Steps

1. Perform transcatheter cholangiography 1 week after external biliary drainage; in this case, we observed complete obstruction of the medial and distal common bile duct.
2. Clear the obstruction using the usual procedure: passing a hydrophilic guidewire and catheter through the stenosis to the duodenum.
3. Check the length of the stenosis with a calibrated catheter and choose the stent with most appropriate length.
4. Place the stent; this means going past the papilla and leaving a sufficiently large margin in the duodenum and adopting smooth angles over the main biliary tract to avoid future kinks. In this particular case (though it is not always necessary), we completed the initial insufficient expansion with the help of a balloon-angioplasty catheter, which yielded good results.

Equipment

(1) 150 cm long 0.035 in. Teflon exchange guidewires; (2) 7F or 8F introducer sheath; (3) 40 cm long multipurpose catheter; (4) 150 cm long 0.035 in. hydrophilic guidewire; (5) 145 cm long extra-stiff guidewire; (6) biliary stent; (7) 40 cm long variable caliber (6–8 mm) angioplasty balloon catheter; (8) Manometer

Case 9.8

A Single Stent to Treat a Type Ii Hilar Tumor from the Right Side

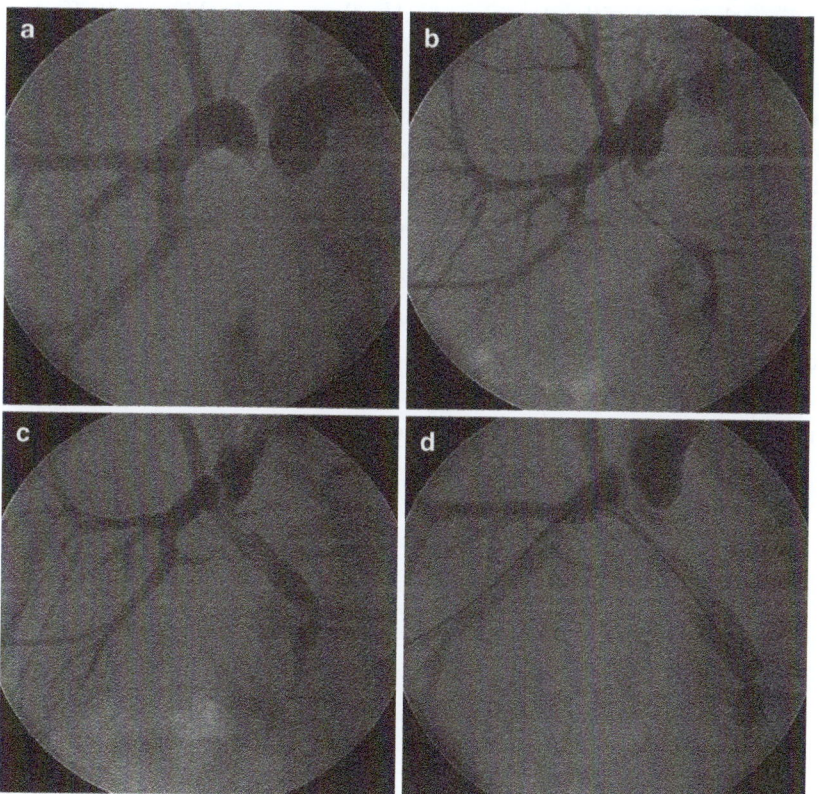

Fig. 9.8.1

Figure 9.8.1 (**a**) Cholangiogram obtained through a 4F multipurpose catheter delimits the stenoses in both hepatic ducts (B-II); (**b**) passing a hydrophilic guidewire and catheter from the *right* side through the obstruction to the duodenum; (**c**) initial deployment of the metallic Wallstent; (**d**) situation, expansion, and appropriate functioning of the stent in the suprapapillary position

An 82-year-old-male patient presented intense jaundice due to an adenocarcinoma of the gallbladder that had infiltrated both main biliary ducts (right and left); surgery was ruled out because of his advanced age and family opposition due to his poor clinical situation and reduced life expectancy.

Comments

It would have been equally possible and correct to place two stents, one for each liver lobe, but due to the clinical circumstances, in this particular case we preferred to avoid a second biliary access (left) and hope that the blood bilirubin levels dropped enough with a single stent. If the patient needed left drainage in the coming weeks, he would return and we would place a second stent at the same time, crossing the meshwork of the first stent and positioning the stents in the shape of a T.

Procedure Steps

1. Advance a multipurpose catheter over a 7F introducer sheath and obtain a cholangiogram to delimit the extent of the stenosis caused by the tumor. In this case, it affected the right and left hepatic ducts, so it was classified as Bismuth-II, and the medial and distal common bile duct were patent to the papilla.
2. In this case, we decided to place a single stent from the right side to the common bile duct without compromising the papilla (suprapapillary position).
3. Use a balloon catheter to complete the initial expansion of the stent; in this case, the final check showed excellent results.

Equipment

(1) 150 cm long 0.035 in. Teflon exchange guidewires; (2) 7F or 8F introducer sheath; (3) 40 cm long multipurpose catheter; (4) 150 cm long 0.035 in. hydrophilic guidewire; (5) 145 cm long extra-stiff guidewire; (6) biliary stent; (7) 40 cm long variable caliber (6–8 mm) angioplasty balloon catheter; (8) Manometer

Case 9.9

■

Stent from the Right Side to Treat a Type B-Iii Hilar Tumor.

Figure 9.9.1 This is a case of severe stenosis of the right hepatic duct and common hepatic duct caused by a type B-III hilar tumor that we treated with a single *right* stent. The images in (**a–c**) come from the case described in the text. Images (**d–f**) come from a similar case treated in the same way. The flexibility of the Wallstent enables it to be easily adapted to fit the anatomy of the biliary tract

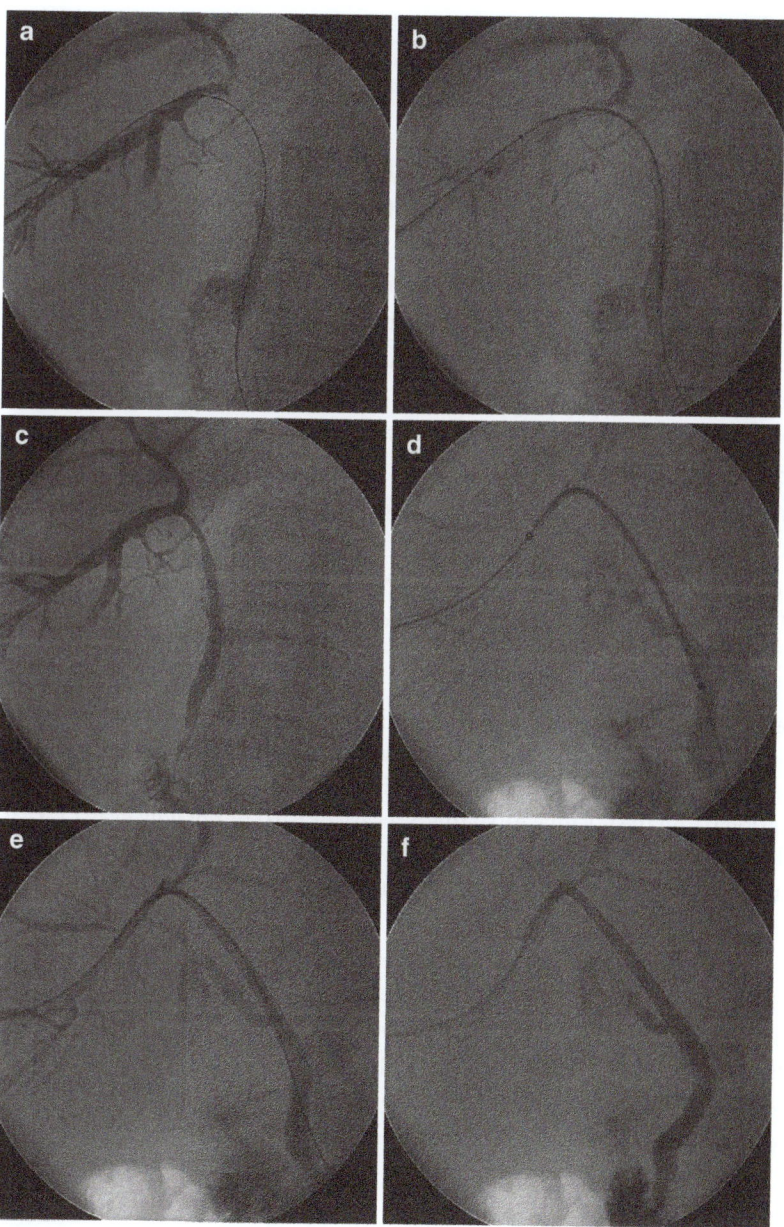

Fig. 9.9.1

A 62-year-old-man with jaundice and dilation of the intrahepatic biliary tract due to metastases from gastric cancer was referred from the oncology department of another hospital with the aim of reducing his high bilirubinemia so that he could resume chemotherapy. After biliary drainage lowered his bilirubinemia considerably, the patient and his family requested that a stent be placed for palliative treatment as he could not tolerate definitive external drainage psychologically.

Comments

Palliative treatment of cancer that affects the biliary tract is a challenge for interventional radiologists because a specific strategy must be designed for each particular case. Although there are general guidelines about how to approach each situation technically, *the best approach is always to consider each case individually to find the best palliative solution for each patient and his or her particular disease.*

As a general rule, it is important to remember that these are patients deemed unsuitable for curative surgery and we should all work toward eliminating palliative bypass surgery from our hospitals (although there are exceptions). Metallic stents are the best approach to manage these situations.

There are two major areas of biliary tract involvement by cancer that require treatment by interventional radiologists: distally located lesions in the biliopancreaticoduodenal junction and proximally located lesions that affect the medial common bile duct, common hepatic duct and its right and left subdivisions, and the first intrahepatic branches of the common hepatic duct. The Bismuth classification divides hilar tumors into four types:

Type B-I: Obstruction of the common hepatic duct

Type B-II: Involvement of the two main biliary ducts (right and left)

Type B-III: Obstruction of the main hepatic duct (right or left) and diffuse involvement of the contralateral lobe

Type B-IV: Diffuse infiltration of the intrahepatic ducts of both lobes

Procedure Steps

1. In the initial cholangiogram, we observed that the common bile duct was patent and that most, but not all, the right intrahepatic biliary ducts filled completely; however, the left ducts were not seen at all. In this case, the left liver lobe is infiltrated by a large space-occupying lesion (from the CT image), so this is a case of B-III or possibly even of B-IV.
2. We decided to place a stent in the suprapapillary position using the usual procedure. The final outcome was good, enabling a large part of the right liver lobe to be drained.

Equipment

(1) 150 cm long 0.035 in. Teflon exchange guidewires; (2) 7F introducer sheath; (3) 40 cm long multipurpose catheter; (4) 150 cm long 0.035 in. hydrophilic guidewire; (5) 145 cm long extra-stiff guidewire; (6) self-expanding metallic Wallstent (variable diameter and length); (7) 40 cm long variable caliber (6–8 mm) angioplasty balloon catheter; (8) 6F or 8F external biliary drainage catheter.

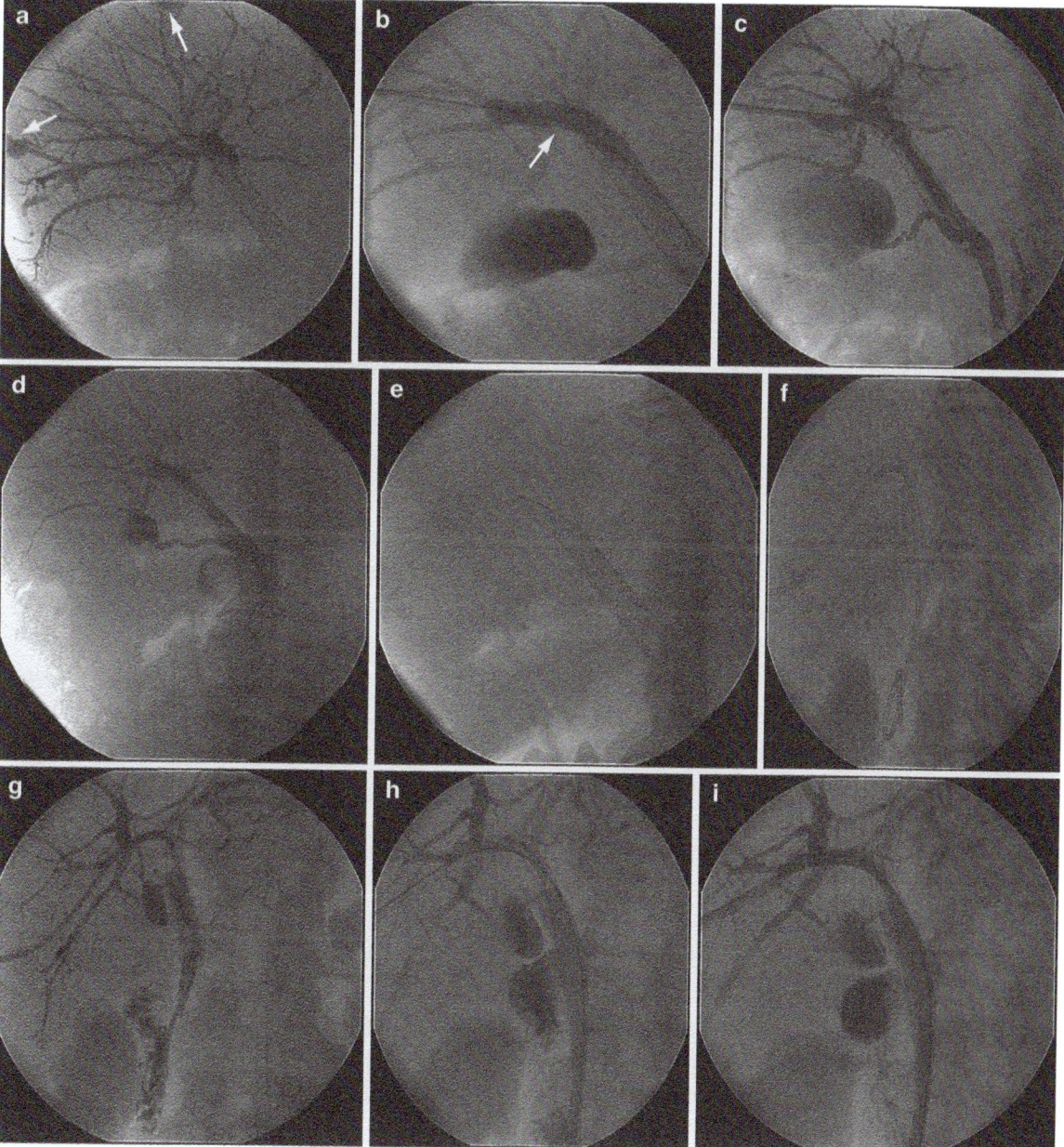

Fig. 9.10.1

Figure 9.10.1 (**a**) Complete obstruction of the two coaxial metallic stents. Biliary abscesses due to cholangitis (*arrows*); (**b**) De novo posterior dilation of the proximal end of the new coaxial stent; (**c**) confirmatory cholangiogram obtained through the introducer sheath shows good patency; (d) follow-up cholangiogram 3 days later (just before withdrawal of the external biliary drainage) shows excellent functioning of the three coaxial stents; (**e**) detail of the three expanded coaxial stents. (**f**) Internal–external biliary drainage a few days earlier for the obstruction of the *right* stent; note the partial obstruction of the proximal end of the *right* stent; (**g–i**) recovery of the patency with a coaxial stent

The patient was a 79-year-old-man who had been treated in our unit 10 months before with biliary drainage and placement of a metallic stent for cholangiocarcinoma involving the common hepatic duct (B-I). Surgery was considered unviable due to vascular infiltration. Three months after the procedure, a second stent had to be implanted after jaundice recurred due to tumor invasion of the first stent. Four months later, he was readmitted for cholangitis. After dilation of the intrahepatic was confirmed, reobstruction of the stents was suspected and he was referred for biliary drainage.

Comments   It is important to recognize the different patterns of biliary obstruction because they will determine the strategy for palliative treatment. Type B-I obstruction can be treated by placing a single stent; its distal tip should be placed above the papilla if there is a margin of 2–3 cm to avoid complications in future reinterventions. In cases in which future reintervention is unlikely, it is better to place the distal tip over the duodenum with smooth angles.

In type B-II obstruction, it is often difficult to decide whether to place two stents (one for each lobe, which then gives rise to different possible configurations: in X – with independent left and right biliary access, in Y – with both through the same access, or in T – with one stent placed through the other side at a later time, which makes it necessary to open the mesh of the initial stent and insert the second stent through it) or whether to drain only one side through a single stent and wait and see whether the patient's jaundice resolves sufficiently. If significant improvement is not seen, consider another biliary drainage of the other lobe (external or by placing a second stent). This strategy is becoming more common.

Type B-III obstructions require very careful management; stents should be placed only in determinate cases (see, for example, case 3), and external biliary drainage alone might be sufficient.

Type B-IV obstructions (with few exceptions) should not be treated by stenting or even by external biliary drainage in most cases.

Finally, there are cases in which tumors, basically pancreatic tumors, obliterate the duodenal lumen and this situation must be solved before or immediately after placing the biliary stent (either with a duodenal stent or biliary bypass surgery (gastrojejunal anastomosis)).

In the natural course of cancer patients treated with stents, the stent will become partially or totally obstructed after a few months due to tumor growth or impaction of biliary sludge. However, these situations are easy to resolve by placing new stents or by balloon dilation, respectively. Placing an internal–external drainage catheter should be reserved for exceptional cases, such as when placing another stent is unjustified (for example, a fourth or fifth stent) because of the patient's reduced life expectancy or when the obstruction occurs over a stent placed for benign disease (indicated a last resort).

(1) 150 cm long 0.035 in. Teflon exchange guidewires; (2) 7F introducer sheath; (3) 40 cm long multipurpose catheter; (4) 150 cm long 0.035 in. hydrophilic guidewire; (5) 145 cm long extra-stiff guidewire; (6) self-expanding metallic Wallstent (variable diameter and length); (7) 40 cm long variable caliber (6–8 mm) angioplasty balloon catheter; (8) 6F or 8F external biliary drainage catheter.

Equipment

1. Perform cholangiography through the external drainage catheter to check for complete obstruction of the stent and intrahepatic biliary dilation with images of small biliary abscesses (cholangitis).
2. In this case, the standard procedure (introducer sheath + multipurpose catheter + hydrophilic guidewire) was able to cross through the obstructed stents with the help of a super-stiff guidewire from the duodenum.
3. Next, dilate the stenosis within the stent using a balloon catheter.
4. After dilation, place a third coaxial metallic stent and dilate it with a catheter balloon once it is in place. Then check that it has been correctly expanded in an immediate cholangiogram.
5. Check the results 1 day later through the external catheter.

Procedure Steps

Further Reading

Books and Chapters in Books

García García L. Radiología intervencionista en Patología Biliar: ¿ Qué hacer, cómo hacerlo, y cúando hacerlo? 2007. *Ed. Elsevier-Doyma*

García García L. Manual Práctico de Radiología Biliar Intervencionista 2001. *Ed.Lab.Rovi SA y Lorenzo García*

García García L, Lanciego C, Rodríguez I. Radiología Intervencionista en la Patología Biliar 1998. *Ed.Izasa SA y Lorenzo García*

García García L, Lanciego C. Radiología Intervencionista en la Patología Biliar en Diagnóstico y terapéutica Endoluminal: Radiología Intervencionista. Tema 18, Cap 18.1 pags 421-443. 2002. *Ed.Masson SA*

Mauro M, Murphy KP, Thomson KR, Venbrux AC, Zollikofer C. Image-Guided Interventions. Section 22: The Biliary Tract Chap-134-138, pags 1425-1490. 2008, Ed.Saunders-Elsevier (ExpertRadiology collection)

Related Articles

Berkman WA, Bishop AF, Pallagallo GL, Cashman MD. Transhepatic balloon dilatation of the common bile duct and ampulla of Vater for removal of calculi. *Radiology* 1988;167: 453-455

Brountzos E, Ptochis N, Panagiotou I et al. A survival analysis of patients with malignant biliary strictures treated by percutaneous metallic stenting. *Cardiovasc Intervent Radiol* 2007;30(1): 66-73

Burke D, Lewis CA, Cardella JF et al. Quality improvement guidelines for percutaneous transhepatic cholangiography and biliary drainage. *JVIR* 2003;14:s243-s246

Chen JH, Sun CK, Liao CS, Chua CS. Self-expandable metallic stents for malignant biliary obstruction: efficacy on proximal and distal tumors. *World J Gastroenterol* 2006;12(1):119-122

Citron SJ, Martin LG. Benign biliary strictures: treatment with percutaneous cholangioplasty. *Radiology* 1991;178:339-341

García García L, Lanciego C. Percutaneous treatment of biliary stones. Sphincteroplasty and occlusion balloon for the clearance of bile duct calculi. *AJR Am J Roentgenol* 2004; 182:663-670

García García L, Venegas JL. Tratamiento percutáneo transhepático de la colédocolitiasis. *Radiologia* 1996;38:179-184

García-Vila J, Redondo-Ibañez M, Díaz-Ramón C. Balloon sphincteroplasty and transpapillary elimination of bile duct stones: 10 years experience. *AJR Am J Roentgenol* 2004; 182:1451-1458

Gibson RN, Adam A, Yeung E et al. Percutaneous techniques in benign hilar and intrahepatic strictures. *JVIR* 1988;3:125-130

Gil S, De la Iglesia P, Verdú JF, España F, Arenas J, Irurzun J. Effectiveness and safety of balloon dilation of the papilla and the use of an occlusion balloon for clearance of bile duct calculi. *AJR Am J Roentgenol* 2000;174:1455-1460

Ho CS, Voss MD. Self-expandable metallic biliary stents with permanent access. *AJR* 2005;184(2):410-414

Isayama H, Kamatsu Y, Tsujino T et al. A prospective randomised study of "covered" versus "uncovered" diamond stents for the management of distal malignant biliary obstruction. *Gut* 2004;53:729-734

Lee MJ, Mueller PR, Saini S et al. Percutaneous dilation of benign biliary strictures: single-session therapy with general anesthesia. *AJR Am J Roentgenol* 1991;157:1263-1266

Lee KH, Lee DY, Kim KW. Biliary Intervention for cholangiocarcinoma. *Abdom Imaging* 2004;29(5):581-589

Muchart J, Perendreu J, Casas JD, Diaz Ruiz MJ. Balloon catheter spinchteroplasty and biliary stone expulsion into the duodenum in patients with an indwelling T-tube. *Abdom Imaging* 1999;24:69-71

Park YS, Kim JH, Choi YW, Lee Th, Hwang CM, Cho YJ et al. Percutaneous treatment of extrahepatic bile duct stones assisted by balloon sphincteroplasty and occlusion balloon. *Korean J Radiol* 2005;6(4):235-240

Park H, Kim MH, Choi JS et al. Covered versus uncovered wallstent for malignant extrahepatic biliary obstruction: a cohort comparative analysis. *Clin Gastroenterol Hepatol* 2006;4(6):790-796

Silva MA, Tekin K, Aytekin F et al. Surgery for hilar cholangiocarcinoma: a 10-year experience of a tertiary referral centre in the UK. *Eur J Surg Oncol* 2005;31(5):533-539

Williams HJ, Bender CE, May GR. Benign postoperative biliary strictures: dilation with fluoroscopic guidance. *Radiology* 1987;163:629-634

Yoon WJ, Lee JK, Lee KH et al. A comparison of covered and uncovered Wallstent for the management of distal malignant biliary obstruction. *Gastrointest Endosc* 2006;63(7):996-1000

Ernesto Santos and Javier Blázquez

J.J. Muñoz and R. Ribes, *Learning Vascular and Interventional Radiology*, Learning Imaging,
DOI: 10.1007/978-3-540-87997-8_10, © Springer-Verlag Berlin Heidelberg 2010

Case 10.1

■ Radiofrequency Ablation of a Renal Mass

Figure 10.1.1 Chest CT shows the pacemaker cables in the chambers of the heart

Figure 10.1.2 Axial CT after intravenous contrast administration shows a hypervascular mass in the upper pole of the right kidney (*arrow*) in contact with the surface of the liver. Fine-needle aspiration cytology showed renal cell carcinoma

Figure 10.1.3 Unenhanced CT shows a renal tumor that is hypodense with respect to the renal parenchyma (*arrows*). The patient is in the supine position, with a wedge to elevate her right side; this makes it easier to introduce the radiofrequency electrode in the horizontal plane

Figure 10.1.4 Axial CT shows the hooked electrode centered within the tumor in two different places. CT-fluoroscopic-guided puncture allows the advancement of the needle to be controlled in real time

An 81-year-old woman with diabetes, hypertension, ischemic heart disease, and a definitive bicameral pacemaker for second-degree A-V block was admitted to another center for urinary sepsis. US detected a 3.4-cm mass in the upper pole of the right

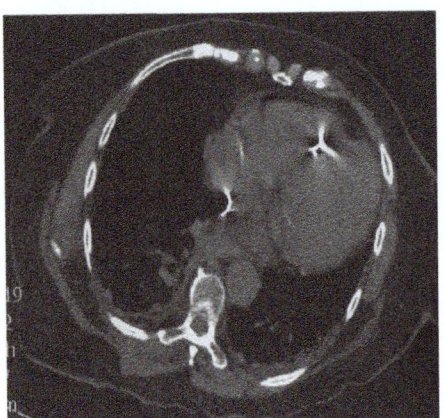

Fig. 10.1.1

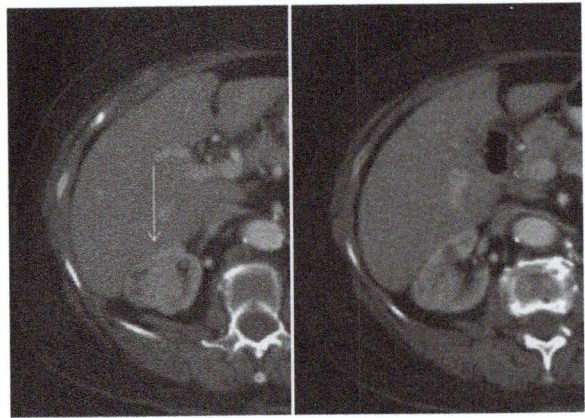

Fig. 10.1.2

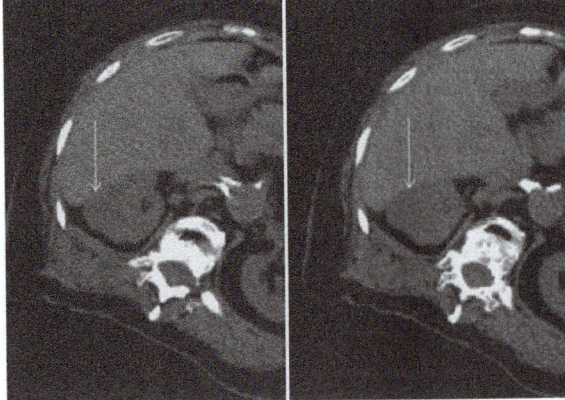

Fig. 10.1.3

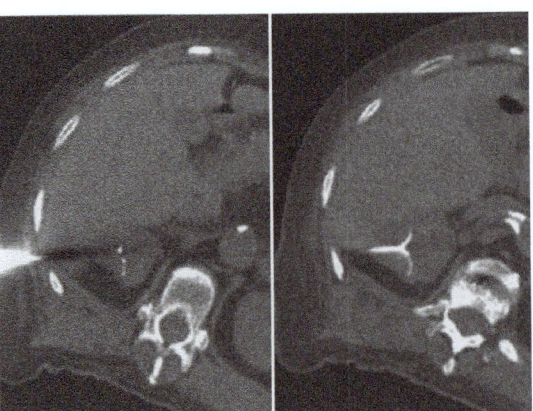

Fig. 10.1.4

kidney. She was referred to our center to evaluate the possibility of resection of the tumor, but due to her comorbidities and baseline condition, the clinical committee decided on radiofrequency ablation of the mass. US revealed the proximity of the costophrenic sinus to the theoretical path of the needle, so the lesion was ablated under CT-fluoroscopic guidance. The procedure was carried out using epidural anesthesia and sedation. Because the patient had a pacemaker, a cardiologist was present to control possible interferences with the device during radiofrequency ablation; no interference occurred.

Comments

Renal cell carcinoma is the third most common cancer of the urinary tract; it accounts for 3.5% of all malignant tumors. Increased imaging in patients with abdominal symptoms has led to a significant increase in the incidental detection of renal masses. Surgical resection (open or laparoscopic) continues to be the standard treatment, whether by radical or partial nephrectomy. The 5-year survival rate is 85–95% for patients with tumors discovered incidentally in stage T1a (<4 cm) and 53% for those with symptomatic renal tumors.

Different minimally invasive techniques based on delivering energy to destroy the tumors have been developed in recent years. These techniques include radiofrequency ablation, cryoablation, microwave ablation, laser ablation, and high-intensity focalized ultrasound ablation. These techniques offer several advantages over surgical resection, including reduced morbidity, the possibility of interventions in patients with severe underlying disease, better preservation of renal function, and faster recovery time.

The established indications for radiofrequency ablation of renal tumors are: patients unsuitable for surgery, single kidney, multiple renal tumors, and von Hippel-Lindau disease. Various metaanalyses have found that radiofrequency has a 90% success rate for the local control of renal tumors with a mean size of 2.6 cm (range, 1.7–5 cm). Enhancement after contrast administration is considered indicative of incomplete treatment.

Procedure Steps and Equipment

1. Select the imaging technique to guide the intervention: US, CT, or MRI.
2. Monitor the patient. Prepare the patient as necessary in function of the type of anesthesia. Place the adhesive grounding pads (monopolar system).
3. Position the patient to facilitate puncture.
4. Obtain axial CT slices. Select a reference slice for CT-fluoroscopy centered on the tumor.
5. Define the trajectory of the electrode to avoid neurovascular structures and intestinal loops.
6. Prepare a sterile field and use leaded gloves, goggles, and aprons.
7. Puncture under real-time guidance (CT-fluoroscopy).
8. Deploy the prongs of the electrode. Use CT-fluoroscopy to check that the prongs are correctly placed and cover the entire lesion.
9. The cardiologist can set the pacemaker in the correct mode to avoid interferences. Connect the radiofrequency generator.
10. Obtain final CT images to detect possible complications (hematoma).

Case 10.2

■

Ureteral Stenosis in a Transplanted Kidney: Treatment with a Metallic Stent

Figure 10.2.1 Pyelogram of the transplanted kidney shows filiform stenosis of the medial and distal thirds of the ureter (*left*). Balloon dilation is not efficacious. A calibrated guidewire is introduced to measure the length of the stenosis (*right*)

Figure 10.2.2 An 8 × 60 mm self-expanding nitinol stent was implanted (*arrows*). Note the ureteral spasms at the proximal and distal ends of the stent (*left*). Pyelogram shows good contrast flow to the bladder (*right*)

Figure 10.2.3 Follow-up pyelogram obtained through the nephrostomy catheter 24 h after the procedure shows minimal ureteral spasm and no filling defects in the urinary tract

Figure 10.2.4 CT reconstructions in different planes 1 year after stenting. The pyelocalyceal system is not dilated, and the patient's creatinine is stable

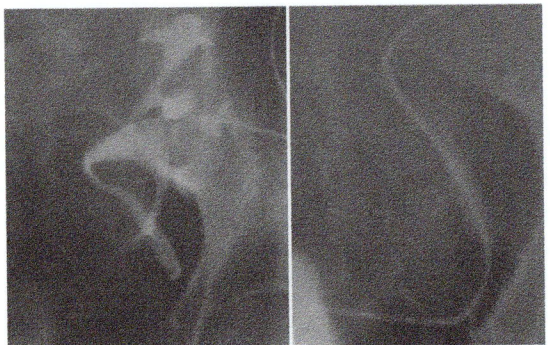

Fig. 10.2.1

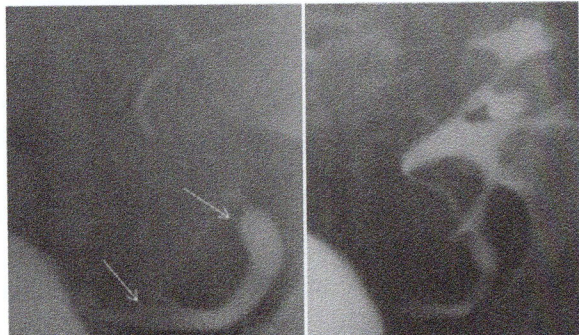

Fig. 10.2.2

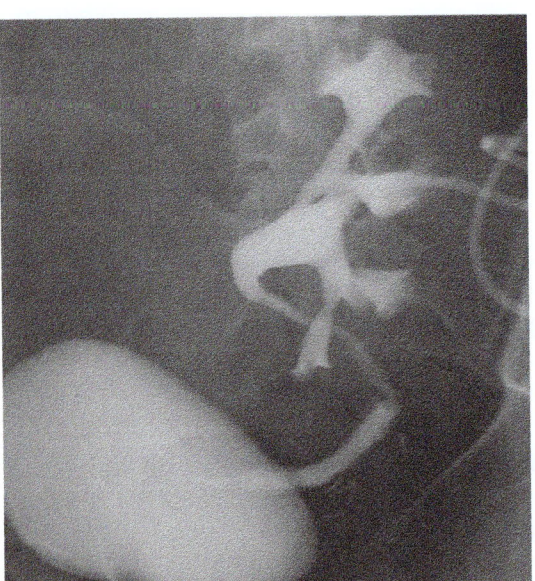

Fig. 10.2.3

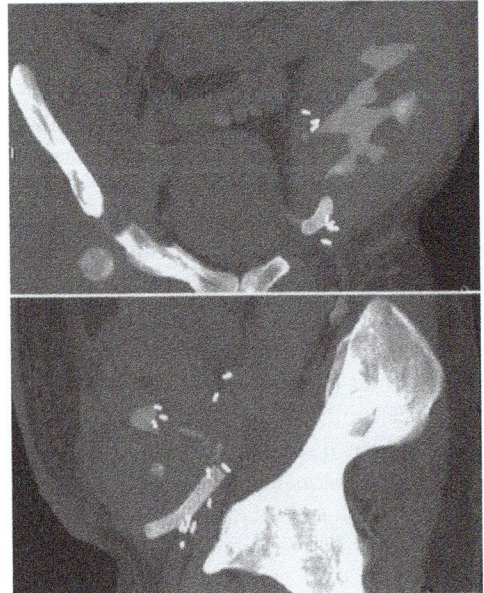

Fig. 10.2.4

A 36-year-old man with chronic renal failure due to rapidly progressing glomerulonephritis and two previous transplants presented with elevated creatinine (1.8–4 mg/dL) 2 months after the third transplant. US detected pyelocalyceal dilation. An urgent nephrostomy catheter was placed under US and fluoroscopic guidance and the patient was scheduled for pyelopyelic reanastomosis, which could not be performed due to the presence of adhesions. Thus, percutaneous treatment was performed, first with balloon dilation (which was not efficacious due to the elastic component of the stenosis) and then by deploying a metallic stent centered within the stenosis. The patient's creatinine stabilized at 2.1 mg/dL.

Comments

Urological complications of kidney transplantation are associated to increased morbidity of the patient and of the graft. Urological complications are second in frequency (after vascular complications) and cause renal dysfunction that can lead to loss of the transplanted kidney or death. The incidence of urological complications varies from 3 to 27%. The most common complications are urine leaks, stenosis or obstruction of the ureterovesical anastomosis, and stenosis or obstruction of the ureter or pyeloureteral junction.

Stenosis of the distal ureter accounts for 13–25% of the urological complications and is usually due to the necrosis of the wall. Implanting a double J stent not only reduces early urological complications (urine leaks and obstruction), but also results in a significant increase in urinary infections. Early diagnosis of complications is essential in the post-transplantation period, and percutaneous treatment has significantly reduced the need for surgical treatment in recent years. The therapeutic arsenal of the interventional radiologist is continually growing, with the introduction of different types of balloons (conventional, cutting, cryoplasty) and stents (uncoated, coated, and recoverable) enabling practically all urological complications to be treated.

Procedure Steps and Equipment

1. Use a 22G needle to puncture a renal pelvis of the graft under US and fluoroscopic guidance. After aspirating urine, inject contrast material and insert a 0.018 in. guidewire.
2. Withdraw the needle and introduce a sheath to enable a 0.035 in. guidewire to be advanced. Insert an introducer sheath to perform pyelography and locate the stenosis.
3. Choose the most appropriate guidewire and shapeable catheter to catheterize the stenosis. Advance a guidewire to the bladder.
4. Select a balloon to dilate the stenosis and then perform pyelography.
5. If the result is satisfactory, leave an internal–external catheter (10F–12F) in place for two to four weeks.
6. If the results are suboptimal, try to dilate the stenosis with "special" balloons or to implant a stent (depending on the team's experience). Place a closed external nephrostomy catheter. Control renal function.
7. Withdraw the external or internal–external catheter.

Case 10.3

■

Wunderlich Syndrome. Spontaneous Extracapsular Renal Hemorrhage Secondary to a Renal Angiomyolipoma

Figure 10.3.1 Urgent US shows a hyperechogenic lesion measuring 11 cm (*arrows*) on the upper pole of the left kidney (superior). US also detected a heterogeneous image that corresponded to a large retroperitoneal hematoma (*asterisks*)

Figure 10.3.2a angiographic study of the left renal artery shows a large tumor with a marked angiogenic component, compatible with an angiomyolipoma

Figure 10.3.2b Selective study of the tumor also shows extravasation of contrast material (*arrow*) related to active bleeding

Figure 10.3.3 Angiogram after embolization with PVA particles and metallic coils demonstrates the occlusion of the vessels of the angiomyolipoma and the preservation of the renal parenchyma

Figure 10.3.4 Follow-up CT 6 months after embolization shows a necrotic mass with a minimal myovascular component

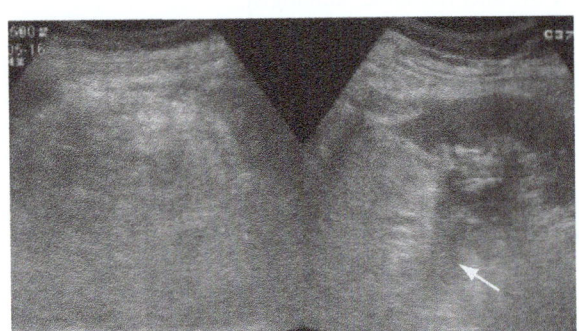

Fig. 10.3.1

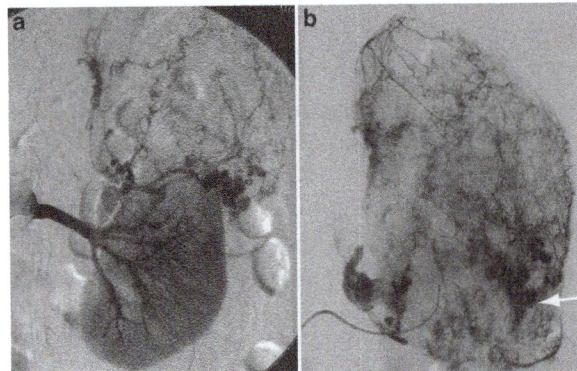

Fig. 10.3.2

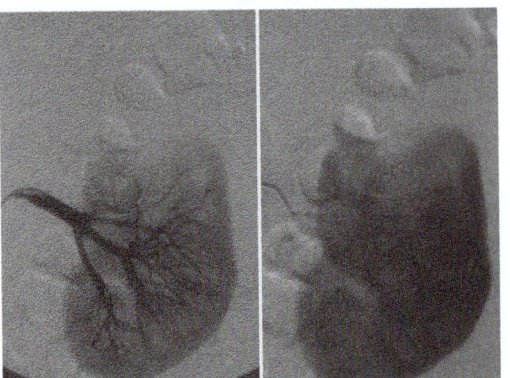

Fig. 10.3.3

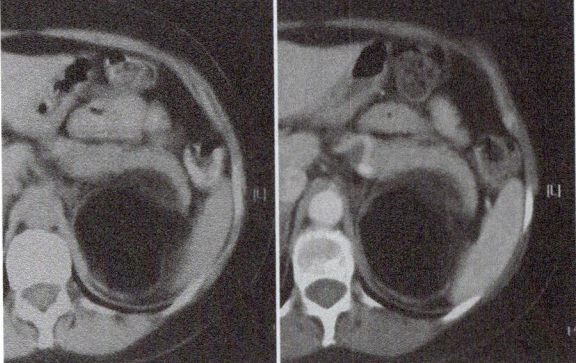

Fig. 10.3.4

A 55-year-old woman with a history of hypertension presented at the emergency department with left renal fossa pain and nausea. Her blood pressure was 90/55 mmHg. Her hemoglobin was 8.4 mg/dL. Abdominal CT showed a large retroperitoneal hematoma with extravasation of contrast material related to active bleeding and a 12-cm tumor with a fatty component in the upper pole of her left kidney, considered to be an angiomyolipoma (AML). Urgent angiography showed the hypervascular renal tumor with a large angiogenic component and extravasation of contrast material. The AML was embolized using 500–700 micra PVA particles and metallic coils. After embolization, the patient remained stable without evidence of new episodes of bleeding. Follow-up CT 6 months after embolization showed a significant reduction in the myovascular component of the tumor.

Comments

Renal AMLs are benign hamartomatous tumors that contain fat, smooth muscle, and anomalous vessels. There are two presentations: a) sporadic or solitary tumors (80%), which are solitary tumors most common in women between 50 and 80 years of age, and b) tumors associated to tuberous sclerosis and other phacomatoses. The typical clinical presentation consists of retroperitoneal bleeding, hematuria, or abdominal mass. No symptoms are present in 40% of cases. Patients with AMLs greater than 4 cm should be treated.

Given the benign nature of AMLs, treatment is based on interventions that preserve the renal parenchyma, such as tumorectomy and selective embolization. Different materials can be used for embolization, including the combination of alcohol with PVA particles, liodol, or Spongostan, or PVA combined with metallic spirals. Embolization is technically successful in 95% of cases, with a mean reduction in the size of the AML of 25%. The angiogenic component is eliminated in 33% of patients and reduced in the rest.

Procedure Steps and Equipment

1. Puncture the femoral artery and introduce a catheter to obtain an aortogram. This will enable anatomic variants like polar arteries to be evaluated and other arteries that can cause retroperitoneal bleeding to be identified (lumbar arteries).
2. Use a cobra or Simmons I catheter to selectively study the renal artery; this will enable the arteries that supply the tumor to be studied.
3. Perform superselective catheterization of the AML's afferent vessels.
4. Confirm that the catheters are in a stable position.
5. First, use particles to embolize the branches within the tumor and then occlude the arterial pedicle with metallic coils.
6. Embolization is finished when arterial stasis is achieved. Obtain a final angiogram to confirm the selective devascularization of the tumor.

Case 10.4
■
Bilateral Renal Fibromuscular Dysplasia

Figure 10.4.1 Initial aortogram obtained with a calibrated catheter makes it possible to identify subtle irregularities in both renal arteries and to confirm the absence of polar arteries

Figure 10.4.2 Selective angiography of the right renal artery shows the typical findings of fibromuscular dysplasia: beaded stenosis of the middle third of the renal artery; the compressive bands cause severe stenosis

Figures 10.4.3 and 10.4.4 Selective study of both renal arteries before (*left*) and after (*right*) angioplasty. After balloon dilation, despite the irregularities in both arteries, no signs of arterial dissection or slowing of flow are seen

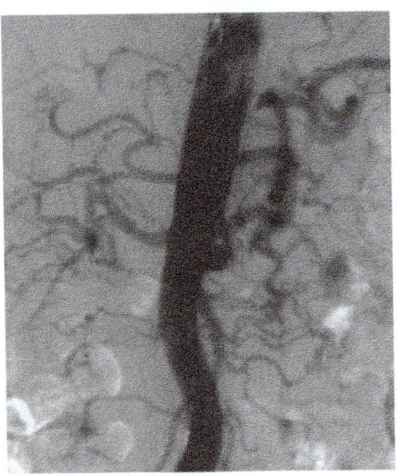

Fig. 10.4.1

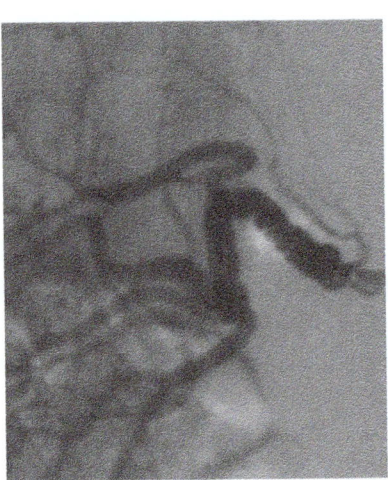

Fig. 10.4.2

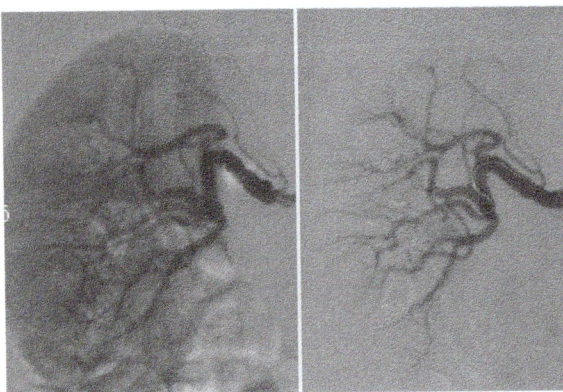

Fig. 10.4.3

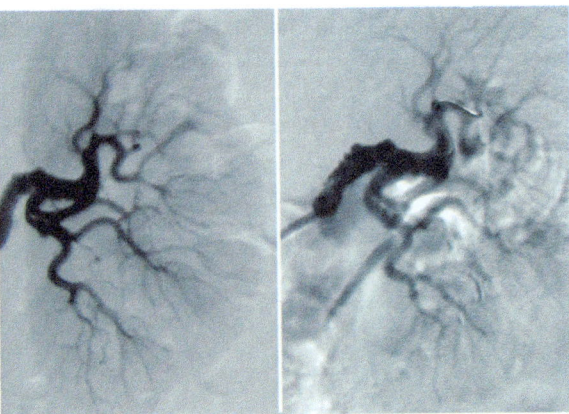

Fig. 10.4.4

A 39-year-old woman with a 9-year history of hypertension progressively worsening in the past year (24-h Holter showed peaks of 190/110 mmHg), despite treatment with three drugs, was referred to the vascular radiology unit from another hospital. Physical examination found an abdominal murmur.

The usual imaging techniques like Doppler US and MRI detected no significant alterations; however, angiography was performed for clinical suspicion of renal artery stenosis. The invasive arterial study revealed classic angiographic findings of fibromuscular dysplasia (FMD) involving the middle third of both renal arteries, where the classic "string-of-beads" image (dilations and bands causing severe stenosis) was seen. Six months after percutaneous treatment (bilateral angioplasty), the patient only required one drug to keep her blood pressure within the normal range.

Comments

FMD is a nonatherosclerotic, noninflammatory arterial disease. It involves the renal arteries in 65% of cases and is bilateral in 35%. FMD normally affects the middle third of the renal arteries, although bands causing stenoses in the segmental arteries are not uncommon.

FMD is more common in women, especially in those between 15 and 50 years of age. FMD accounts for 10% of cases of hypertension due to renovascular causes. FMD progresses in 40% of cases, but does not usually result in occlusion of the artery. The mass of the kidney decreases in 60% of cases, but the incidence of renal failure is low. For these reasons, treatment is based on controlling hypertension.

Percutaneous revascularization (angioplasty) has supplanted surgical revascularization, and the success rates of the two techniques are similar (83–100%). A complete cure is achieved in 14–60% of cases, and clinical improvement is seen in 21–57% of the rest of the patients. Successful angioplasty leads to rapid, substantial lowering of blood pressure with clinical benefits persisting 5 years after the intervention in 80% of cases.

Procedure Steps and Equipment

1. Puncture the femoral artery and introduce a calibrated catheter to obtain an aortogram. This will enable anatomic variants like polar arteries to be evaluated.
2. Use a cobra or Simmons I catheter to selectively study the renal artery to evaluate the extent of the FMD .
3. Place a 6F catheter guidewire in the ostium of the renal artery.
4. Elaborate a vascular map and use a 0.014–0.018 in. guidewire to catheterize the stenoses induced by FMD.
5. Introduce an angioplasty balloon (5–7 mm in diameter and 2–4 cm long) and center it in the lesion using the map.
6. Dilate the stenoses with the balloon.
7. Check the results by angiography: irregularities are usually seen after dilation, but stenting is unnecessary unless there is significant arterial dissection or hemodynamic compromise.

Case 10.5

■

Arteriocalyceal Fistula After Renal Biopsy. Percutaneous Treatment

Figure 10.5.1 Arterial, capillary, and late phase images after selective injection of the left renal artery show the lesion in the lobar artery with progressive filling of a calyx in the lower pole (*arrow*)

Figure 10.5.2 Superselective catheterization using a microcatheter and a vascular map enabled the damaged artery to be embolized with metallic coils

Figure 10.5.3 Final angiographic study of the left kidney shows the result of the embolization; the fistula has disappeared and loss of renal parenchyma has been kept to a minimum

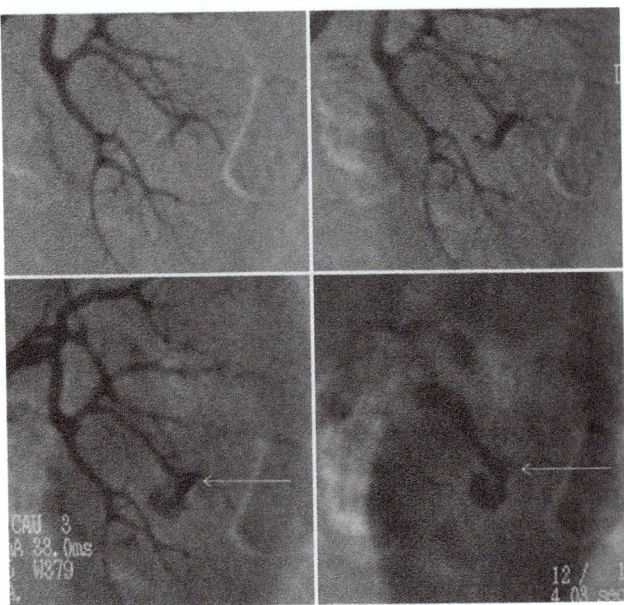

Fig. 10.5.1

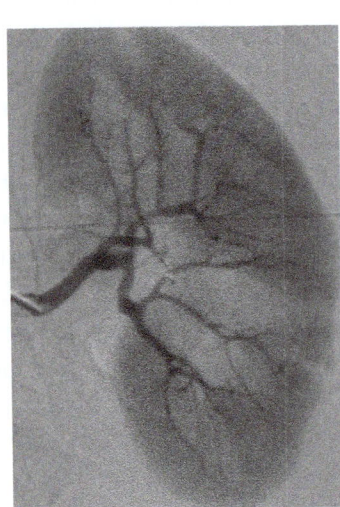

Fig. 10.5.2

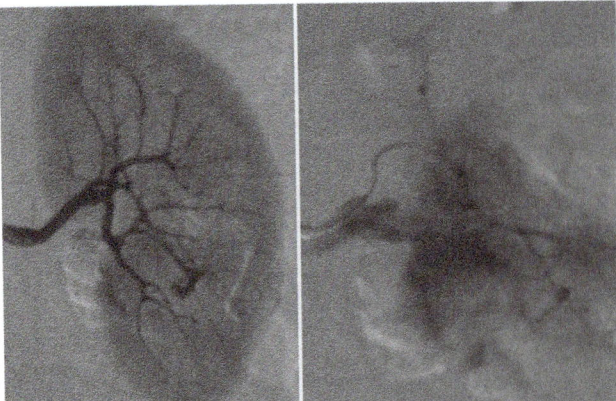

Fig. 10.5.3

A 29-year-old woman with hypertension and proteinuria progressively developed renal failure (creatinine 2.2 mg/dL). Thirty minutes after US-guided biopsy performed to rule out glomerulonephritis, she developed pain in her left renal fossa, hematuria, and hypotension with loss of consciousness.

Once the patient was stabilized, she was referred to the vascular radiology suite with a suspected vascular lesion. After obtaining an aortogram, we identified the lesion in a small arterial branch of the left kidney with posterior filling of a calyx in the lower pole of the kidney. Selective study of the renal artery confirmed the findings. We proceeded to selectively catheterize the damaged lobar artery with a microcatheter and embolized it with metallic coils measuring 3 mm in diameter. The fistula disappeared and the outcome was satisfactory.

Comments

In recent years, kidney biopsy has become an essential procedure in the diagnostic workup of both kidney disease and kidney transplants. After biopsy, patients must rest for 6 h. During this period, blood pressure and pulse should be checked often, and the first urine should be tested to rule out hematuria. Patients should refrain from vigorous exercise for 1 week after the procedure.

Complications after kidney biopsy are rare. The most common complication is bleeding (3–5%), which is normally limited to perirenal hematoma or hematuria. Less than 1% of patients require transfusion or angiography to detect a vascular lesion. Pseudoaneurysms and arteriovenous fistulas are the most common lesions in this group, and fistulas between arteries and the urinary tract are extremely rare. The main risk factor is hypertension.

Lesions are usually located in the lower pole and embolization with microcatheters is very efficacious in their exclusion. The procedure usually leads to a loss of 10–30% of the renal parenchyma.

Procedure Steps and Equipment

1. Puncture the femoral artery and introduce a pigtail catheter to obtain an aortogram. This will make it possible to evaluate the renal vascularization and occasionally to identify the arterial lesion.
2. Selectively study both renal arteries with a cobra or Simmons I catheter; this will enable you to diagnose the lacerated artery and decide whether to use a microcatheter.
3. Elaborate a vascular map and use a microcatheter to selectively catheterize the damaged artery.
4. Estimate the size of the artery to choose the size of the metallic coils. Given the terminal character of the renal circulation, proximal embolization is efficacious. Other materials, like bucrylate or Spongostan, can also be used.
5. Minimize the loss of renal parenchyma.
6. Obtain an angiogram to check the results of the embolization and ensure that the pseudoaneurysm and extravasation have disappeared.

Case 10.6
Stenosis of an Ureteroileal Anastomosis: Treatment with a Temporary Metallic Stent

Figure 10.6.1 After nephrostomy, a 7×40 mm balloon was antegradely centered in the ureteroileal anastomosis; the narrowing in the center of the balloon corresponds to the area of the stenosis

Figure 10.6.2 The balloon was dilated to 8 atmospheres and the area of stenosis disappeared

Figure 10.6.3 After withdrawing the balloon, we placed a self-expanding coated metallic stent in the stenosis. Note the radiopaque marks used to implant the stent under fluoroscopic guidance (*arrows*)

Figure 10.6.4 Antegrade pyelography shows the good flow of contrast material from the ureter to the ileum

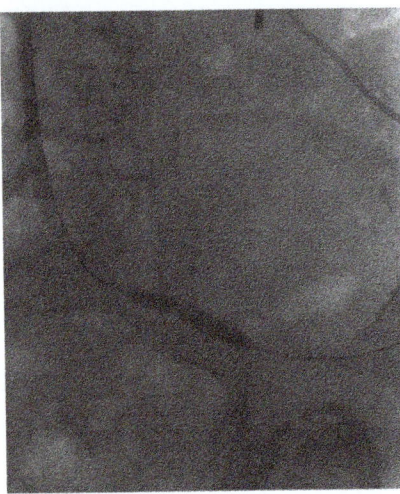

Fig. 10.6.1

Fig. 10.6.2

Fig. 10.6.3

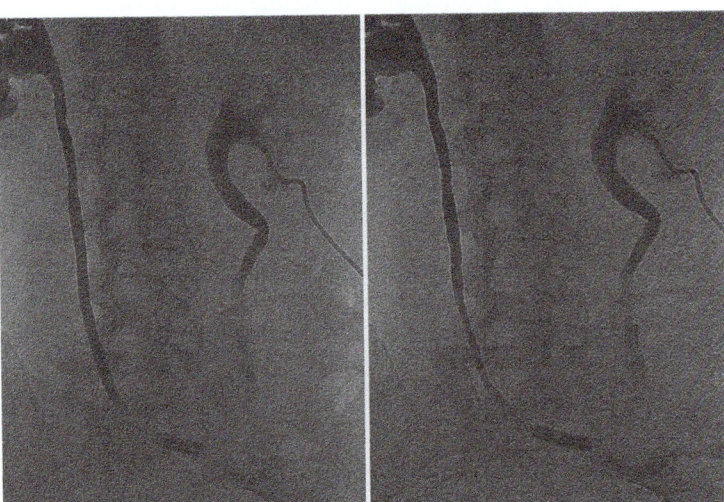

Fig. 10.6.4

A 69-year-old man with a history of hypertension, hepatitis C, and high-grade urothelial carcinoma treated with radical cystectomy, Bricker ileal conduit (Wallace I), and chemotherapy in 2005 presented at the emergency department in July 2008 with fever and deteriorating renal function. CT showed significant left pyelocalyceal dilation and mild right pyelocalyceal dilation. Relevant blood test results were creatinine 2.3 mg/dL and leukocytes 17,000 with a left shift.

After bilateral nephrostomy, descending urography showed a filiform stenosis of the left ureteroileal anastomosis. After dilation with a balloon (7 mm in diameter), a temporary coated metallic stent (Allium) was implanted to be left in place for 6 months. The idea was to withdraw the stent through the cutaneous stoma using a cystoscope.

Comments

Bricker ileal conduit surgery is normally performed in patients with underlying tumors (bladder, prostate, colon), although 20% of these procedures are performed in patients with benign disease (neurogenic bladder, radiation cystitis, bladder exstrophy).

Postoperative mortality is 7% and is especially common in patients with cancer. Immediate morbidity is related to intestinal complications like ileus, fistulas, and evisceration. Late morbidity (18%) is related to parietal complications like incisional and parastomal hernias, stenosis of the stoma, and urological complications like pyelonephritis (11%), ureteroileal stenosis (6–10%), and lithiasis.

Ureteroileal stenoses can be managed surgically or endourologically. Between 50 and 75% of cases are managed endourologically with internal–external catheters and stents, resulting in 60% secondary patency 4 years after the procedure.

Procedure Steps and Equipment

1. Perform nephrostomy and use a 22G needle to puncture a calyx of the graft under US and fluoroscopic guidance. After aspirating urine, inject contrast material and advance a 0.018 in. guidewire.
2. Withdraw the needle and introduce a sheath to enable a 0.035 in. guidewire to be inserted. Insert an 11F introducer sheath to perform pyelography and locate the stenosis in the ureteroileal anastomosis.
3. Choose the most appropriate shapeable catheter for the catheterization of the stenosis. Advance a rigid guidewire to the bowel loop.
4. Use a 7-mm diameter balloon to dilate the stenosis and perform pyelography.
5. Withdraw the balloon and implant an 8 × 60 mm temporary coated metallic stent, centered within the stenosis.
6. Obtain a pyelogram to check that contrast flows freely from the ureter to the small bowel loop. Leave an internal–external safety catheter in place.
7. Withdraw the internal–external catheter and check renal function.

Case 10.7

■

Intrarenal Saccular Aneurysm. Treatment by Embolization

Figure. 10.7.1 Aortogram and selective study of the left renal artery show a 3-cm intrarenal saccular aneurysm in subsegmental artery

Figure. 10.7.2 Aneurysmogram obtained through a microcatheter does not show the arteries that the aneurysmatic sac is derived from. The aneurysm was embolized with mechanically released microcoils, and no significant residual neck was observed

Figures. 10.7.3 and 10.7.4 Follow-up CT (axial slices and coronal reconstruction) 3 years after embolization shows the metallic coils. The aneurysm has not grown and does not fill with contrast material. Selective embolization made it possible to preserve all of the parenchyma of the left kidney

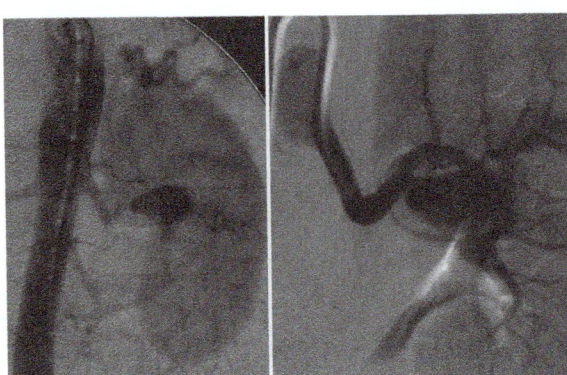

Fig. 10.7.1

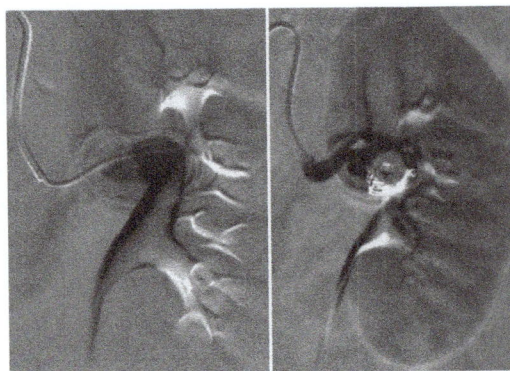

Fig. 10.7.2

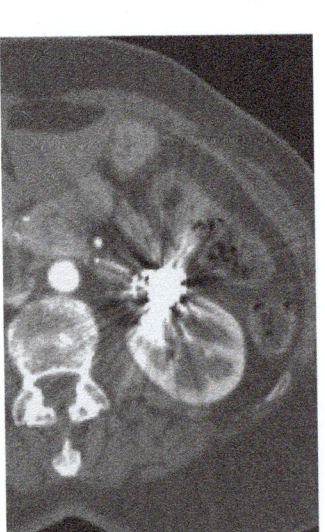

Fig. 10.7.3

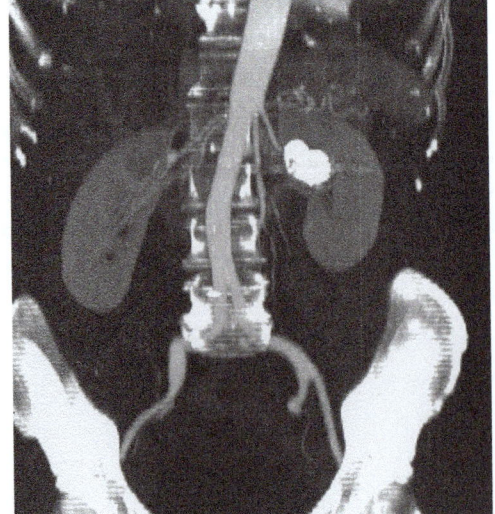

Fig. 10.7.4

A 61-year-old woman with a history of thyroidectomy presented with a 3-month history of low back pain. Spinal X-ray and CT examinations detected an intrarenal aneurysm measuring 3 cm in diameter.

Owing to the location of the aneurysm, angiography was performed to evaluate the arterial anatomy and determine whether embolization was possible. Given the saccular morphology of the aneurysm, the sac was embolized using a microcatheter and mechanically released metallic coils until the aneurysm was packed. After embolization, no loss of renal parenchyma was seen.

Comments

Renal aneurysms are uncommon; their incidence in autopsy series is 0.01%. Women are affected in 68% of cases and the mean age of presentation is 45 years. Renal aneurysms have been associated to fibromuscular dysplasia, Ehlers-Danlos syndrome, pseudoaneurysms, polyarteritis nodosa, tuberculosis, and neurofibromatosis. Renal aneurysms are often discovered incidentally in asymptomatic patients. Symptomatic patients present hypertension, abdominal pain, hematuria, renal infarction, or rupture.

Treatment is indicated in symptomatic patients, in pregnant women or those who wish to become pregnant, in patients with aneurysms larger than 2 cm, and in those in whom the aneurysm is seen to grow.

It is essential to perform CT or MRI prior to the intervention. The treatment options depend on the number and location of the aneurysms and are based on chemical repair (patch and bypass), nephrectomy, and percutaneous treatment using either metallic spirals or stent-grafts.

Procedure Steps and Equipment

1. Introduce a pigtail catheter to obtain an aortogram. This will enable the appropriate catheter to be selected for the selective renal study, especially in cases involving the descending arteries (Simmons I catheter).
2. Selectively study the relevant vessels until you find the best projection to enable the aneurysm and its neck to be visualized. Ideally, you should perform a 3D study to find the best projection.
3. Elaborate a vascular map and use a microcatheter to selectively catheterize the aneurysm. Obtain an aneurysmogram to exclude the presence of arteries that might originate from the aneurysm of its neck.
4. Check the stability of the system, start embolizing with mechanically released metallic coils in a way that enables them to be recovered before release if they are not in the right position.
5. Obtain an angiogram to check whether the embolization has excluded the aneurysm from the circulation.
6. Follow-up the patient with CT.

Case 10.8
■
**Angioplasty
of the Renal Artery
in a Patient with
Takayasu's Arteritis**

Figure 10.8.1 Arteriogram of the supraaortic trunks shows stenoses at various levels in the carotid arteries, in the right brachiocephalic trunk (in the origins of the vertebral, subclavian, and carotid arteries), in the left subclavian artery (both at its origin and in the middle third), a very long stenosis in the right subclavian artery, and hypertrophy of the right internal mammary artery

Figure 10.8.2: Angiogram of the abdominal aorta shows a delayed flow to the left kidney, stenoses of the renal arteries, and hypertrophy of Riolan's arch

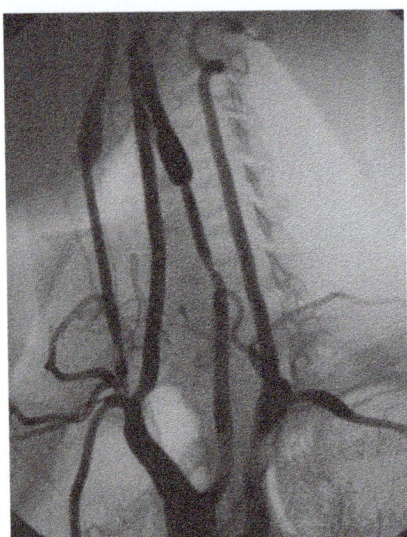

Fig. 10.8.1

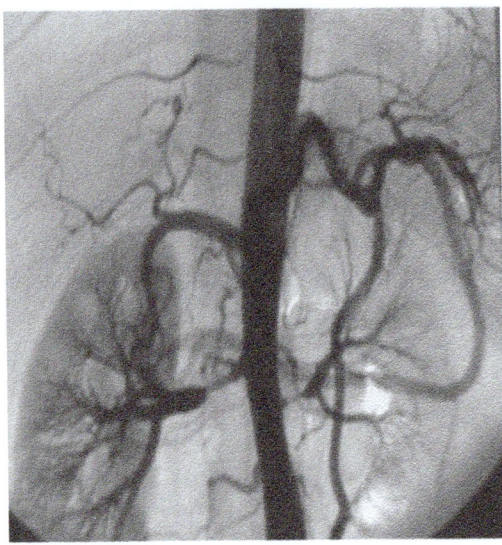

Fig. 10.8.2

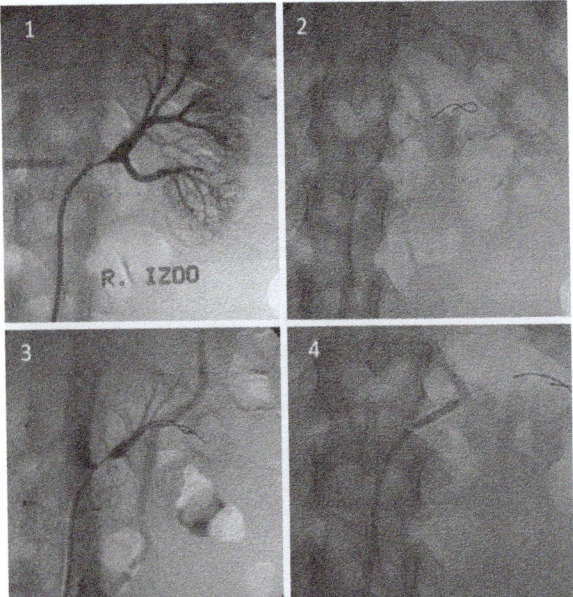

Fig. 10.8.3

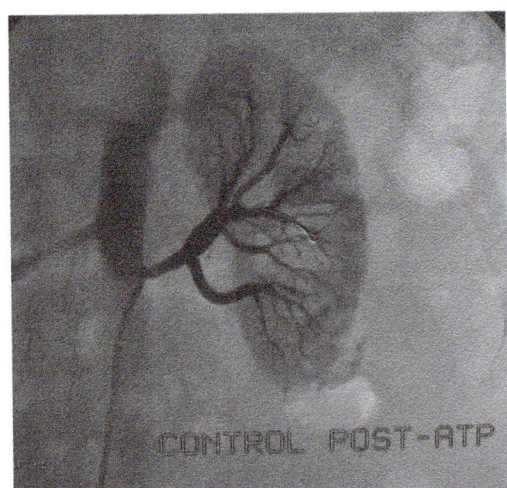

Fig. 10.8.4

Figure 10.8.3 *1.* Selective arteriogram of the left renal artery obtained with a guiding catheter; this image makes it possible to calculate the diameter and the length of the balloon to be used. *2.* Catheterization of the stenosis with a 0.014 in. guidewire. *3.* Selective arteriogram of the left renal artery with the guidewire distal to the lesion to confirm the absence of dissection and to enable the angioplasty to be correctly positioned. *4.* Dilation of the lesion with a balloon
Figure 10.8.4 Angiographic confirmation of the results showing the vessel has recovered its normal caliber and the absence of intimal dissection

A 24-year-old woman was referred to the nephrology department for hypertension after presenting at the emergency department on two occasions with an intense headache. Doppler US confirmed marked stenosis of the renal arteries.

Angiography showed compromise of the medial portion of both subclavian arteries, of the medial portion of the left common carotid artery, and a distal lesion of the brachiocephalic trunk. The imaging findings together with the obligatory criterion and other minor clinical/laboratory criteria, like elevated erythrocyte sedimentation rate, arterial hypertension, or carotid hypertension, were sufficient to establish the diagnosis of Takayasu's arteritis.

Immunosuppressor treatment with corticoids (Prednisone 60 mg/day) was initiated and a joint committee of the vascular surgery, interventional radiology, and nephrology departments decided to try to save the left kidney by restoring the patency of the arteries supplying it by percutaneous transluminal angioplasty as a first step in the management of the disease in its phase of established arterial stenosis.

We confirmed the critical stenosis of the left renal artery with angiography and then dilated it with a balloon.

The angiographic findings after the angioplasty and the improvement in the patient's hypertension enabled clinical follow-up.

Comments

Takayasu's arteritis is a vasculitis defined by the American College of Rheumatology as an idiopathic chronic inflammatory vasculopathy that affects the large elastic arteries. It is an uncommon disease that predominantly affects young women (10–40 years old) and Asians.

The definitive diagnosis is confirmed by histologic study of the compromised arterial segment. Due to the difficulty of obtaining a specimen from the affected artery, Ishikawa proposed a set of criteria for the diagnosis of Takayasu's arteritis.

- Obligatory criterion: Age of onset <40 years.
- Major criteria: Involvement of the left or right subclavian artery.
- Minor criteria: Arterial hypertension, elevation of the erythrocyte sedimentation rate, pain in the region of the carotid artery, and arterial compromise in the left carotid artery, in the brachiocephalic trunk, in the thoracic or abdominal aorta, aortic insufficiency, or lesion of the pulmonary artery.

The diagnosis is established by fulfillment of the obligatory criterion and two major criteria or of the obligatory criterion and one major and two or more minor criteria, or of the obligatory criterion and four or more minor criteria.

Treatment basically depends on the patient's clinical symptoms:
- Asymptomatic patients call for observation and periodic follow-up.
- Symptomatic patients should receive immunosuppressor treatment.
- Revascularization should be considered in patients with symptoms of ischemia.

Percutaneous transluminal angioplasty in these patients is controversial because the inflammatory nature of the disease results in a high rate of restenosis (50–70%).

Procedure Steps and Equipment

1. Use a 5F pigtail catheter to perform angiography of the supraaortic trunks and of the abdominal aorta.
2. With a 45-cm long 6F introducer sheath and with the help of a 4F cobra catheter, introduce a 0.014 in. nitinol guidewire to the lobar branch of the left kidney.
3. Administer sodium heparin whenever an intervention (angioplasty or stenting) is carried out in the arterial lumen. In this case, we also administered spasmolytic medication (nitroglycerine 0.1 mg).
4. Use a 5 × 20-mm low-profile monorail balloon; this can be very useful in cases of critical stenosis like this one.
5. After the dilation, check the results by angiography; in cases of unsatisfactory results (intimal dissection or arterial rupture) a stent must be placed.

Case 10.9

Embolization of an Arteriovenous Fistula in a Renal Graft

Figure 10.9.1 Doppler US shows a vascular anomaly, with turbulent flow, compatible with an arteriovenous fistula

Figure 10.9.2 *Left*: Arteriogram of the distal aorta and iliac arteries obtained with a pigtail catheter after puncturing the left femoral artery. There is a renal graft in the right iliac fossa. *Right*: Selective catheterization of the artery of the graft shows an arteriovenous fistula in the lower pole

Figure 10.9.3 Selective catheterization of the arterial component of the arteriovenous fistula with a microcatheter

Figure 10.9.4 Arteriogram after embolization with metallic coils shows that the arteriovenous fistula has been occluded and that the renal parenchyma has been preserved

A 64-year-old woman treated in the nephrology department presented with increased edema in her lower limbs and worsening dyspnea, which at that time was present on moderate effort.

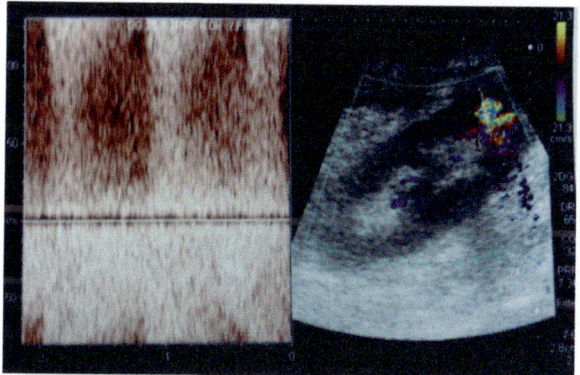

Fig. 10.9.1

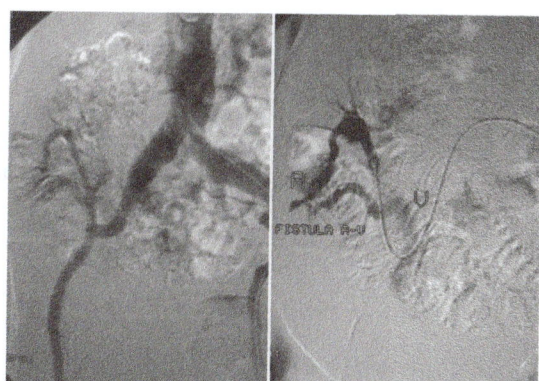

Fig. 10.9.2

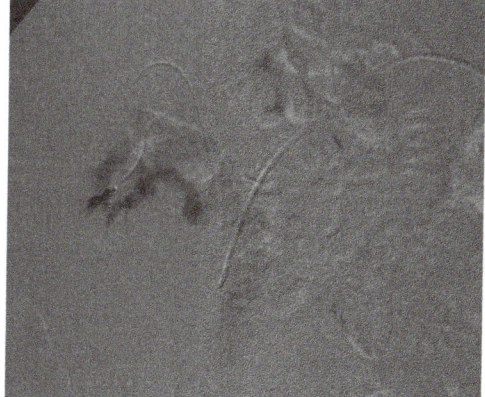

Fig. 10.9.3

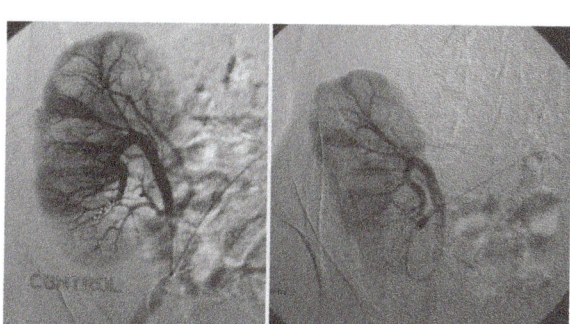

Fig. 10.9.4

Her personal history included aortic and mitral valve replacement with biological prostheses and kidney transplant in the right iliac fossa 1 year before. Two and a half months after the kidney transplant, the graft was biopsied due to suspected rejection. Histologic study revealed minimal, nonspecific changes.

Renal US showed a graft in the right iliac fossa with normal parenchyma and smooth cortex; the urinary tract was not dilated. Doppler study showed an image 2 cm in diameter with increased, turbulent flow, and an arteriovenous fistula secondary to renal biopsy was suspected.

The angiogram showed a pathological communication between an artery and a vein in the lower pole of the renal graft. The fistula was embolized with metallic coils and postprocedural angiography showed the occlusion of the pathological communication and the preserved vascularization of the kidney, with a normal nephrogram.

Blood test before and after the procedure showed creatinine 1.8 mg/dL without significant increases.

Comments

The incidence of arteriovenous fistulas after renal biopsy is about 0.1% in native kidneys, but generally higher in transplanted kidneys (1–15%).

Renal arteriovenous fistulas are generally asymptomatic, although they may manifest clinically depending on their size and location.

Symptoms can include hematuria, deterioration of renal function, or hypertension. High-flow fistulas can have repercussions on the systemic circulation (in our case, worsening of heart failure).

Arteriovenous fistulas are diagnosed by Doppler US, which can also be used for follow-up in cases with expectant management. Angiography should be reserved for planning endovascular treatment.

The treatment of small, asymptomatic fistulas is controversial as they close spontaneously in 70–95% of cases. Nevertheless, in cases with clinical repercussion, surgical or endovascular treatment is indicated.

Procedure Steps and Equipment

1. Confirm that an arteriovenous fistula is present with Doppler US before deciding whether to perform angiography.
2. Use a 5F pigtail catheter to perform angiography of the distal aorta and iliac arteries through the contralateral femoral artery. This will enable us to confirm the fistula and plan the approach to the artery of the graft, usually through the contralateral artery.
3. Selectively catheterize the artery of the renal graft with a curved 4F Simmons I hydrophilic catheter.
4. Use a 2.8F microcatheter to perform superselective catheterization of the arterial component of the fistula and try to embolize as little of the healthy renal parenchyma as possible and to avoid infarction of the lower pole of the kidney.
5. Place metallic coils of the appropriate caliber in the artery to be embolized and in the catheter being used. In our case, we used coils measuring 3 and 4 mm in length and 0.018 mm in diameter.
6. Check the results with angiography: confirm the occlusion of the fistula and the degree of embolization of the healthy renal parenchyma.
7. Follow-up the patient after the procedure (clinical and laboratory tests).

Case 10.10

■

Presurgical Embolization of Renal Cell Carcinoma

Figure 10.10.1 *Left*: Abdominal CT shows a tumor with a cystic component arising from the right kidney; it displaces the liver and colon. *Right*: Arteriogram of the abdominal aorta obtained with a pigtail catheter shows a large hypervascular mass

Figure 10.10.2 *Left*: Selective catheterization of the right renal artery shows hypertrophy of the right renal artery and multiple branches feeding the tumor. *Right*: Selective catheterization of a lumbar artery that also supplies the tumor

Figure 10.10.3 *Left*: Angiogram after embolization of the right renal artery with particles and coils shows the absence of filling of the kidney and of the tumor. *Right*: Angiogram after embolization of the lumbar artery shows the absence of flow

Figure 10.10.4 Angiogram of the abdominal aorta for a final check shows the total absence of vascularization of the tumor

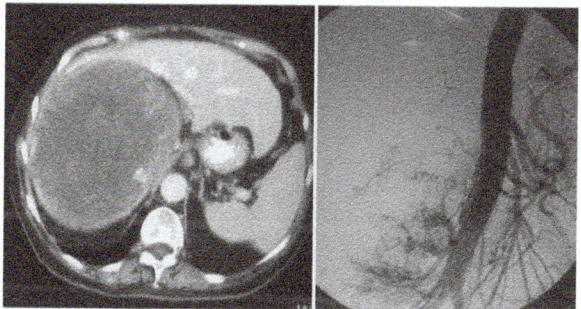

Fig. 10.10.1

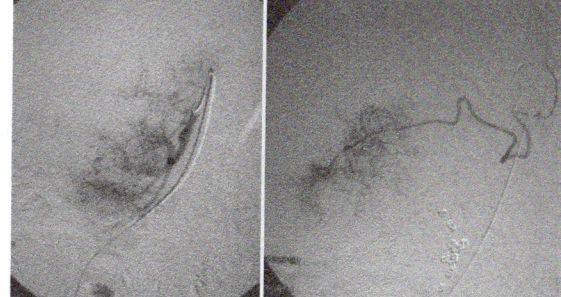

Fig. 10.10.2

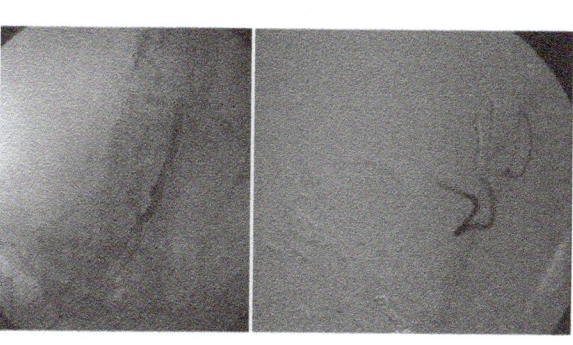

Fig. 10.10.3

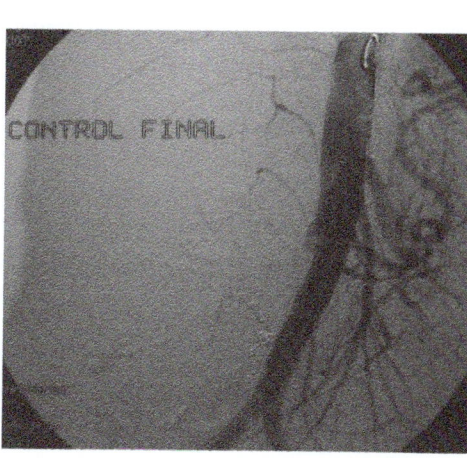

Fig. 10.10.4

A 78-year-old woman was attended at the digestive disease department with a 2-month history of asthenia, anorexia, and enlargement of the right abdomen.

Abdominal US detected a mixed lesion that appeared to be connected to the liver rather than to the kidney.

Abdominal CT showed a solid mass on the right kidney displacing the ascending colon and liver.

Due to the size of the tumor and its arterial hypervascularization, the team decided to embolize the tumor before surgical treatment (right radical nephrectomy with lymph node dissection).

Histologic study after nephrectomy showed clear-cell renal cell carcinoma.

Comments

Clear-cell renal cell carcinoma is the most common malignant kidney tumor, accounting for about 80%. Its causes include hereditary genetic factors (Von Hippel-Lindau disease), tobacco use, and exposure to asbestos or heavy metals. In general, because it grows slowly without causing noteworthy symptoms, it is often very large or has already metastasized when it is discovered. This tumor often leads to paraneoplastic symptoms like hypertension, hypercalcemia, hyperprolactinemia, altered hepatic function, neuropathy, or Cushing's syndrome, among others. Clear-cell renal cell carcinoma is characterized by marked angiogenesis.

The main treatment is surgical excision, either by conventional open surgery or laparoscopic surgery, although in recent years techniques like radiofrequency ablation, cryoablation, microwave ablation, or high-intensity focused ultrasound ablation have also proven efficacious.

The angiogenic capacity of these tumors often results in hypertrophy of the renal arteries; however, sometimes it leads to arterial neovascularization that can supply the tumor from other arteries. Thus, it can be very useful to elaborate a vascular map for large tumors prior to surgery.

The arteries that feed the tumor are often selectively embolized prior to surgery (even including the main renal artery when radical surgery is planned) because when the vascular supply is reduced the transfusion requirements and operating time are also reduced.

This technique is also used in cases with unresectable tumors or intractable hematuria.

Procedure Steps and Equipment

1. Prepare the patient for the procedure and monitor vital signs.
2. This is a potentially painful procedure, so it must be done under adequate anesthesia.
3. Perform aortography to locate the branches that supply the tumor.
4. Using an appropriate catheter (often microcatheters to preserve healthy renal parenchyma), selectively catheterize the branches that supply the tumor.
5. Choose the material for embolization (metallic coils, microparticles, gelfoam, alcohol, cyanocrylates, etc.
6. Check the results by angiography to ensure adequate embolization with total occlusion of the embolized arteries.
7. Control the postembolization syndrome (nausea, pain, and fever).

Further Reading

Alhadad A et al. Revascularisation of renal artery stenosis caused by fibromuscular dysplasia: effects on blood pressure during 7-year follow-up are influenced by duration of hypertension and branch artery stenosis. J Hum Hypertens 2005; 19:761–767.

Arend W, Michel B, Bloch D, Hunder G, Calabrese L, Edworthy S, et al. The American College of Rheumatology 1990 criteria for the classification of Takayasu arteritis. Arthritis Rheum 1990; 33(8):1129–1134.

Bali H, Jain S, Jain A, Sharma B. Stent supported angioplasty in Takayasu arteritis. Int J Cardiol 1998; 66(suppl 1): S213–S217.

Bilge I, Rozanes I, Acunas B, Minareci O, Nayir A, Oktem F, Tonguc Kozok Y, Emre S, Ander H, Sirin A, Poyanli A. Endovascular treatment of arteriovenous fistulas complicating percutaneous renal biopsy in three paediatric cases. *Nephrol Dial Transplant* 1999; 14:2726–2730.

Bookstein JJ, Goldstein HM: Successful management of post biopsy arteriovenous fistula with selective arterial embolization. *Radiology* 1973; 109:535–536.

Boss A, Clasen S, Kuczyk M, Schick F, Pereira PL. Image-guided radiofrequency ablation of renal cell carcinoma. Eur Radiol 2007; 17:725–733.

Casey RG, Murphy CG, Hickey DP and Creagh TA. Wunderlich's syndrome, an unusual cause of the acute abdomen. Eur J Radiol 2006;57(3):91–93.

Dalgic A, Boyvat F, Karakayali H, Moray G, Emiroglu R, Haberal M. urologic complications in 1523 renal transplantations: the Baskent University experience. Transplant Proc 2006; 38: 543–547.

DeSouza NM, Reidy JF, Koffman CG. Arteriovenous fistulas complicating biopsy of renal allografts: treatment of bleeding with superselective embolization. AJR Am J Roentgenol 1991; 156:507–510.

Donohoo JH, Anderson, Mayo-Smith WW. Pacemaker reprogramming after radiofrequency ablation of a lung neoplasm. AJR Am J Roentgenol 2007; 189:890–892.

Dorffner R, Thurnher S, Prokesch R, Bankier A, Turetschek K, Schmidt A, Lammer J: Embolization of iatrogenic vascular injuries of renal transplants: immediate and follow-Up results. *Cardiovasc Interv Radiol* 1998; 21:129–134.

Ettorre GC, Francioso G, Francavilla I, Di Giulio G, Vinci R, Esposito T, Campobasso N. Reanl arteriovenous fistulas after renal biopsy. Percutaneous embolization. Radiol Med 2000; 100:357–362

Fichtner J, Swoboda A, Hutchenreiter G, Neuerburg J. Percutaneous embolization of the kidney: indications and clinical results. Aktuelle Urol 2003; 34(7):475–477.

Fürhman SA, Lasky LC, Limas C. Prognostic significance of morphologic parameters in renal cell carcinoma. Am J Surg Pathol 1982; 6:655–663.

Gonzalo Rodríguez V, Rivero Martínez MD, Trueba Arguiñarena FJ, Martín Martín S, De Castro Olmedo C, Fernández Del Busto E. Empleo del catéter doble J para la prevención de las complicaciones urológicas en el trasplante renal. Actas Urol Esp 2008; 32(2):225–229.

Hegarty NJ, Gill IS, Desai MM, Remer EM, O'Malley CM, Kaouk JH. Probe-ablative nephron-sparing surgery. cryoablation vs radiofrequency ablation. Urology 2006; (Suppl 1A):7–13.

Henke PK, Cardneau JD, Welling III TH, Upchurch GR, Wakefield TW, Lloyd A. Jacobs LA, Proctor SB, Greenfield LJ, Stanley JC. Renal artery aneurysms. A 35-Year clinical experience with 252 aneurysms in 168 patients. Ann Surg 2001; 234(4):454–463.

Hétet JF, Rigaud J, Karam G, Glémain P, Le Normand L, Bouchot O, Le Néel JC, Buzelin JM. Complications of Bricker ileal conduit urinary diversion: analysis of a series of 246 patients. Prog Urol 2005; 15(1):23–29.

Ishikawa K. Diagnostic approach and proposed criteria for the clinical diagnosis of Takayasu's arteriopathy. J Am Coll Cardiol 1988; 12(4):964–972.

Kothary N, Soulen MC, Clark TWI, Wein AJ, Shlansky-Goldberg RD, Crino PB, Stavropoulos SW. Renal angiomyolipoma: long-term results after arterial embolization. J Vasc Interv Radiol 2005; 16:45–50.

Kunkle DA, Uzzo RG. Cryoablation or radiofrequency ablation of the small renal mass: a meta-analysis. Cancer 2008; 113:2671–2680.

Lehman DS, Landman J. Kidney cancer ablative therapy: indications and patient selection. Curr Urol Rep 2008; 9:34–42.

Liatsikos EN, Kagadis GC, Karnabatidis D, Katsanos K, Papathanassiou Z, Constantinides C, Perimenis P, Nikiforidis GC, Stolzenburg JU, Siablis D. Application of self-expandable metal stents for ureteroileal anastomotic strictures: long-term results. J Urol 2007; 178(1):169–173.

Maturen KE, Nghiem HV, Caoili EM, Higgins EG, Wolf JS, WoodDP, Renal mass core biopsy: accuracy and impact on clinical management. AJR Am J Roentgenol 2007; 188: 563–570.

Mostofi FK, Davis CJ. "Histological typing of the kidney tumours". World Health Organization. International classification of tumours. 2nd Ed. Springer, New York; 1998.

Motze RJ, Barder RH, Nancis DM. Renal cell carcinoma. New Engl J Med 1996; 335:865–875.

Munro NP, Woodhams S, Nawrocki JD, Fletcher MS, Thomas PJ. The role of transarterial embolization in the treatment of renal cell carcinoma. BJU Int 2003; 92(3):240–244.

Mwipatayi B, Jeffery P, Beningfield S, Matley P, Naidoo N, Kalla A, et al. Takayasu arteritis: clinical features and management: report of 272 cases. ANZ J Surg 2005; 75(3):110–117.

Numano F, Okawara M, Inomata H, Kobayashi Y. Takayasu's arteritis. Lancet 2000; 356(9234): 1023–1025.

Parrish AE. Complications of percutaneous renal biopsy: a review of 37 years experience. Clin Nephrol 1992; 38: 135–141.

Radeleff BA, Heye T, Lopez-Benitez R, Grenacher L, Hosch W, Haferkamp A, Kauffmann GW, Richter GR, Hallscheidt P. Interventional management of acute bleeding giant renal angiomyolipoma: report of three cases and review of the literature. Eur J Radiol 2007; 61(3):119–128.

Rutherford EE, Cast JEI, Breen DJ. Immediate and long-term CT appearances following radiofrequency ablation of renal tumours. Clin Radiol 2008; 63: 220–230.

Sato E, Lima D, Espirito Santo B, Hata F. Takayasu arteritis. Treatment and prognosis in a university center in Brazil. Int J Cardiol 2000; 75(suppl 1): S163–S166.

Slovut DP, Olin JW. Fibromuscular dysplasia. N Engl J Med 2004, 350:1862–1871.

Surowiec SM, Sivamurthy N, Rhodes JM, Lee DE, WaldmanD, Green RM, Davies MG. Percutaneous therapy for renal artery fibromuscular dysplasia. Ann Vasc Surg 2003; 17(6):650–655.

Tavakoli A, Surange RS, Pearson RC, Parrott NR, Augustine T, Riad HN. Impact of stents on urological complications and health care expenditure in renal transplant recipients: results of a prospective, randomized clinical trial. J Urol 2007; 177:2260–2264.

Yigit B, Tellioglu G, Berber I, Aydin C, Kara M, Yanaral F, Titiz I. Surgical treatment of urologic complications after renal transplantation. Transplant Proc 2008; 40:202–204.

Zavos G, Pappas P, Karatzas T, Karidis NP, Bokos J, Stravodimos K, Theodoropoulou E, Boletis J, Kostakis A. Urological complications: analysis and management of 1525 consecutive renal transplantations. Transplant Proc 2008; 40: 1386–1390.

SPRINGER NATURE

GPSR Compliance

The European Union's (EU) General Product Safety Regulation (GPSR) is a set of rules that requires consumer products to be safe and our obligations to ensure this.

If you have any concerns about our products, you can contact us on ProductSafety@springernature.com

In case Publisher is established outside the EU, the EU authorized representative is:

Springer Nature Customer Service Center GmbH
Europaplatz 3
69115 Heidelberg, Germany

The manufacturer's authorised representative in the EU is Springer
Nature Customer Service Centre GmbH, Europaplatz 3, 69115 Heidelberg,
Germany. If you have any concerns regarding our products, please
contact ProductSafety@springernature.com

Printed and bound by CPI Group (UK) Ltd, Croydon, CR0 4YY
27/04/2026
02097672-0001